# CONQUERING CANCER

*Dr. Joel Berman's Integrative Guide to Prevention and Treatment*

## JOEL BERMAN, M.D., F.A.C.S.

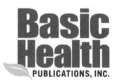

Basic Health
PUBLICATIONS, INC.

The information contained in this book is based upon the research and personal and professional experiences of the author. It is not intended as a substitute for consulting with your physician or other healthcare provider. Any attempt to diagnose and treat an illness should be done under the direction of a healthcare professional.

The publisher does not advocate the use of any particular healthcare protocol but believes the information in this book should be available to the public. The publisher and author are not responsible for any adverse effects or consequences resulting from the use of the suggestions, preparations, or procedures discussed in this book. Should the reader have any questions concerning the appropriateness of any procedures or preparation mentioned, the author and the publisher strongly suggest consulting a professional healthcare advisor.

**Basic Health Publications, Inc.**
28812 Top of the World Drive
Laguna Beach, CA 92651
949-715-7327 • www.basichealthpub.com

**Library of Congress Cataloging-in-Publication Data is available through the Library of Congress.**
Berman, Joel A.
  Conquering cancer : Dr. Joel Berman's integrative guide to prevention and treatment / Joel Berman, M.D.
    pages cm
  Includes bibliographical references and index.
  ISBN 978-1-59120-309-4
  1. Cancer—Alternative treatment. 2. Integrative medicine. I. Title.
  RC271.A62B47 2013
  616.99'406—dc23

                                                      2013029743

Editor: Roberta W. Waddell
Typesetting/Book design: Gary A. Rosenberg
Cover design: Mike Stromberg

Printed in the United States of America

10   9   8   7   6   5   4   3   2   1

*For Suzanne*

*Affirmation of life is the spiritual act by which man ceases
to live unreflectively and begins to devote himself to his
life with reverence in order to raise it to its true value.
To affirm life is to deepen, to make more inward,
and to exalt the will to live.*

—ALBERT SCHWEITZER, *OUT OF MY LIFE AND THOUGHT* (1949)

*There is a principle which is a bar against all information,
which is proof against all argument, and which cannot fail
to keep a man in everlasting ignorance. This principle
is contempt prior to investigation.*

—WILLIAM PALEY (1794)

# OTHER BOOKS BY
# DR. JOEL BERMAN

## Fiction

A Few Loose Screws

A Greek Tragedy

An Alphabetic Collection of
   Ridiculous Medical Poetry

Circle in the Water

Destiny Obscure

Fifty-Two Pieces: Short Stories

Floating World

Murder by Design

Scalpel

Something of the Old

The Cloak of Hippocrates

The Human Machine

The Oldest Sins

## Nonfiction

Comprehensive Breast Care and Surviving Breast Cancer

Love Letters from the War 1942–1945 (An American Surgeon
   Writes Home)

Slave Labor

The Death of America (The Deterioration of Ethics, Character,
   and Education in the United States)

Understanding Surgery

# CONTENTS

# ACKNOWLEDGMENTS

THIS BOOK IS A REFLECTION of my growth as a practicing surgeon and individual who, through his personal professional communications, readings, and patient contacts, has been able to change his view of the art of healing. Of course I owe a great deal to my formal medical teachers, but in the past few years this knowledge has been broadened and enhanced by my introduction to the many aspects of alternative medicine I have now sought to incorporate into my own surgical practice. In addition to my patients and many alternative healthcare professionals, I am indebted to my wife, Suzanne, who has been a strong advocate of dietary, spiritual, and exercise therapies, and has stimulated my interest in these modalities. In addition, I have certainly opened the door to a more spiritual life through works by Eckhart Tolle, Deepak Chopra, Richard Carlson, Shakti Gawain, and many others, and have sought to broaden my understanding of the many healing modalities presented in this book.

I am thankful to publisher Norman Goldfind of Basic Health Publications for giving me the opportunity to present this book to the public. I owe much thanks to my editor Roberta (Bobby) Waddell for her enlightening, if critical, comments. She has taken the M-deity bias and prejudice out of the manuscript and made it into the book it is today.

# INTRODUCTION

I AM A SURGEON. My father was a surgeon. His father owned Jake's Delicatessen on Grape Street in Syracuse, New York and my great-grandfather was allegedly a cavalry officer in the czar's army. So I guess my heritage is that men in my family have been making a living with knives or swords for many generations. I was an English and American Literature major in college, was urged into medicine by my father, following in my older, internist brother's footsteps, and went on into postdoctoral training in surgery in the twentieth-century tradition of the famous surgeons Dr. William Halsted and Dr. Alfred Blalock. I also received a masters degree for breast cancer research along with my surgical fellowship and training. I spent a couple of years as a surgeon in the U.S. Air Force and since then have been in the private practice of general and vascular surgery in Southern California. I have been director of a breast center and taught at a major university as an associate professor; my training and heritage is based in traditional* (*standard*) medicine and surgery. In my spare time I have written two medical books (*Understanding Surgery* and *Compre-*

---

* A note about the word *traditional* here. It has been brought to my attention that, in the alternative/complementary world for whom this book is written, the word *traditional* refers to medicine going back centuries *before* the era of drugs and mainstream allopathic medicine. In the twentieth century, however, the word was co-opted by conventional mainstream medicine, so please bear this in mind concerning the alternate ways of referring to the establishment form of medical practice throughout the book, using such words as *conventional, standard, mainstream,* etc., instead of the misnomer *traditional.* (This explanation is also in the Glossary.)

1

*hensive Breast Care and Surviving Breast Cancer*), as well as thirty fiction and nonfiction books.

As a surgeon, I have dealt predominately with the treatment of cancer *after* it has developed. Although my focus as a conventional medical specialist has rarely been on the prevention of cancer, in the course of writing *Conquering Cancer,* this has all changed.

## Cancer Prevention Means Understanding What Causes the Disease

As I researched prevention, admittedly a subject I was not completely familiar with, it was eye-opening for me to realize that upwards of 80–85 percent of cancer was the result of conditions over which most people have a significant degree of control. As of now, you cannot influence your genes or your heritage, of course, so for the other 15–20 percent of the population, at least, there is an inherited potential placing them at a greater risk for developing cancer. For these people, science is right at the threshold of testing for the genes that can promote cancer, and perhaps developing the ability to anticipate the onset of cancer and thereby take steps to prevent it.

Even more important to preventing cancer is understanding that almost 90 percent of the cancers are attributed to environmental factors. These include tobacco—it causes 90 percent of lung cancer; alcohol, diet, and obesity contribute 30–35 percent of the deaths from cancer in several different organs; infections contribute about 15 percent; and radiation is responsible for another 15 percent of the deaths from cancer. Add to this list environmental pollutants, inactivity, and stress, and you can see how many external factors directly affect whether or not cancer develops during a lifetime. Naturally, these factors are not isolated causes of the disease, and it is now well understood that *many* conditions have to coexist for an individual to develop cancer. Not all heavy smokers get lung cancer and not all obese women with a family history of breast cancer who are taking estrogens will develop breast cancer. But the idea that people do have a significant amount of control over whether they are at a high or low risk for cancer is a factor that should be understood and evaluated in the designing of lifestyles. Suffice it to say that people are not just victims, and they can be proactive in leading lifestyles that intelligently protect them from exposure to cancer-causing substances and environments.

In 1931, Dr. Otto Warburg won a Nobel prize, in part for demonstrating that some cancers are caused by a lack of oxygen respiration in cells. His theories have been tried and tested and questions about their universal validity still remain. However, if you pay attention to the chatter in the media, you will hear people stating categorically that *all* cancer is caused by denying a cell its oxygen requirements. This spurious reasoning makes scientists shudder because such claims are inaccurate and exaggerated for effect.

There is no doubt that a whole host of preventive measures may be effective in reducing cancer risk, and this book will examine many of them, including alkaline conditions in the body, antioxidants, detoxification treatments, energetic therapies, enzymes, immune-system alterations and augmentation, oxygenation therapies, psychological approaches, and others. But it will approach these therapies in a scientific manner, not just an anecdotal one. The best way to combat cancer is to use both modalities intelligently, combining the best of both to achieve the optimum outcome.

### Seven Tips for Cancer Prevention from the Mayo Clinic

Here is a list of seven tips put out by the Mayo Clinic to help reduce the risk of cancer.[1]

1. Do not use tobacco.

2. Eat a healthy diet.

3. Maintain a healthy weight and include physical activity in your daily routine—this lowers risk of breast, colon, kidney, lung, and prostate cancers.

4. Protect yourself from the sun—this helps prevent skin cancer from overexposure to the sun.

5. Get immunized—hepatitis B and HPV vaccines are recommended.

6. Avoid risky behaviors—practice safe sex and avoid sharing needles.

7. Take early detection seriously by screening for breast, cervical, colon, prostate, and skin cancers.

## A Brief Look at Advice and Information
## Concerning Treatments

In both conventional and traditional medicine, there is a superfluity of inexpert expert advice in amongst the valid advice . . . many suggested paths, with a few leading down blind roads and others steering people away from currently valid medical and surgical therapies. Hopefully, from the material I offer, you can design a healthy lifestyle that is both preventive and compatible with your desires for a fulfilling and happy existence.

In the mid-1900s, there was a concerted effort to find a cure for cancer, to find the *magic bullet* that would either prevent cancer or eliminate it once it had occurred. Many experiments and trials were initiated and millions of dollars were spent in this pursuit until it became clear that cancer is not just a single disease but is many diseases lumped under a similar heading. Similar to infection, where there are many sources (bacterial, viral, fungal etc.), and where many different types of antibiotics are needed, cancer treatment is multidimensional.

This point, that there are many approaches to dealing with cancer, is one I particularly want to stress. And in that context, it is very important to understand that one approach is not exclusive of another and that standard Western medicine must be combined with complementary medicine to offer the individual the best of both worlds of therapy. The conventional medical and surgical communities have tested modalities of prevention and treatment, most of which are based on clinical trials conducted on thousands of individuals using the scientific method, and they show the complications and shortcomings of the approaches. Alternative to this is the entire school of complementary medicine, which often has not been subjected to the same exhaustive clinical trials; in many instances, the results are anecdotal, which I have heretofore considered of no validity, or even harmful. Examples of how one individual was treated and cured are of little value to a conventional practitioner evaluating a mode of treatment, and unfortunately there are advertisements on television and the Internet that have unfounded, biased, and frankly inaccurate information. In amongst these, however, I have found many modalities that should be examined, and, in addition to anecdotal reports, these include valid accounts of treatments with complementary medicine that are supported by trials and have long documented histories of successful achievement in preventing or treating cancer.

The National Cancer Institute emphasizes that complementary medicines are methods *used in conjunction* with standard treatment, whereas alternative medicines refer to treatments that are used *instead* of standard treatment. I should make it clear that I am for complementary medicine, but not in favor of alternative medicine that steers patients away from medical and surgical management proven to prevent, cure, and treat cancer. This is my bias as a long-practicing physician. I view these forms of treatment as luring people with cancer away from standard accepted diagnostic and therapeutic cancer treatment, and by their avoidance of such proven methods, often losing their only opportunity for prevention or cure of their cancer. I do know, however, that there are many who see it differently, who do not see conventional mainstream treatment as the only valid way to approach cancer.

Randomized, controlled trials, not only in the standard medical community, but also in the complementary medical world, lend credence and validity to the myriad of nonconventional methods available to the public. But this same public must, in my opinion, take responsibility and examine, not just the standard, conventional methods, but also the alternative and complementary programs that are widely advertised and discussed in the media. In the course of this book, I will list most of the complementary medical approaches cancer by cancer, so you can combine both modalities to arrive at the most effective way of dealing with cancer.

There is no question in my mind that the many-centuries-old Indian Ayurvedic or millennia-old Chinese herbal treatments are effective, and that standard medical practitioners and complementary and herbalist practitioners can and should work together for the common good. The modalities are not, and should not be, exclusive of one another.

In connection with this, the M. D. Anderson Cancer Center in Houston, Texas, has a helpful website that gives definitions from various authoritative sources for many alternative/integrative methods.[2]

## How I Came to Write This Book

In light of my background, the question remains: Why on earth would I want to write a text on cancer, stressing prevention, medical, surgical, and, yes, complementary treatments? As a mainstream conventional surgeon, based in a tradition that usually abhors all so-called nonconventional medical care (alternative, complementary, Eastern, holistic, and a whole host of other ancient traditions), why write such an iconoclastic book? After all, don't most surgeons and internists basically look upon these complementary routes as snake-oil science?

The answer is that my mainstream medical training experienced a jolt several years ago when a Chinese woman brought her eleven-year-old son to see me. He had a pathologically diagnosed cancer on the skin of his right chest wall. As I reviewed the x-rays and the pathology report, I saw this was a rather nasty looking five-centimeter tumor that, under standard care, would require a fairly extensive surgical removal of skin, underlying muscle, and possibly even ribs. The boy's mother refused to subject her son to this treatment and left the office saying she would seek out help from her Chinese herbalist practitioner. I lost track of them for a while, until they reappeared one morning six months later. She wanted to show me the results of what she was sure I thought was her *quack doctor's* treatment. And on examining the boy, I discovered that his tumor had completely disappeared. He had been treated and cured by some strange, centuries-old, traditional Chinese medicine I had no knowledge of. I was dumbfounded. And from that watershed moment on, my outlook was never the same.

Over many years of practice, I have been exposed to a number of so-called nonstandard modes of therapy, often untested by clinical trials, and usually looked upon with great skepticism by conventional medicine. And through it all, I have prided myself on being an honest man—open-minded and willing to at least look at alternative modes of treatment. (As you may surmise, my thought processes have evolved and are still evolving.)

But unfortunately, if you delve into the standard medical texts used by United States internists and surgeons, only lip-service is paid to a whole host of these therapies. At a recent Congress of the American College of Surgeons I attended, not a single session was given over to alternative, complementary, holistic, naturopathic, or similar philosophies. And in perusing the major medical oncology texts, including the voluminous, almost 3000-page standard text on cancer by Dr. Vincent DeVita et al., *Cancers, Principles and Practice of Oncology,* fewer than twenty pages out of the three thousand are devoted to complementary, alternative, and integrative therapies.[3] And in these few pages, the subjects are dealt with in a negative, often condescending tone. Perhaps this is because, although many of these have been practiced successfully for well over a thousand years or more, conventional mainstream medical care in the United States does not even deign to consider these modes of treatment worth evaluating.

So I have taken the liberty of writing this book, not for the physician, but for the layman, to explain mainstream-medicine's management of cancer and give an intelligent overview of the ancient traditional therapies. In spite of the disaffection and arrogance of many of my colleagues, it behooves me to look seriously at all the modes and theories of cancer prevention, surgery, medicine, and complementary care, and present as unbiased an assessment and offering as I can, through which patients and their families can make an informed decision about their own, or a family member's, management of cancer.

I began to look into the voluminous literature of the alternative philosophies of medicine and was both impressed and unimpressed by the nature of what I saw. There were many sensible therapies and others which I, at that point, would have relegated to the *snake-oil* variety. In both traditional and Western medicine, there are financially motivated, ineffective treatments, but there are also those in both the alternative and allopathic world that appear to have great historical presence, validity, and efficacy. Unfortunately, there is such a strong and sometimes violent animosity of one group of practitioners toward the other that, instead of integrating the best of both worlds, they are often mutually exclusive. It's time to look at the field of cancer management with respect for differing traditions—Eastern, Western, and other forms of alternative therapies—offering the best of all prospects in a universal desire to prevent cancer, diagnose and treat all individuals with this disease, or ameliorate and deal sensibly and compassionately with the incurable situations.

PART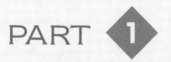

# THE BASICS

# 1

# CANCER THROUGHOUT HISTORY

I T WAS ONCE THOUGHT THAT cancer was primarily a disease of the modern industrial age. In reality, there is good indication that cancers have been present in man since the dawn of the hominids; the famous anthropologist Louis Leakey found evidence of lymphoma tumors in the remains of homo erectus and homo Australopithecus dating back millions of years.

The oldest descriptions of human malignancy were found in Egyptian papyri written around 3000 BC, and the well-known Edwin Smith and George Ebers documents contain details about cancers of the breast treated surgically and with medications, including castor oil, poultices, and medications made from animal parts, barley, and other substances. The hieroglyphics and papyri are replete with descriptions of tumors, benign and malignant, that were not uncommon in the populace. Several Egyptian cases of ulcerated breast cancer were treated by cauterization almost 3600 years ago, using a tool called the *fire drill*, but no cures were described. Treatments for skin tumors, including cauterization and attempts at complete excision, were apparently a common practice. The Egyptians believed cancer was caused by the gods.

Cancer has been found in fossilized bone, human Egyptian mummies, and ancient skulls from all over the world. It's a disease as old as man. Sushruta (circa 800 BC), the ancient Indian surgeon, sometimes known as the father of surgery, listed various types of tumors in his text *Sushruta Samhita* and described surgical and medical treatments from more than 2500 years ago.

Hippocrates (ca. 460 BC–ca. 370 BC), the father of Western medicine, is credited with being the first to describe the difference between benign and malignant tumors and his discourses include many descriptions of cancer throughout the body. It was he who noted the serpentine nature of blood vessels around malignant tumors, which so reminded him of crab claws that he called the disease *karkinos* (crab in Greek), which translates into *carcinos,* or carcinoma in English. The Roman physician Celsus (ca. 25 BC–50 AD) translated carcinos into the Latin *cancer,* which also means crab. In his day, Greek physicians believed that the body was composed of four humors: blood, phlegm, yellow bile, and black bile. And for almost 1500 years, cancer was attributed to an excess of black bile. Another Roman physician, Galen (130 AD–200 AD), used the word *oncos* that has been expanded into oncology, the word now used to define the name for the study of cancer.

Very little was done to advance the knowledge about cancer, or for that matter medicine, for almost a thousand years, and the theories and practices promulgated by the ancient Greeks and Romans held sway until the beginning of the Renaissance in the fifteenth century. The understanding of disease began to show progress with the beginning of knowledge about the human body. Prior to this time, dissection, or any type of internal examination of the human body, was considered sacrilegious and was banned by the religious and governmental authorities. With the development of the scientific method, and the scientific experiments of Galileo and Newton, came more enlightenment and tolerance. The first accurate anatomy atlas was published in 1543 by Andreas Vesalius, with diagrams of the human body, including veins, arteries, organs, and a skeletal system that, prior to this, had only been crudely demonstrated. The great universities and medical schools began allowing dissection of cadavers and, in doing so, elucidated many diseases, including cancer, in a scientific, clinically accurate fashion for the first time.

Still, Western medicine was in its infancy and it was not until 1761 that Dr. Giovanni Morgagni of Padua (1682–1771), the father of modern anatomical pathology, began doing regular autopsies on cadavers to determine their cause of death. His findings laid the groundwork for the science of oncology, the study of cancer. It was partially through his insights that surgeons, such as Scotsman John Hunter (1728–1793), began suggesting that some cancers might actually be cured by surgery. He felt that if the tumor was moveable and had not invaded nearby tissue, "There is no impropriety in removing it." Of course, surgery in this period was fraught with danger from infection, bleeding, morbidity, and death, not to mention terrible pain for the patient who underwent these procedures without anesthesia.

After William Harvey (1578–1657) accurately described the circulation of blood (1628) in his seminal treatise, *De Motu Cordis* (*On the Motion of the Heart*), further discoveries were quick in coming, with Italian Gaspare Aselli's (1581–1686) discovery of the lymphatic system that eventually led to the end of the old theory of black bile as the cause of cancer. The major milestone in identification and classification of the disease of cancer actually started after the discovery of the microscope by Dutchman Anton Leeuwenhoek (1632–1723), the father of microbiology. Although he never wrote a book, his letters and lectures were credited with providing the first microscopic descriptions of microorganisms, the cellular structure of organs, and the abnormalities seen in pathological specimens, such as those connected with cancer. He and others in his generation began to describe the differences between normal and cancerous cells.

Francisco Redi (1626–1697), an Italian, performed experiments that laid to rest the previous philosophies of spontaneous generation, which held that organisms could arise spontaneously from nonliving matter . . . i.e., that maggots could spontaneously appear in decaying meat. This led to the theory that certain diseases, including cancer, were aberrant developments from normal tissue and not *de novo* occurrences. He is credited with the maxim *Omne vivum ex ovo* (every living thing comes from a living thing—literally from an egg).

With the more acceptable dissection of bodies came a flourish of theories, most of them spurious, about the cause of diseases, including cancer. A German, Dr. William Fabry (1560–1634), often called the father of German surgery, was a noted scholar and author of twenty medical books. His *Observationum et Curationum Chirurgicarum Centuriae* was considered the best collection of medical case records of the time, yet in it, he described breast cancer as being caused by a milk clot in a mammary duct. Nicolas Tulp (1593–1674), a Dutch surgeon (also a mayor of Amsterdam), and perhaps best remembered by Rembrandt's portrait of him, "The Anatomy Lesson of Dr. Tulp," postulated that cancer was a poison that spread and could be contagious.

In England, in 1775, Dr. Percival Pott accurately described how chimney sweeps exposed to soot had a high incidence of scrotal cancer, and this lent early support to environmental causes for cancer.

Another Dutch professor, Francois de la Boe Sylvius (1614–1672), made many accurate descriptions of anatomical parts (Aqueduct of Sylvius, Sylvian Fissure) but was offbase when he declared that acidic lymph caused cancer. In the 1600s, a Dutch surgeon, Adrian Helvetiu, claimed cures for breast cancer with lumpectomies and mastectomies, but these operations, performed without general anesthesia, must have been terrifying, painful, and treacherous.

He was followed years later by the famous German physician, Rudolf Virchow (1821–1902), not only a doctor, but also the father of modern pathology, the founder of cellular pathology, an anthropologist, pathologist, biologist, prehistorian, and a politician, who, among his many discoveries, elucidated the theory that "every cell originates from another existing cell like it." The literature was still replete with many unproved philosophies about the cause of cancer, including trauma, chronic irritation, and infection, both bacterial and viral (the latter later proving to have some validity).

The surgical treatment of cancer and many other diseases took a giant step forward with the discovery of anesthesia, initially by Dr. Crawford Long (1815–1878), who did not gain priority because he did not write the first account, and by Dr. William Morton (1819–1868), the dentist who used ether to extract teeth. Shortly thereafter, Dr. John Collins Warren (1778–1856) painlessly removed a tumor from a man's neck, with ether, heralding a new era in cancer treatment. A milestone in the management of breast cancer was described in articles by William Halsted who devised the radical mastectomy entailing removal of the breast, its underlying muscles and axillary lymph nodes (under the arm), and achieved a remarkable advance from almost no cures to 72 percent in those whose disease had not yet spread beyond the chest.

From there, the progression of cancer diagnosis and treatment in the Western tradition advanced rapidly with the discovery of x-rays by the German physicist, Willem Roentgen (1845–1923). Cancer surgery expanded during the twentieth century, and, after the discovery of radiation by Marie and Paul Curie, treatment was augmented by the development of radiation therapy, as well as later discoveries of a whole host of chemotherapeutic, hormonal, and other therapies.

More recently, the 1952 explanation of the structure of DNA by Watson and Crick, and a whole host of genetic studies and discoveries, led to a greater understanding of what happens to normal cells when they transform into cancerous cells. Studies of cancer caused by chemicals, radiation, viruses, and even familial genetic tendencies were undertaken. Today's equipment allows a study of individual genes and locates the exact site of damage, for both the cause and the treatment of the disease. Later chapters will talk about oncogenes, tumor-suppressor genes, and other causes of cancer.

Along with the development of Western medicine's diagnoses and treatments have been a whole host of other modalities. This book will discuss many alternative and integrative therapies, including dietary, environmental, holistic, qigong, Chinese, Indian Ayurvedic, and a number of others that have arisen and survived, some for over a thousand years. Many of these play a significant part in the history of cancer and cancer treatment.

# WHAT IS CANCER?

CANCER, DESCRIBED AS a malignant neoplasm, is a generalized term given to a large group of diseases characterized by an abnormal, autonomous, uncoordinated, uncontrolled growth of cells in any organ or tissue of the body. Cells that divide and proliferate in this way eventually form a growth, or tumor, which may have the capacity to spread locally or distally in a process called metastasis. Cancer preys on the host and continues to grow indefinitely, competing with normal cells and tissues for nutrition and eventually, if unchecked, leading to the death of the host.

Cancer is not a single disease. So talking about cancer, its etiology, progression, cure, or treatment is in effect a discussion of many different diseases that have been lumped together by their natural propensity to grow indiscriminately and eventually lead to the destruction of tissue and death. In fact, malignant tumors can be found in all forms of higher organisms, including plants.

Tumors may be benign or malignant, the latter cancerous. Benign tumors are usually self-limiting and do not invade neighboring tissue or spread throughout the body. Normal, healthy cells control their own growth, and, if they become unhealthy, they will die. In a complex process called cell division, the growth and development of cells and tissue is controlled by their genetic makeup, which is carefully regulated and demands internal controls to prevent indiscriminate growth and spread. When something leads to an alteration of the genes, cell development gets altered and cancer cells may evolve. The damage to the gene may come from various sources, inside and outside the cell, and the exact nature of the genetic damage is complex and beyond the scope of this writing. The causes may stem from inherited abnormalities (heredity is 5–10 percent), or environmental and behavioral matters, such as diet, infectious agents, lack of physical activity, obesity, pollutants, radiation, tobacco, and even psychological, spiritual, or other causes, depending on the culture, belief set, and background of the person.

## A Brief Understanding of the Biology of Cancer

Cancer is a generalized word that is used to characterize a disease where cells divide in an out-of-control manner and may form tumors that have the potential to spread throughout the body, eventually leading to death. There are more than 100 different types of cancer and each is classified according to the type of cell initially affected and/or the original location of the cancer.

Cancers can grow and produce hormones, interfere with the blood-producing, circulatory, digestive, metabolic, nervous, and respiratory systems. Cancers have the potential to move from their primary location to other parts of the body, either by direct extension or through the blood or lymphatic systems; this is called invasion and can lead to the destruction of normal tissue. Often, in a process called angiogenesis, the cancer cell and/or tumor stimulates the growth of new blood vessels, thus allowing itself to be nurtured and thereby continue its rampant, uncontrolled growth. As you will see, one of the newer methods of controlling cancer is aimed at inhibiting the growth of these tumor blood vessels. Tumors that spread to other parts of the body are said to have metastasized, making treatment and cure much more difficult.

### Classifying Cancers

There are basically five groups of cancers.

1. **Adenomatous.** These are tumors that arise in glandular tissue, such as the brain (pituitary gland), the adrenal gland, and the pancreas.

2. **Carcinomas.** These are cancers of epithelial cells, or cells that line or cover the internal or external parts of the body, such as the lung, the colon, or the breast.

3. **Sarcomas.** These occur where the cells are primarily located in bone, cartilage, connective tissue, fat, and other supportive tissues.

**Lymphomas.** These are cancers arising in the lymphoid system, including bone marrow, the immune system, the nodes, and the spleen.

 **Leukemias.** These are cancers arising in bone marrow or blood-producing organs (hematopoietic system).

### How Cancers Are Labeled

The prefix is related to the cell type of origin and the suffix denotes the type of cancer, as listed above. These are the common prefixes and their meanings, along with some examples.

**Adeno-gland.** Adenocarcinoma, could be cancer of the breast

**Anaplastic.** A reversion to a more primitive cell type—anaplastic carcinoma

**Angio.** Relating to blood vessels—angiosarcoma

**Astro-star-shaped.** As of brain and spinal cord cells—Astrocytoma

**Basal cell.** A base layer of skin—basal-cell carcinoma

**Broncho.** Relating to the breathing tube—bronco-alveolar carcinoma

**Cholangio.** The biliary system–cholangiocarcinoma

**Chondro.** Cartilage—chondrosarcoma

**Embryonal.** Early stage, developing—embryonal-cell carcinoma

**Erythro.** Red blood cells

**Hemangio.** Relating to blood vessels—hemangiosarcoma

**Hepato.** The liver—hepatocarcinoma

**Lipo.** Fat—liposarcoma

**Lympho.** Lymphoid cells—lymphoblastoma

**Melano.** Pigmented cells—melanoma

**Myelo.** Bone marrow—myeloma

**Nephro.** Kidney—nephroblastoma

**Neuro.** Nervous system—neuro-endocrine carcinoma

**Myo-muscle–leiomyosarcoma.** Cancer of smooth muscle

**Osteo.** Bone—osteosarcoma

**Retino.** Eye—retinoblastoma

**Rhabdo.** Skeletal muscle—rhabdomeiosarcoma

With certain cancers and cancer syndromes, the names of individuals who discovered the disease are used. Here are a few of the more common ones.

**Barrett's esophagus.** An abnormal process in the esophagus that is precancerous

**Burkitt's lymphoma.** An aggressive B-cell tumor

**Ewing's sarcoma.** A bone cancer

**Hodgkin's lymphoma.** A lymphoma, very treatable, with high cure rates

**Kaposi's sarcoma.** A skin malignancy often associated with AIDS

**Paget 's disease.** A cancer of the nipple

**Wilm's tumor.** A kidney tumor

And there are several eponyms used in strange places.

**Cloquet's nodes.** Cancer involved in nodes in the abdomen

**Gleason's score.** Rating the severity of prostate cancer

**Papanicolaou (Pap) test.** A test for cervical cancer

**Reed Sternberg cells.** Refers to certain cancer cells found in Hodgkin's disease

**Sister Mary Joseph Nodes.** Referring to cancer in lymph nodes around the umbilicus

## The Increased Incidence of Cancer

One hundred years ago the incidence of cancer was much lower than it is today. It is now recognized that almost 30–40 percent of people will develop cancer during their lifetime. Cancer-causing agents, known as carcinogens, are now found in the water you drink, the air you breathe, the food you eat, as well as in insecticides and herbicides. People are now relentlessly exposed to electromagnetic radiation from cell phones, computers, and television and have become subjected to the stress that affects all immune systems.

### The Human Cell—The Root of Cancer in Humans

Since the human cell is the structure at the basis of all organs, and since its transformation from a normal cell to a cancerous cell is the basis for this entire text, it will behoove you to have at least a basic understanding of its structure and function.

The cell is generally the smallest unit of life that is classified as a living thing. Humans, then, are multicellular organisms. The cell was first described by the English natural philosopher and architect Robert Hooke (1635–1703) who, in his book *Micrographia* (1665), described what he saw in plant cells, using the word cell because he thought the structure of the plants looked like monks' cells—thus the word *cell*.

Cells vary in size and shape—the largest known cell, in fact, is that of an ostrich egg, and it can weigh 2–3 pounds. Human cells contain several structures. Although a detailed analysis of these is not necessary for an understanding of this text, I am listing here the more basic structures or organelles: the cytoplasm (the *soup* in which everything rests), lysosomes, vessicles, centrosome, ribosomes, cytoskeleton Golgi apparatus, endoplasmic reticulum, centrioles, mitochondria, and nucleus.

The nucleus contains DNA and the mitochondria contain RNA. Both these substances are important in cell development and, conversely, their mutations can lead to a cancerous conversion of the cell. The nuclei of all animal cells have structures called chromosomes where replication of DNA (this is the hereditary material of genes) and RNA (this processes information necessary to build certain proteins, such as enzymes) takes place. A kind of nuclear envelope protects the DNA and RNA from accidental damage in the replication process, but outside or inside influences causing mutations in the DNA or RNA may lead to malignant transformation.

The chromosomes have twenty-three pairs of linear DNA molecules. When other foreign genetic material is artificially (or otherwise) introduced into the cell by a process called transfection, strange DNA with other information may be inserted into the cell's genetic makeup, such as occurs with AIDS, and can cause damaging or even malignant developments.

And finally, a brief discussion of cell division. In this process, one cell (the mother cell) divides into two daughter cells, which leads to the growth of tissue. In humans, this process, known as mitosis, is where a complete replication of the cell occurs and where the cell's genome, or DNA, is duplicated.

## The Eight Stages of Cell Division

**1** Interphase

**2** Preprophase

**3** Prophase

**4** Prometaphase

**5** Metaphase

**6** Anaphase

**7** Telophase

**8** Cytokinesis

Each of these has a distinctive appearance and a pathologist looks for the presence of these various stages in cancer cells. Highly active, aggressive cancers have more of these stages visible and they are called mitotic figures. Usually in normal, noncancerous tissue, the pathologist would only see a rare mitotic figure. In cancers, there are many of them and their presence is often pathognomonic (characteristic) of malignancy.

## Immunology and Cancer

The body's immune systems are designed to destroy cancer cells by producing substances called cytokines, which have numerous capabilities, and among these are such things as colony-stimulating factors, interferons, tumor necrosis factors, and interleukins. The adult human body has about 80–100 trillion cells organized into different tissues in the body. All of these originated from a single cell, or zygote, at the time of conception. This single cell multiplies and subsequent cells go through a process of differentiation to form the different organs. Every day the body produces more than a trillion cells and a similar number of cells die each day in a controlled suicide process called apoptosis. Skin is replaced by new skin every two to three months, and blood is replaced every 120 days. The production of new cells is called cell division, a well-regulated process controlled by genes known as DNA (deoxyribonucleic acid). If the DNA is damaged by internal or external factors, including, for example, radiation, bad diet, or carcinogens in the environment, normal cell division may be interrupted and the new cell may become malignant. This change in the DNA is known as mutation.

The human body and its cells have a remarkable ability to destroy aberrant cells or repair abnormal DNA and thereby prevent the development of cancerous growths. This process is carried out by detoxifying the enzymes that destroy tumor-promoting factors or even cells. Malignant transformation is a rare event because of the wonderful ability of the body to correct errors in DNA or destroy abnormal cells. Most newly formed cancer cells in the body never grow beyond the microscopic stage because the body's immune system produces cytokines, substances that recognize cancer cells and destroy them. Among the cytokines you may hear mentioned are interferons (alpha, beta, and gamma), interleukins (1–15), or colony-stimulating factors. When the immune system is suppressed by poor diet, radiation, drugs, stress, or a disease, such as AIDS, the risk for developing cancer is multiplied many times.

When the body, and thereby the cells, are affected by the influences mentioned above, new genes may be produced that lead to cancer production. These are called oncogenes and suppressor genes, and they act on the DNA in the cells and transform them into cancer cells. HER-2/neu oncogene, associated with breast cancer, and c-Myc oncogene, associated with Burkitt's lymphoma, are among the many that have been recognized. It is noted, however, that at least three oncogenes in a cell are usually required before a malignant transformation takes place.

Another set of genes called mutator genes have the function of repairing or destroying damaged DNA, but, if a mutation occurs in these mutator genes, they are unable to do their jobs and tumors may arise. Still another group, tumor-suppressor genes, inhibit the development of cancer by producing certain proteins that suppress cellular proliferation. As with the mutator genes, mutation in a suppressor gene may allow unregulated growth of a cell. One example is the p53 gene that acts to regulate apoptosis (programmed cell death) as well as suppress the uncontrolled proliferation of cells. A mutated p53 gene is found in 40–50 percent of all human cancers. Many of the tumor-suppressor genes are highly specific for certain tumors, such as the WT-1 gene associated with Wilm's tumor and the APC and DCC genes associated with colon cancer.

All in all, the process of cancer development is a complex and multi-stepped one. At any given moment the human body is producing cancer cells, but these are usually rapidly destroyed by the body's own inherent immune system. This text will not only discuss the measures used by conventional medicine to treat cancers with surgery and allopathic medicines but will also carefully examine the environmental, dietary, radiational, and psychological aspects, plus any other causes that affect the body's ability to prevent or destroy cancer.

Many of the chemotherapeutic agents used by oncologists are aimed at hindering or incapacitating oncogenes, or assisting the immune system in clearing away damaged DNA or cancerous tumors that have gone beyond the body's ability to respond and eliminate them.

## Causes of Cancer—An Overview

The many diseases that fall under the heading of cancer have several things in common. They all have cells that grow out of control, eventually forming a mass called a tumor that can invade locally or spread to other parts of the body, and they all have the potential to destroy the host in which they have grown. Cancer-cell growth is not like normal cell growth—instead of having a normal lifespan and then dying (apoptosis), cancer cells continue to grow, forming more abnormal cells. Why does this happen? There are many reasons, but the basic one is that normal cells become cancer cells because of changes and damages to DNA that is in every cell and essentially controls all the actions of every cell. In the normal cell, damaged DNA is either repaired or the cell dies. In the cancer cell, the damaged, abnormal DNA is not repaired and the cell doesn't die, instead it just goes on to reproduce, causing more cancer cells to grow with the same damaged DNA. Damaged DNA can be inherited from parents, but more often the damage is due to external factors that will be examined in this chapter.

There are several well-known causes of cancer, as in the relationship between smoking cigarettes and lung cancer, but many more etiologies (causes of a disease or condition) are obscure and involve several combining causes. Environmental factors, diet, obesity, medication, exposure to radiation have been studied. Also it is known that several substances affect the body's, and therefore the cell's, ability to fight off cancer, and this is where an intelligent understanding of complementary medicine can sometimes collide with mainstream medical and scientific data.

Cancer is believed to develop in two stages, initiation and promotion. The initiator is the substance or environmental factor that affects the DNA and promotes the development of the genetic material called an oncogene, which plays a major role in causing the cancer or the carcinogenic process. Among the initiators we know today are radiation, tobacco smoke, pesticides, hormones, poor diet, viruses, toxic metals, obesity, and also just getting older (for those who don't use preventive measures).

An oncogene may remain dormant in a cell and never cause cancer. Apparently, other factors, called promoters, can work to *turn on* the oncogene and cause the development of the malignant cell. These promoters may be complex, involving many of the initiators, such as genetics, toxins, illnesses that inhibit the body's ability to protect itself, or it may be stress. It could also be damage to one of the normal body's defense systems—the immune system.

The standard, mainstream, and the time-honored traditional and nontraditional philosophies about the cause of cancer will be examined. In addition to standard therapy once a cancer has developed, it will be of benefit to examine the holistic, complementary, herbal, or other common alternative methods, as well as lesser known ones, which may actually eliminate the causes and augment the body's ability to prevent or destroy existing cancer cells.

Tobacco smoke, either through smoking or through second-hand exposure, causes cancer; in fact, tobacco smoke produces more than 2000 chemical compounds, many of which are carcinogenic. Nicotine, a very addictive substance, acts as the promoter and, in addition to lung cancer, it has also been connected with cancer of the breast, cervix, esophagus, kidney, mouth, pancreas, and stomach. It is now known that many chemicals, such as DDT and PCBs, cause cancer, and in places where these chemicals and other toxins have been reduced or eliminated, the cancer rate has declined.

Hormones, especially BCP (birth control pills) that contain estrogen, are responsible for an increased risk of breast cancer, and postmenopausal women who take HRP (hormone replacement pills) have a significantly higher incidence of breast cancer. Taking this into consideration can explain why overweight women have a higher incidence of this cancer, since fatty tissue has components that break down into estrogen.[1]

Dietary considerations are important, since a poor diet and poor general health set the stage for diminished functioning of the immune system and genetic repair.[2]

Environmental substances, such as radon gas, have been implicated[3] and, although not yet proven, many suggest that excessive chlorine (that can produce trichloroethylene and chloroform) and fluorine can cause cancer in laboratory animals and possibly increase the risk in humans.

Newer studies have shown some increased cancer risk in individuals exposed to excessive electromagnetic fields around electric wires and high-power installations. A study in Loma Linda, California, showed that EMFs (electromagnetic fields) stimulate the activity of the enzyme ornithine decarboxylase, which promotes the growth of cancer. EMFs may be generated by proximity to electrical wires, television, heaters, hair dryers, vacuum cleaners, fluorescent lights, *cell phones*, and video terminals—in other words, contemporary society is conducive to an increased risk of carcinogenesis.[4]

Several reports have linked the loss of a loved one, with its incumbent stress and emotional upheaval, to an increased risk for malignancy.[5] Conversely, a study at Stanford found that women with advanced breast cancer who participated in a support group live twice as long as those who did not.[6]

And it should be noted that as people grow older, the incidence of DNA abnormalities and need for genetic repair increases, and with this comes the potential for an increase in the incidence of cancer. It is postulated, for example, that every man, who lives long enough will develop prostate cancer. It is also known that men can live with this cancer for a long time and die of other, unrelated causes.

Chemical carcinogens have been widely studied since the 1915 experiments of the Japanese who showed that exposing rabbits to coal tar, or rats to butter yellow (dye used to color butter), caused cancer, and that certain aniline-dye factory workers developed a much higher incidence of bladder cancer. Vehicle fumes, including carbon monoxide, nitrous oxide, benzene, lead, and many complex organic compounds, can increase the risk of cancer.[7] Industrial toxic wastes may build up in the body causing DNA damage, aluminum, cadmium, lead, and mercury, being among these.[8]

Most people have heard the reports about farmers and agricultural workers being more prone to developing cancer after exposure to pesticides, herbicides, and insecticides, such as chlordane DDT (dichloro-diphenyl-trichloroethane), lindance, alar, and malathione. These substances get into the foods and then the general public becomes at risk.

Most food additives, including colorants, preservatives, and sweeteners have shown an increase in carcinogenic activity—saccharin and cyclamate in bladder cancer, and aspartame can possibly cause some brain tumors. And there are also potential dangers from blue dye #2, red dye #3, nitrofurans, and gentian violet.[9]

Physical carcinogens include x-rays, gamma rays, and other particle radiation sources. Their ionizing radiation causes direct DNA damage even at low levels. In susceptible people (sick, old, undergoing chemotherapy), even small doses may be harmful. People who experience low-level radiation from working or living around nuclear reactors, and radiologists with constant exposure to radiation may be at increased risk for thyroid cancer and leukemia. The incidence of thyroid cancer in individuals exposed to radiation at Hiroshima, Nagasaki, and Chernobyl was over 100 times the normal rate.[10]

Ultraviolet rays from the sun cause changes in the cancer-suppressor gene p53 and can lead to a higher incidence of skin cancer. And now, with a hole in the ozone layer, everyone is increasingly more exposed to these damaging rays.[11]

Biological carcinogens are coming under increased scrutiny. Scientists have shown that certain viruses (a virus is essentially a strand of DNA or RNA in a coating known as a capsid) cause cancer in laboratory animals. Obviously, direct human experimentation is not feasible, but there is ample evidence to infer that certain viruses cause human cancers. The EBV (Epstein-Barr virus) has been associated with 90 percent of nasopharyngeal cancers, and with Burkitt's lymphoma and testicular cancer. HPV (human papillomavirus) is associated with cervical cancer and the herpes virus is often seen with multiple myeloma and Kaposi's sarcoma. There is a much higher incidence of liver cancer with patients who have hepatitis B and C virus, and the HIV virus is associated with Kaposi's sarcoma, non-Hodgkin's lymphoma, and cancers of the anus and cervix.

Genetic abnormalities are present in many cancers and in some instances certain chromosomal abnormalities are identified and named, such as the Philadelphia chromosome in chronic myeloid leukemia. Chromosomal abnormalities with such descriptive names as duplication, insertion, translocation, and deletion are studied and can often help in diagnosis and prognosis of a cancer.

What about the hereditary factor in cancer etiology? Much of the work in this area has been done with the BRCA1 gene. This is found predominately in Ashkenazi Jewish women and confers an 85-percent lifelong risk of breast cancer and a 50-percent risk of ovarian cancer in carriers. Other familial cancers include retinoblastoma, multiple endo-crine neoplasia, adenomatous colon polyps, and non-BRCA breast and ovarian cancers. A strong family history of a given cancer must be seri-ously followed by the patient and her/his physician.

What about geographical location? It's known that the incidence of stomach cancer is very high in Japan compared with Western countries and breast cancer is higher in the United States than in Japan. After a Japanese woman comes to the United States, within five years her inci-dence of breast cancer rises to that of Americans.[12] The incidence of malignant melanoma increases appreciably as you approach the equa-tor where exposure to ultraviolet rays is much greater.

The more prevalent usage of chemotherapy and radiation therapy in the treatment of cancers has led to a higher incidence of certain leukemias, and over many years a higher incidence of solid tumors.

Holistic, herbal, complementary, Ayurvedic, and Chinese practi-tioners, as well as many Western physicians, are convinced that diet and nutrition play a large role in the development of human cancers. Many of the preventive and therapeutic treatments are based on this theory and the truth behind this philosophy is beginning to make its way into standard Western medicine, and each cancer discussed will examine these approaches. It is proposed that fast foods high in sodium and cholesterol but low in fiber, vitamins, and calcium may lead to cancer. Stomach cancer is higher in China where pickled and smoked foods are eaten. Certain grilled and Tandoori Indian foods contain hydrocarbons that may damage DNA and cause cancer. Fried and broiled meat contain a higher content of mutagens (substances prone to cause DNA mutations), and excessive eating of animal pro-tein leads to larger nitrogenous wastes in the colon, which can be converted into carcinogenic compounds called nitrosamines, known to be causes of colon, pancreatic, prostate, and breast cancers.

The problem with excess fat intake has been discussed, and the sub-stances in what is called the omega-6 class (saturated fat . . . oily food, meat, eggs, dairy products) are thought to promote cancer growth.[13] Conversely, the omega-3 class of fats (safflower, sunflower, sesame, walnut, corn, and pumpkin seed) are beneficial to health.[14,15] The dietary group of potential carcinogens is very long and includes contaminated fish from industrial pollutants, methyl mercury from manufacturing plants, and agricultural pollutants such as PCBs (poly-chlorinated biphenyls).

Cows receiving rBGH (recombinant bovine growth hormone) to increase production may produce milk that leads to breast cancer, and meat contaminated with steroids may also be carcinogenic.[16,17] Too much iron intake may produce free radicals that increase the risk for cancer. Some researchers postulate that alcohol stimulates the formation of breast, throat, pancreas, and liver cancer by suppressing natural killer cells. Another study blames caffeine for some urinary tract cancers by damaging DNA and impairing natural DNA repair.

Lastly, and more specifically, there is the connection between immuno-suppression and cancer. The immune system operates through two basic modes: one is humoral- or antibody-mediated immunity, and the other is cell-mediated immunity.

Antibody mediated immunity produces specific antibodies through B-lymphocytes (B-cells). The cell-mediated immunity consists of T-lymphocytes (T-cells) and natural killer (NK) cells, macrophages, and lymphokine-activated killer (LAK) cells that eliminate viruses, bacteria, and toxic molecules, either by engulfing and devouring them, or by producing specific proteins called cytokines that destroy them.

When cancer cells form in the body, they develop antigens (certain proteins) on their surface that are recognized as foreign by the body's immune system and are rapidly destroyed. Natural killer (NK) cells have over a hundred biochemicals that destroy these foreign proteins; they also kill circulating cancer cells in the blood and lymphatic system, preventing metastases. Macrophages destroy and devour cancer cells, as well.

In the immune system there are certain agents called cytokines that destroy cancer cells. Other names used by oncologists for these substances are interleukin 1 through 15 (IL1–15), interferons (alpha, beta, and gamma), colony-stimulating factor (CSF), and tumor necrosis factor (TNF). When the cytokines completely kill a tumor, it is said that the cancer has spontaneously regressed—that is the miracle cure physicians have all seen in their practices.

This basic understanding of the human body's immune system, leads to a discussion of standard and complementary modalities of treating cancer, bearing in mind the many causative bases for cancer development.

## Invasion, Metastasis, Angiogenesis

These are frightening words for a person to hear from his or her physician. *Invasion,* the spread of cancer cells into adjacent tissue, is one of the distinguishing features of cancer malignancy. It means the tumor has the capacity to grow in an expansive manner, invading the surrounding tissue of its own original organ, or extending into nearby tissues of different organs, for example, a breast cancer extending into the underlying pectoralis muscle. The cancer cells become able to break away from the primary tumor, develop pseudopods (false footlike projections to the cells) that enable them to crawl through surrounding tissue. In the course of this migration, the cells can reach blood vessels and lymphatic channels and lead to near and distant metastases.

The earliest cancers in the body are called in situ, meaning that the cancer can grow in place but does not have the potential to spread. These are usually called stage 0 cancers. Diagnosis and treatment at this stage result in near 100-percent cure rates. However, when the cancer demonstrates the ability to be invasive, the prognosis becomes much more ominous, the treatment more severe, and the outcome less favorable.

Metastasis is the word indicating that the cancer cells have moved from the primary site of origin to another site. The cancer cells travel to other parts of the same organ, or to other organs by way of the bloodstream or the lymphatic system. Breast cancer may metastasize to local lymph nodes or to the liver, bone, or lungs, and those cancer cells seen in the lung, for example, would have the appearance of breast cancer cells and would be called metastatic cancer, not lung cancer.

The mechanism of invasion and metastasis is complex and involves changes in the cell's behavior and in the surrounding tissue. All cells in the body exist in surrounding tissue called the extracellular matrix (ECM), a soft-tissue connective substance made up of a complex gelatinous material called glycoaminoglycans (GAGS). Most normal cells need this ECM to survive, and, if they are removed from their position in the matrix, they will undergo apoptosis (self-death) and self-destruct. A healthy matrix actually prevents cancer-cell extravasation, acting as a barrier to invasion and metastasis. However, cancer cells don't care about ECM and can live without it. The cancer cells produce their own matrix that helps them proliferate and migrate, and can produce other substances that upset the normal matrix. These cancer cells produce enzymes (protease that dissolves protein, and glycosidase that digests glycosides) that allow the cancer cells to digest and dissolve the ECM, and at that point the cancer cells can spread, become invasive, and eventually metastasize.

Many conventional and herbal compounds are used to destroy or hinder the cancer cell's ability to destroy the ECM. One substance making up the ECM is hyaluronic acid, and the enzyme that destroys it is called hyaluronidase (*ase* being the suffix applied to most enzymes). There are many substances that retard the action of hyaluronidase—among these are vitamin C, a flavonoid called apigenin, escin from horse chestnuts, and many others.

Another component of ECM is collagen, broken down by collagenase. Many natural substances can inhibit collagenase activity, or increase collagen synthesis, or stabilize the existing collagen. A few of these are curcumin, genistein, green tea extracts (EGCG–epigallocatechin gallate), luteolin, vitamins A and C, and others.

In addition to the proteases that damage or destroy the surrounding ECM, the tumor cell develops the ability to move in what has been found to be a very complex biological mechanism. Many therapies are being designed to impede this mode of spread.

When a cancer metastasizes, it often seeks out an area of the body that has at least some similarities to its site of origin, or some underlying metabolic similarity. It's a complex system. Prostate cancer usually spreads to bones; colon cancer to the liver; breast cancer to bone; and, peculiarly, stomach cancer to the ovary (a Krukenberg tumor). Melanoma often spreads to the brain, probably because brain tissue and melanocytes (the cells where melanomas originate) arise from the same cell line. In exciting new research, scientists are now able to detect certain genes in a cancer and thereby differentiate between the primary tumor and the metastasis, and also determine the propensity for the primary tumor to spread. By studying these genes (as with the Oncotype DX test that tests for twenty-one genes), the oncologist can be guided toward the appropriate management of a cancer and also have a better knowledge of the potential for metastasis.

Another area of study is Angiogenesis. To grow locally or in an invasive or metastatic fashion, tumors need nourishment. In this regard they have the potential (using a substance called vascular endothelial growth factor—VEGF) to induce the formation of blood vessels to bring in food and oxygen and discard waste. This process is angiogenesis (birth of new blood vessels), or neovascularization, and much research has been targeted toward impeding this development. Angiogenesis inhibitors (such as a VEGF inhibitor), invasion inhibitors (anti-adhesive agents—monoclonal antibodies, such as vitaxin), and metastasis protease inhibitors, as well as anti-VEGF drugs, are being developed. All of these are at the forefront of cancer research and their development is a highly complex field. This is a very superficial treatment of a very complex subject, but I wanted to give you at least an overview of the kind of problems facing cancer researchers.

What are the most common signs and symptoms of invasion and metastasis? Usually a cancer will spread into its surrounding tissue and then to local lymph nodes and this is behind the theory of treatment called sentinel-node biopsy where the surgeon seeks out the most probable lymph node for cancer spread, identifies it using radioisotopes or certain blue dye (lymphazurin or methylene blue), and then performs a biopsy to evaluate whether or not there is cancer in the node. So the earliest sign of spread may be node enlargement (although cancer cells can be present in small nodes and clinical identification is not possible by palpation).

Other signs relate to specific organs.

◇ **Liver.** Enlargement (hepatomegaly), pain, and jaundice

◇ **Bones.** Fracture, pain

◇ **Brain.** Neurological symptoms, such as intellectual and memory deficits, headaches, seizures, dizziness

◇ **Breast.** Ulceration through skin

◇ **Lymph nodes.** Enlargement of nodes, pain

◇ **Lungs.** Coughing up blood (hemoptysis), cough, shortness of breath (dyspnea)

It is important to emphasize that, although several years ago, metastatic disease was felt to be incurable and was a sign of impending doom, today there are new and improved therapies that can eradicate metastases medically or surgically, and can, if not cure the disease, significantly impact its growth and development. Many people with metastatic disease live productive lives for many years.

# **3**

# METHODS OF DIAGNOSIS

## Signs and Symptoms

In many cases, the earliest diagnosis of cancer may come from the individuals themselves. Being aware of the signs and symptoms of the disease may be the first indication that something has changed in a person's body homeostasis, and this often leads to earlier detection of a tumor. The general symptoms of cancer can include pain, fatigue, loss of appetite, loss of weight, fever, generalized weakness, pallor from anemia, bleeding (in urine, stool, vomit, or cough). There may be coughing in lung cancer, swallowing difficulty in esophageal cancer, obstruction or bleeding in colon cancer, a change in the breast with breast cancer (a lump, a depressed area, nipple discharge, or pain), blood in the urine with bladder cancer, paralysis with spinal-cord cancer, and a headache with a brain tumor. Of course, these symptoms can also occur with a host of other, noncancerous, diseases, but the presence of one of them, or an increasing symptomatology (set of symptoms exhibited) should alert the person to seek out professional help.

## Physical Examination

A complete history and physical examination by a professional is usually the next step. The examiner will normally have the person completely undressed in a covering gown and will check for abnormalities in each area of the body. A pelvic exam with a Pap test is often done by a family physician but may be done by a woman's gynecologist.

It is important for the physical exam to include careful observation of the skin, looking into the mouth, listening to the heart and lungs, and manually examining the abdomen as well as areas that might make the person uncomfortable, areas such as the penis and testicles of men, or the vagina and breasts of women, plus a rectal examination. This is no time to be shy, or do only a cursory checkup.

## Laboratory Studies

Several blood and urine tests will be helpful, though often not diagnostic. A routine CBC (complete blood count) can detect anemia (from blood loss or poor blood production), urine studies may show blood or abnormalities indicative of kidney, bladder, liver, or other cancers, and a comprehensive metabolic screening has a whole host of possibilities for detecting signs of possible malignancy.

Certain tumor markers may be ordered if specific markers are suggestive of cancer, though not definitively diagnostic. Here are a few of the more common ones.

### *Tumor-Marker Sites as Possible Cancer Locations*

◇ **Alpha fetoprotein (AFP).** Blood test for cancers of the liver, lung, ovary, pancreas, stomach, and testis

◇ **Bence Jones protein.** Urine test for multiple myeloma

◇ **CA 15–3.** Blood test for cancers of the breast, lung, ovary, and prostate

◇ **CA 19–9.** Blood test for colorectal and pancreatic cancer

◇ **CA 27–29.** Blood test for cancers of the breast, colon, kidney, stomach

◇ **CA 72–4.** Blood test for stomach cancer

◇ **CA 125.** Blood test for ovarian cancer (also cancer of the cervix, colon, liver, lung, pancreas, uterus, et al.)

◇ **Carcino-embryonic antigen (CEA).** Blood test for cancers of the bladder, colon, kidney, liver, lymphoma, melanoma, and pancreas

◇ **Catecholamines.** Blood/urine tests for pheochromocytoma (adrenal gland tumor)

◇ **5 Hydroxyindoleacetic acid (5HIAA).** Blood test for a carcinoid tumor

◆ **Human chorionic gonadotrophin (HCG).** Blood test for testicular tumors

◆ **Pancreatic oncofetal antigen (POA).** Blood test for cancer of the pancreas

◆ **Prostate specific antigen (PSA).** Blood test for prostate cancer

## CAUTION

The word *caution* is a mnemonic to note many of the warning signs of cancer.

C = Change in bowel or bladder habit

A = A sore that does not heal

U = Unusual bleeding or discharge

T = Thickening or lump in the breast or skin

I = Indigestion or problem swallowing

O = Obvious change in skin lesion

N = Nagging cough or hoarseness

### X-Rays

Since the discovery of radium by the Curies at the beginning of the twentieth century, tremendous advances have been made in the ability to look inside the body. Many times the simplest x-rays will show cancer even before other more sophisticated imaging systems are needed for further clarification. Chest x-rays are excellent for identifying lung cancers and metastatic disease, as well as visualizing tumors of the thymus gland, mediastinum (central portion of the chest), and ribs. Abdominal x-rays will show evidence of obstruction due to cancer, as well as many tumors that displace the intra-abdominal structure. Bone x-rays will show bone cancer. Breast imaging is called a mammogram and can pick up 85–90 percent of breast cancers. However, for better evaluation, many women also need ultrasound and MRI studies of the breast. Standard x-rays do emit radiation and give only a limited amount of detail.

Most cancers are better visualized and seen earlier in their development by the use of a CAT scan (computerized axial tomography), but this exposes the person to much more radiation. PET (positron emission) scans and MRI (magnetic resonance imaging) are also used. An MRI is excellent for brain cancer and some lymphomas. These modalities offer very clear pictures of the anatomy in many different views, even elucidating the blood supply and very early tumor growth.

Techniques that use a large amount of radiation must be avoided during pregnancy, and in rare cases, repeated exposure can eventually lead to the development of cancer where there was none before. Each technique has its strengths and weaknesses, and the physician has to weigh the importance of the test against its risks. Ultrasound is one test that has no increased risks but has the ability to illuminate testicular cancers and certain breast cancers.

### Instrumentations

For many years doctors have been using rigid scopes for looking at the gastrointestinal tract. With the development of fiber optics, however, specialists can look into the colon (colonoscope), esophagus, stomach (gastroscope), and even parts of the small intestine, using endoscopes, and they can perform biopsies. Orthopedists regularly use arthroscopes to look into joints and may even find rare synovial cancers. Interventional radiologists can biopsy most areas of the body using imaging techniques, eliminating the need for open surgical biopsies in many cases.

Internists perform spinal taps to remove spinal fluid and test for a metastatic malignancy. Many of these modalities will confirm the presence of an abnormality.

### Surgical Biopsies

In many cases the definitive diagnosis can only be achieved by taking a piece of the suspected neoplasm (tumor) and showing it to a pathologist. It will usually take one to two days for the pathologist to complete the process of making a slide of the tissue sample and examining it under a microscope.

### Other Diagnostic Methods for Cancer

◇ **Colposcopy.** To examine the vulva, vagina, and cervix

◇ **Cystoscopy.** To examine the bladder and urethra

◇ **Dilation and curettage.** To examine the uterus and biopsy

◇ **Endoscopic biopsy.** Fiberoptic examination of many parts of the body

◇ **Endoscopic retrograde cholangiopancreatography (ERCP).** To examine ducts of the biliary tract and pancreas

◇ **Laparoscopy.** For examining the abdomen with a fiberoptic scope through a small opening

◇ **Lumbar puncture.** A needle into the back to evaluate spinal fluid

◇ **Sentinel-node biopsy.** A biopsy to examine the first lymph nodes draining a tumor area

Using all these modalities, the contemporary physician will have an excellent idea as to the type, location, staging, and treatment of newly diagnosed or recurrent cancer.

## Cancer Conferences and Committees

Every major hospital and medical institution in the United States is urged to have a series of Cancer Conferences and Cancer Evaluation Committees. They are also called working tumor boards and are usually composed of oncologists, surgeons, radiologists, radiation therapists, pathologists, oncology nurses, infusion center nurses, social workers, and often plastic surgeons and other medical and surgical specialists. Meetings are usually held in a conference room on a weekly basis and case presentations are followed by discussion of the management suggestions by all of those present.

The patient is, in effect, receiving many second opinions. The conferences not only benefit the person whose condition is being evaluated but they also keep all members of the team abreast of the most up-to-date therapies and diagnostic modalities. Neither the public nor the patient is allowed at these conferences, in order for the members to have a free flow of ideas and comments concerning treatment and prognosis that is unhindered by any sensitivity to the presence of the person whose case is being reviewed. It is important to discuss the reality of a situation without being concerned about hurting anyone's feelings or frightening the person involved. After the conference, the patient's physician(s) (surgeon, oncologist) will have a meeting and discuss the outcome and the recommendations of the committee. The patient always has the last word in determining the care she or he wants. And in the coming years the hope is to incorporate more complementary modalities into the discussions at these meetings. This will necessitate inviting practitioners with alternative modes of therapy to the conference, and for the mainstream Western physician to have an open mind with regard to other forms of therapy. In several of the tumor conferences at my hospital, we are instituting nonconventional modes of therapy for discussion, including herbal, dietary, psychosocial, meditational, and spiritual approaches to the management of cancer.

### Second Opinions

In most major surgical situations, I recommend that my patients get a second opinion before subjecting themselves to a given procedure. In most instances the person is satisfied with the course of treatment recommended, but, especially with cancer cases, he/she and the family may feel more comfortable when the recommended treatment is concurred with by another specialist (or specialists). There also may be a difference of opinion about treatment, and they may opt for a different course of action.

Be aware, however, that while the Internet can provide excellent overall information, it is not a good source for a second opinion. It is not edited and anyone can say just about anything without any evidence to back up their statements, so it is better to have a face-to-face visit with a physician than to get a second opinion online. When seeking out a second opinion, in addition to consulting with another physician or healthcare practitioner, a good place to go is a major medical institution. Be sure to take complete copies of your records so the second-opinion doctor has the same information as your primary doctor.

The second opinion may result in three options. The second doctor may agree with the diagnosis and course of action, she/he may agree with the diagnosis, but recommend another course of action, or he/she may disagree with both the diagnosis and the course of treatment. At the last two junctures, the patient will have to make a decision or seek out yet another opinion. It should be understood that getting happier news, or the expectation of a better outcome doesn't mean the second opinion is necessarily the correct one. Don't just assume the second-opinion doctor is correct as opposed to your own first doctor. And perhaps most important and more difficult, don't assume that the doctor with a better bedside manner is the better physician. Of course it's important to have a doctor with whom you can develop a rapport, but equally important is the accuracy of her or his diagnosis and treatment plan and how this impacts your concept of adequate and excellent care, and your care itself.

It's important for you to be comfortable with the treatment that's offered. You can start by asking your own doctor whom to go to for a second opinion. Any doctor worth his or her salt will welcome a second opinion. You can also get names through a medical center or from another physician (ask your family practitioner or a gynecologist—doctors know doctors). Be careful about getting information from other patients or family members who have the same disease, without knowing the details of their problem. Best to go to a medical library or discuss the case with other caregivers. And remember that physicians are not perfect.

A very fine doctor with excellent skills, judgment, and outcomes will always have a few patients who will denigrate her or his services. Hitting 500 percent is great in baseball but patients expect their physicians to be batting 100 percent all the time and that's just not possible.

As outlined, when dealing with cancer, there will usually be a team approach and the patient will often have the benefit of a tumor board or tumor committee to back up the treatment being offered. Still, go seek out valid and legitimate second opinions, and when combining standard and complementary medicine, be sure to inform each practitioner of the therapy the other is providing, as well as the credentials of the individuals involved.

Be wise and educated when offered unfamiliar therapy, as you want to be sure of a successful outcome without any waste of your time and money.

# METHODS OF TREATMENT— MEDICAL, SURGICAL, AND COMPLEMENTARY

## MEDICAL TREATMENT—MEDICAL ONCOLOGY

This is the conventional Western treatment of cancer. It involves several modalities to reach a diagnosis and staging of cancer and then a design for treatment of the disease. The medical oncologist cares for the patient in a comprehensive fashion by treating the disease, the pain and suffering, and the emotional and familial problems. As well, this doctor keeps abreast of the newest advances in his/her field. After medical school (usually four years), and three years of internal medicine fellowship, the medical oncologist must take two or three years training in oncology and pass examinations in the specialty, enabling her or him to have a Board Certification in Oncology. (Many of these physicians take an extra year and also become board-certified in hematology.)

When is an oncologist needed? When the diagnosis of cancer is suspected or confirmed.

### Examining the Signs and Symptoms of the Disease

The individual usually goes to the family physician or gynecologist (and, in the case of women, also gets a screening mammogram) on a regular basis. In some cases, a routine examination by a physician or practitioner indicates that cancer may be present. In other instances, the person him-/herself notices a lump or a change in bowel habits or diet, weight loss, or other symptoms that necessitate a visit to the family physician. After a complete physical exam, several tests may be run, including a chest x-ray, a computerized axial tomography (CAT) scan, ultrasound, and blood and urine tests.

Cancer symptoms are usually divided into three groups.

1. There are systemic symptoms usually related to the presence of cancer in the body, but not directly caused by the cancer itself. These include poor appetite, weight loss, cachexia (wasting syndrome), night sweats, fatigue, and anemia (low blood count). They are vague and generalized symptoms, termed paraneoplastic phenomena, and mediated by the body's response to the presence of the cancer, although they may also occur when there is no cancer. They are, however, salient enough to alert a physician to do further tests and exams.

2. A second group, local symptoms, can include enlargements, swellings, or lumps (tumors), pain, bleeding (hemorrhages or vomiting up blood—hematemesis), coughing up blood (hemoptysis), blood in urine or stool (hematochezia), physical deformity, and change in bowel habits (constipation or diarrhea).

3. Or, when cancer has spread to other parts of the body, there can be a third group, metastatic symptoms, with findings of enlarged lymph nodes, hepatomegaly (enlargement of the liver), splenomegaly (enlargement of the spleen), bone pain and/or fractures, and neurological changes (confusion, memory loss, weakness, paralysis).

When the individual comes to the oncologist, she/he will have a complete physical examination and a workup that can include x-rays, an EKG, blood and urine studies, and possibly bone-marrow biopsies. After that, the physician may send the patient on to other specialists for more specialized studies, such as colonoscopy, bronchoscopy (examining the trachea and bronchi, the breathing tubes), or send for radiological or surgical biopsies. The oncologist will become the person in charge, coordinating the workup and treatment of the patient. Eventually, he/she may decide on a course of pharmacological treatments, depending on the diagnosis and stage of the disease. In many cases, patients will need to have venous access devices (Port A Cath, PIC line—peripherally inserted catheters) for the delivery of chemotherapeutic agents.

The oncologist essentially engages in compassionate care of people with cancer, involving many ancillary services, including cancer-support groups, the American Cancer Society, hospice, referral to tertiary treatment centers for more advanced or complex treatments, including bone-marrow transplants, and psychiatric support. She/he will usually follow the patients through the complete eradication of the cancer (or for the rest of their lives, in the case of systemic cancers) and will meet with family members to discuss the various therapy options, including radiation, chemotherapy, surgery, or cessation of treatment. The oncologist will have an overview of the patient's status and will be able to decide, along with the patient and the family, when, or if, hospice care should be offered. This specialist will also be knowledgeable in all aspects of supportive care and referral to other centers for new and more technical treatments and will have access to research protocols. Since this oncologist will have access to the latest information about treatment, which can change rapidly for common malignancies (such as those in the lung, breast, and colon), he/she can, in many instances, offer experimental treatments where standard therapy has failed.

The enlightened oncologist will also make full use of complementary therapies and will utilize many dietary, holistic, or other modalities that can benefit the patient. More and more, oncologists are becoming aware of the benefits of alternative and ancient traditional therapies that can be of significant help in dealing with cancer.

### Radiation Therapy

It has long been known that radiation can cause cancer, as evidenced by the sequelae of the dropping of the nuclear bombs on Hiroshima and Nagasaki in 1945. The therapeutic effects of this same modality have been known and used for almost a century, since the original discoveries by Marie and Pierre Curie at the beginning of the twentieth century. Radiation medicine is a highly complex field combining the intricacies of physics and ionization with the experience of radiology and internal medicine. This brief summary will not attempt to describe the principles of radiobiology, namely dosage, treatment time, positioning, or the specifics of agents used by radiotherapists to increase effectiveness or decrease complications. But it will discuss how radiation works and also how it is delivered.

Radiation is used to cure a cancer (skin cancer), prevent a recurrence of cancer (i.e., breast cancer after a lumpectomy), or as a palliative measure to shrink tumors in the brain, spine, and esophagus, or to alleviate symptoms caused by a primary tumor or a metastasis.

After the radiation therapist has consulted with the patient and determined the location and dosage, tattoos (small skin marks) are placed to allow exact positioning for treatment. The number and length of treatments are individualized and discussed with the person receiving them.

Another form of radiation treatment is called brachytherapy in which the radiation source is in direct contact with the tumor, in contrast with external beam therapy where the source is 80–100 cm away from the person. Brachytherapy may be performed with temporary or permanent implanting of isotopes, using catheters to deliver the radioactive material or seeds, ribbons, or needles. There is low-dose-rate (LDR) and high-dose-rate (HDR) brachytherapy. Brachytherapy has become common in prostate and certain gynecological cancers as we shall see later. Other advances in radiation treatment include IMRT (intensity-modulated radiation therapy), conformal therapy, and tomotherapy proton therapy. Stereotactic radio-surgery with cobalt (called the gamma knife) is used in treating certain brain tumors. An HDR treatment for breast cancer called MammoSite is being used in some patients with breast cancer who have undergone breast-conserving surgery. The side effects and complications of radiation therapy can be minimal or severe depending on the location, dosage, and time of exposure, and the patient is warned in advance about these aftereffects.

In many instances, complementary medicine, such therapies and supplements as acupuncture, antioxidant and anti-inflammatory compounds (found, for example, in the curry spice turmeric), ginkgo biloba, massage therapy, probiotics, reiki, and selenium, are highly useful and effective in alleviating many of these symptoms and are being used more and more by knowledgeable therapists.[1,2,3,4] There is, in fact, an entire text, *Alleviating the Side Effects of Cancer Treatment,* written by a well-respected oncologist in China, Dr. Zhang Dai-zhao, that focuses on the usage of integrative medicine to relieve the side effects of cancer (available on Amazon.com).

The most common aftereffects of radiation may be nausea, weight loss, general malaise, burning of the skin, itching, and localized temporary pain and swelling. Head and neck treatment can lead to hair loss, injure the salivary glands, and lead to dry mouth, which, in some cases, is long-lasting. Lower body radiation can lead to urinary problems.

Late side effects include damage to the bowels (causing diarrhea, bleeding, and even obstruction), fibrosis (scarring), memory loss (with brain radiation), infertility (pelvic radiation), and, on rare occasions, a second cancer. (Children treated for Hodgkin's may develop cancer later in life.) There are radiosensitizers that make cancer cells more sensitive to radiation, such as 5-FU (5-fluorouracil) and cisplatin, and radioprotectors that protect normal cells, such as amifostine (Ethyol), that can protect the salivary glands.

Another form of treatment, systemic radiation, is delivered intravenously, by mouth, or bound to a monoclonal antibody (an antibody produced by a laboratory-grown immune cell that is a clone of a unique parent cell). After some types of systemic radiation or brachytherapy, a person can be minimally radioactive for a few weeks and might be advised to stay away from children and pregnant women.

## Cancer and Drugs—A Brief Overview

Chemotherapeutic agents are divided into several groups depending on how they attack the cancer cell. I will very briefly describe what the agents do and then list some of the more common drugs in each group.

### Chemotherapy

**Alkylating agents** work by forming bonds or connections with certain portions of the tumor DNA or RNA that lead to tumor death.

- Alkyl sulfonate (busulfan)
- Aziridine (thiotepa)
- Nitrogen mustards (chlorambucil, cyclophosphamide, melphalan, ifosphamide)
- Nitrosoureas (streptozosin, carmustine)
- Platinum complexes (carboplatin, cisplatin, oxyplatin)

**Antimetabolites** work by competing with normal metabolites in DNA and RNA in rapidly dividing tumors.

- Adenosine analogs (cladribine, pentostatin)
- Purine analogs (mercaptopurine, thioguanine, fludarabine)
- Folate analogs (methotrexate)
- Pyrimidine analogs (capecytabine, floxuridine, fluorouracil, gemcitabine)
- Urea substitutes (hydroxurea)

**Targeted Agents** are relatively newer substances—antibodies that target specific tumor antigens.

◇ Monoclonal antibodies (mAbs) have the ending mab for monoclonal antibody (alemtuzumab, bevacizumab, cetuximab, rituximab, trastuzumab)

◇ Molecularly targeted therapies (botezomib, dasatinib, lapatinib, sunitinib)

**Natural products** are agents from plants, bacteria, and fungi that have anticancer activity. Many synthetics are manufactured with similar chemical compositions. Manufactured compounds include the following.

◇ Antitumor antibiotics—bleomycin (from cultures of the bacterium streptomyces verticillus), dactinomycin, doxorubicin, epirubicin, mitomycin)

◇ Camptothecin analogs (irinotyecan, topotecan)

◇ Enzymes (aspariginase)

◇ Epipodophyllotoxins (etoposide, teniposide)

◇ Microtubule agents (docetaxel, pacletaxil, vinblastine, vincristine, vinorelbine)

"Throughout history, natural products have afforded a rich source of compounds that have found applications in the field of medicine, pharmacy, and biology. Within the sphere of cancer, a number of important new commercialized drugs have been obtained from natural sources, by structural modification of natural compounds, or by the synthesis of new compounds, designed following a natural compound as model."[5]

The pharmaceutical industry proposes that their agents are *improved* over the natural product and can off more cytotoxic activity with fewer side effects. The alternative medical field questions this philosophy and offers many natural anticancer substances, such as pterostilbenes and other compounds from phytochemicals, or natural anti-breast-cancer drugs, such as chrysin or cytochrome p450 (found in grapefruit), which are natural substitutes for aromatase inhibitors.[6,7]

### Angiogenesis Inhibitors

When a cancer starts to grow, it produces substances that initiate the growth of blood vessels. These have the complex names VEGF/VPF ligand-receptor, and the tyrosine kinases PDGFR systems. The latest research has found drugs that target and destroy these substances, thereby decreasing or completely inhibiting the cancer's ability to develop blood vessels and feed itself. By starving the tumor, you can essentially limit its growth or destroy it.

There are several natural substances in the human body that act to destroy this VEGF/VPF and PDGFR, among them thrombospondin, interferon A, B, and G, endostatin, vasostatin, and angiostatin. Many of the complementary approaches to therapy are focused on augmenting this system.

There are many anti-angiogenic drugs (angiogenesis inhibitors) on the market and they are all in clinical trials to determine their effectiveness. Among these are bevacizumab (Avastin), IMC 1121, VEGF trap, CEP-7055, SU11248, ZD6474, and many others. Compared with standard chemotherapy, these drugs have relatively little toxicity, but many who take them still have headaches, high blood pressure, some nausea, and increased blood clotting. This therapy is at the front line of research.

### Hormone Therapy

Several cancers originate in tissue that is hormonally dependent, such as prostate, breast, endometrium (lining of the uterus), and thyroid tissue. The tumor tends to retain some of the hormone dependency of its original normal host. Hormone therapy can be very effective in curing or palliating these cancers. The physician can prescribe anti-estrogens, anti-thyroid drugs, and similar substances that block the effects of the hormone. Surgeons can remove the hormone-producing glands (adrenals, ovaries, testicles), or radiation therapy can destroy them. Unfortunately, as drastic as these procedures may sound, with my extensive knowledge of breast-cancer treatment, the use of anti-estrogen drugs, though preferable, is sometimes inadequate and surgery or radiation is necessary.

Many breast cancers need estrogen to grow, and an anti-estrogen compound called Tamoxifen can be used to treat the disease. There are, however, negative side effects, including heart problems, that need to be taken into consideration. An oophorectomy, a surgical removal of the ovaries, can be done to stop the growth of hormone-dependent breast cancers.

| TABLE 4.1. THE MORE COMMON ANTI-HORMONE DRUGS AND THEIR TARGETS | |
| --- | --- |
| AGENT | TARGET CANCER |
| Adrenal steroids (prednisolone) | Lymphatic leukemia |
| Aminoglutethamide (aromatase inhibitor hormone) | Prostate cancer |
| Dexamethasone | Breast cancer |
| Diethyl stilbesterol (estrogen hormone) | Prostate cancer |
| Luprolide and buserelin | Prostate cancer |
| Medroxyprogesterone | Endometrial carcinoma |
| Megestrol (progestin hormone) | Breast |
| Methyl prednisolone | Lymphoma |
| Octreotide | Metastatic carcinoid tumors |

## Immunotherapy

Cancer immunotherapy is the use of the human immune system to fight cancer. Immunization can be accomplished by administering a cancer vaccine or through the administration of drugs that function as antibodies. In the latter, each person's own immune system is augmented to destroy tumor cells, using the lymphocyte-activated killer cells, natural killer cells, dendritic cells, and cytotoxic lymphocytes. Using a process called recombinant DNA technology, alpha interferon was manufactured in 1981. Interferons are the most commonly used immune cytokines, but, when used in the most effective high doses, the side effects are significant and include liver damage, depression of white blood cells, (granulocytopenia, leucopenia), fatigue, vomiting, neuropsychiatric effects, and muscle pain, to name a few. In view of this, many regimens stay with low-dose therapy over a longer duration.

Holistic treatments that can often diminish these effects will be discussed, as will the many natural products that stimulate the immune system, such as Reishi mushrooms and the Agaricus blazei mushrooms.

Dermatologists are now using topical immunotherapy, such as imiquimod, an immune-enhancement cream, to destroy basal and squamous-cell cancers, cutaneous T-cell lymphoma, and superficial spreading melanoma.

Several of the antibodies are listed under the heading of monoclonal antibodies and molecularly targeted therapies. Among these are the following.

### TABLE 4.2. MONOCLONAL ANTIBODIES AND MOLECULARLY TARGETED THERAPIES

| ANTIBODY | BRAND NAME | TARGET DISEASE |
|---|---|---|
| Alemtuzumab | Campath | Hematologic cancer<br>T-cell lymphoma |
| Bevacizumab | Avastin | Vascular endothelial/colorectal/lung cancer |
| CD20 | Rituxan | Non-Hodgkin's lymphoma |
| CD52 | | Chronic lymphocytic leukemia |
| Cetuximab | Erbitux | Epidermal growth/colorectal cancer |
| Iritumomab | Zevalin | Lymphoma |
| Trastuzumab | Herceptin | Erb 2 Breast cancer |

### Bone-Marrow Transplantation

Bone marrow is the spongy tissue found inside bones containing stem cells that produce blood cells (red cells that carry oxygen, white cells that fight infection). In such diseases as leukemia, the marrow stem cells malfunction and form cancer cells. To destroy these cells requires high doses of radiation, which destroys normal as well as cancerous cells.

Developed in the 1950s, bone-marrow transplantation (BMT) is a procedure that replaces a cancer patient's bone marrow with marrow from a donor. A bone-marrow transplant allows the physician to treat the diseases by first killing the cancer and then repopulating the bone marrow with normal, nonmalignant cells. The donor marrow is extracted, usually from a hip bone (iliac crest), under anesthesia in the operating room, and then stored until reimplantation occurs after the recipient's treatment is successfully completed.

There are three kinds of donors: syngenic, allogenic, and autologous.

 In syngenic, the donor is an identical genetic match with the recipient, as with identical twins,

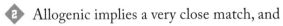 Allogenic implies a very close match, and

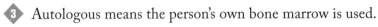 Autologous means the person's own bone marrow is used.

First, the patient is given high doses of chemotherapy or radiation therapy that essentially destroys the bone marrow. Following this, the saved, or new, marrow is (re)injected intravenously and makes its way to the bones over a period of a couple of weeks. Between the time when the malignant marrow has been destroyed and the time when the reinfusion and repopulation of clean, new, nonmalignant marrow cells has taken place, the intended recipient is at extreme risk for infections and complications and must be keep in isolation.

Bone-marrow transplantation is used for acute leukemias and lymphomas.

### Stem-Cell Transplantation

Similar in many ways to bone-marrow transplantation, this procedure involves transplanting stem cells (an early developmental form of cells that have the possibility to form many different kinds of cells—multipotential cells). These cells may be harvested from bone marrow, from peripheral blood (venous blood), the umbilical cord, or amnionic fluid. As with bone-marrow transplants, the graft types may be autologous (from the sick individual, then stored), or allogenic (from a donor). The latter need to be carefully matched, using a matching system called HLA, and race and ethnic background seem to play heavily in finding a suitable donor.

Stem-cell transplantation is used in diseases of the blood or bone marrow (Ewing's sarcomas, neuroblastomas, and certain other cancers). This is a very high-risk procedure reserved only for extreme cases and has a high risk for fatal complications. It is used in those who are extremely sick with leukemias or lympho-proliferative cancers (multiple myeloma) where other treatments have failed.

### Gene Therapy

Oncolytic gene therapy involves the use of viruses that have been genetically engineered to destroy cancer cells. These drugs and procedures, such as using adenoviral therapy (ONYX-015) for squamous-cell cancers of the head and neck, and altered herpes simplex virus

(HSV-1 as G207 and NV1020) for colorectal cancers and certain brain tumors, are still in clinical trials. There are also experiments to actually transfer portions of genes into cancer patients in an attempt to correct the DNA defects that are causing cancer. This experimental work is in its early phase, but gendicine (a Chinese FDA-approved p53 gene therapy that can restore the normal p53 gene function in cancer cells) has been used for squamous-cell neck cancers.

## Your Oncology Team

### National and International Organizations

To lend validity to a given specialty in medicine, organizations have been established in many countries to oversee and standardize the qualifications, training, and certification of their members. These organizations or fellowships are academic in nature and bring attention to the studies and continuing education of practitioners in a given area of expertise. While membership in these organizations is often not required for individual practice in a given specialty, most academic and public institutions and hospitals require at least basic assurances that those practicing in their facility have been adequately trained, and continue to upgrade the credentials, which are reviewed every few years. Continuing education courses are offered, and in many states in the United States, documentation is required on a regular basis as part of the relicensing process for physicians.

When a physician graduates from medical school, she/he receives a medical degree, an M.D. or a D.O., which allows him or her to apply for a medical license in the state or states in which she/he wishes to practice. Further training, whether in general surgery, surgery subspecialties, internal medicine, oncology, or other areas, requires other documentation to practice that particular specialty in hospitals, or to qualify for certain national or insurance reimbursements.

In regard to the traditional medical specialties that predate Western allopathic medicine, such as Ayurveda, traditional Chinese medicine (TCM), naturopathy, and other nonconventional Western and Eastern medical practices, specialty boards have been established to ascertain the adequacy of the practitioner from the point of view of Western medicine.

In the United States, the *American College of Physicians,* the *American*

*Medical Association,* the *American College of Surgeons, Certification Boards in Surgery, Obstetrics and Gynecology, Oncology, Hematology, Orthopedics, Vascular Surgery, Radiation Therapy, Radiology,* and so forth (the list is extensive), all quantify and qualify what their members should know and also lay down a basis for ethical and moral conduct in their practice of medicine.

### The Pathologist

Pathology derives its name from the Greek pathos (suffering) and logos (study) but is essentially the study of the structural and functional changes in cells, tissues, and organs that cause diseases (dis-ease).

A pathologist is a physician who specializes in the study of diseases, either clinical, surgical, or postmortem. He/she is a fully trained doctor with four years of medical school and at least four years of postdoctoral training in pathology, who may decide to continue studies in a subspecialty, becoming an expert in a narrow field within the larger field of pathology. Most pathologists work in hospital laboratories or reference laboratories, where they spend time directing the operation of the laboratory, examining biopsies for diagnosis of disease, and in many instances being directly involved in tumor board conferences, educating other physicians, and, in medical centers with students, educating the students.

The pathologist uses molecular, immunologic, microbiologic, and morphologic techniques to explain disease and to help other physicians in treating cancer and other illnesses. Pathology has two major divisions, clinical and anatomic. Clinical pathology deals with the performance and interpretation of laboratory tests (blood, urine, spinal fluid, cultures, etc.). Anatomical pathology deals with tissue diagnosis. Most pathologists are board certified by the American Board of Pathology in both major divisions of their specialty. Coroners and medical examiners (like Quincy on TV) study forensic pathology. Other specialties are dermatopathology (skin pathology), transfusion medicine (blood bank and donating blood products), cytopathology (Pap smears and needle biopsies), hematopathology (diseases of blood cells), and molecular pathology (a molecular and genetic approach to pathology).

The pathologist is the physician who performs the microscopic and gross examination of tissues to make the diagnosis of cancer. She or he may recommend further studies to elucidate the diagnosis, especially when dealing with cancers that have many subgroups, such as lymphoma, leukemias, and breast cancers (that have many different cell types). Special staining methods and immunological techniques are used to further categorize the cancer diagnosis.

The pathologist may be given tissue from surgical specimens and these may need to be placed in special preservatives (fixed), cut (sectioned), and implanted in paraffin wax so the fixed tissue can be placed in a machine called a cryostat or microtome that makes tiny slices of the tissue. These slices are placed on slides to be examined under a microscope. The tissue can be stained with a whole host of special dyes that will elucidate different characteristics of the cells and help the pathologist further diagnose the disease.

The pathologist will be present at conferences where groups of physicians assemble to discuss all the aspects of managing people who have cancer. The group will usually be shown slides by the pathologist who also gives a description of the findings as the basis for understanding how to treat a given patient with a given disease. This skilled specialist is the one who supplies the basic information necessary to make intelligent plans for therapy. In the course of any given treatment, further biopsies may be needed to evaluate the cancer tissue and determine what effect the treatments are having on the progression or elimination of the disease. In some cases, the pathologist will send tissue to another pathologist or another institution to get a second opinion. There are many centers of excellence, especially when dealing with difficult diagnoses or the complex pathological problems that may be seen with cancer. Some pathologists are renowned in their own very narrow area of specialization, and these individuals are sought out for their opinion on difficult cases. The patient may confer with the pathologist, although this is not a usual occurrence.

In the United States, well over a million people are diagnosed with cancer each year and most of them are cured of their disease. Still, cancer accounts for about 23 percent of all deaths, second only to heart disease, so an accurate diagnosis of cancer is of major importance to the appropriate management of the disease.

### Dermatopathologist

Specializing in the cancer of the skin, the physicians in this subspecialty diagnose conditions like squamous-cell and basal-cell cancers and the more dangerous malignant melanoma. They also have the ability to identify the many obscure and rare cancers that can involve the skin and other conditions of the skin and may give a clue about other underlying malignancies. Patients need to be aware that dermatologists will often make a visual diagnosis of skin cancer and rush toward removing a skin lesion that might not need extensive excision. Patients should always demand to see biopsy results performed by a pathologist, and not by the dermatologist, unless this doctor has taken a fellowship or advanced training in pathology.

When dealing with serious skin cancers like melanoma, an accurate diagnosis and the extent of the disease are important in treatment. Some melanomas can be locally excised with free margins and be cured. Others may need very wide excisions and sentinel-node biopsies and subsequently require immune therapy to prevent metastatic disease. The pathologist is of key importance in determining the severity of the condition and in planning the therapy for it.

### Hematopathologist

The field of hematopathology has become so complex in the last twenty years that the pathologist often defers to this specialist when diagnosing certain leukemias, lymphomas, or other hematological cancers. The hematopoietic system refers to those areas of the body that produce blood cells (hematopoietic cells) and includes bone marrow, lymph nodes, lymphoid tissues, the spleen, and the thymus. In addition to being a specialist in diagnosing this area of cancer, he or she is familiar with other technical studies as well, including molecular hematopathology (arriving at a diagnosis through studying the cancer patient's blood).

Another area of great interest, and at the forefront of contemporary pathology, is the field of flow cytometry or FCM. This technique is used for counting and examining microscopic particles, such as chromosomes, cells, and a large number of cellular components, and is used in the diagnosis of many blood cancers. The physics and biology behind flow cytometry, a technique used to identify and separate different types of cells based on detecting and measuring the fluorescence emitted with a laser light beam, is extremely complex. Briefly, the cytometer has five main components: a flow cell, a measuring system, a detector, an amplification system, and a computer to analyze the data collected. If this sounds complicated, it is, but it has enabled the pathologist to measure many parameters of cellular micro-anatomy and function.

Below are facts about cancer tissue that the pathologist determines through chemical tests or examination with a microscope.

◇ Apoptosis and cell viability

◇ Cell adherence

◇ Cell surface antigens

◇ Chromosome analysis

◇ DNA and RNA content of cells

◇ Enzymatic activity

◇ Multidrug resistance in cancer cells

◇ Nuclear antigens

◇ Protein modifications and expression

◇ Volume and morphological complexity of cells

The pathologist has become an integral part of the cancer diagnostic and treating team.

### Nursing—Oncology and Infusion Centers

With the advances in cancer therapy in the second half of the twentieth century, the role of the nursing support teams changed. When cancer was formally recognized as a major chronic health problem and the National Cancer Act was instituted in 1971, a comprehensive approach toward the management of people with cancer was developed. This had, as one of its foci, a change in the nature and implementation of nursing care. Whereas cancer treatment in the United Stated had previously been relegated only to surgical removal, new oncology advances allowed for a whole set of new parameters in patient care. Special cancer units were set up and these required a new approach, not only by physicians, but also nurses.

A new approach required a change in the perception of cancer, and specific education of nurses toward better management of cancer-related problems was developed. Not only were these nurses the caregivers for the cancer patients, but they also had to be able to educate and support the families, learn about the administration of chemotherapy, and understand the complications and side effects of this new therapy. Today, all major hospitals have a separate unit or floor designated as the cancer ward where patients may feel more comfortable because they know they are in a specialized care area and their needs will be met.

Nurses were offered advanced education in this specialty, often receiving masters or doctorate degrees. They became cancer-care coordinators for cancer units, or administrators, and many opted for work in research, assisting with the development and carrying out of protocols. The important principle is that a person with cancer often requires very different management than the individual who has had a hernia or gallbladder operation, or who has heart or lung disease. The problems, complications, and side effects of the treatments are often complex and different from the noncancer patient. Because these nurses are working in this field on a regular basis, they become very familiar with the diseases and can manage situations more quickly and effectively.

Oncology nurses in hospital settings often obtain certification from the Oncology Nursing Certification Corporation, receiving basic degrees such as OCN (Oncology Certified Nurse), CPON (Certified Pediatric Oncology Nurse), or CBCN (Certified Breast Care Nurse). Many go on to become AOCN (Advanced Oncology Certified Nurses or AOCNP (Advanced Certified Oncology Nurse Practitioners), with more patient responsibility and legal abilities. These nurses attend conferences with other nurses or with physicians and assist in many decision-making plans for cancer patients.

Infusion therapy is the intravenous delivery of fluids and medications. A doctor will write a prescription (order) for chemotherapy and the nurse will check the order with a pharmacist to ensure correct dosage before proceeding with the infusion. In some cases, if the person is very sick, this is done in a hospital inpatient setting, but more and more outpatient infusion centers have been developed where patients come in for an hour or two, have their treatments, and are discharged home, with less disruption of the normal life routines, and at a significantly lower cost to the patient and to the insurers. Some patients have special infusion pumps that deliver a continual infusion of medication, and these need to be examined and refilled on a regular basis. Patients who need frequent treatment, and those whose veins collapse or become thrombosed (blocked) may need to have special intravenous access ports (Port A Cath) or PIC (peripherally inserted catheters) placed.

### Psycho-Social Support

Coping with the physical and medical challenges of having cancer creates the need for special emotional support groups. They are established to provide comfort, reduce anxiety, supply information, and extend therapeutic coping skills in a comfortable setting with other individuals who have similar cancer diagnoses. Dealing with specific problems related to their disease by talking with others has a supportive, even therapeutic, effect. Several studies have shown that those with advanced cancer who participate in support groups have a better quality of life and in many cases live longer. Whether or not this has to do with emotional stability affecting the immune system is under study, but the example followed with women who have breast cancer seems to bear out the premise that those who work a program of support do much better than those who do not participate. The groups meet in hospitals, community centers, school classrooms, offices, or members' homes. Although there are online support groups, they should be used with caution because privacy and confidentiality cannot be assured.

The groups are led or facilitated by cancer survivors, other group members, or trained professionals. Certain support groups are listed as therapy sessions and will be led by psychologists, psychiatrists, social workers, nurses, or specialized therapists. There is usually little or no cost for most of these sessions.

Discussing common issues, such as breast prostheses, reconstruction, sexual problems, and familial interactions are important for those with breast cancer. Patients with colon cancer who have temporary or permanent colostomies need information and support that they can get from others with similar problems. But the support groups are not only available for the patient, but also for the family and even the caregiver. I recommend these groups to all my cancer patients . . . they are upbeat, not morose or depressing. Frequently these groups are visited by medical professionals, such as oncologists, surgeons, plastic surgeons, and members of the American Cancer Society, who answer questions and speak about their area of expertise.

### Cancer Centers

This topic is an important yet difficult one to discuss because in many ways it places certain cancer centers in conflict with others. As a physician, it is incumbent upon me to recommend places and physicians who have a proven track record of honesty, proven therapy results, and quality medical care. After all, cancer medicine is big business and many smaller organizations want to get a small piece of the financial pie as well. Be very careful when listening to advertisements on television or in other news material about centers that profess extraordinary results in curing late-stage cancers. If it sounds too good to be true, it probably is. Most accredited cancer centers have access to, and utilize, many complementary medical programs along with their standard therapy. Rather than spend time and money at questionable clinics, seek out well-respected cancer foundations, and, if you desire additional complementary medical treatment, obtain it through them. There are many well-advertised cancer clinics in Tijuana and Sonora, Mexico, almost never covered by insurance (although the wording in their ads suggest that after you pay up front, you'll probably be reimbursed—wrong), offering ineffective treatment and touting outstanding results. You may have heard of them through famous actors with cancer who have wasted time and money in their frightened attempts to save themselves. Best to spend your time and money where it will do some good. When you're reaching for straws— that's exactly what you'll get—straws.

I have listed a few of the most prestigious cancer centers in the United States that are looked upon as the pinnacle of cancer treatment. They are comprehensive centers, approved and respected across the country, and their websites will provide complete outlines of what they offer. What you should be looking for is a therapy combining the best of standard medical care with complementary care. The major medical centers offer you the best possible approach for treatment of your cancer. Those with NCI CCC (Comprehensive Cancer Centers by the National Cancer Institute), all generally have the same types of facilities and expertise.

◇ **Memorial Sloan-Kettering Cancer Center (NCI CCC).** This center is located in Manhattan, New York, and includes the Rockefeller Outpatient Pavilion, the Evelyn Lauder Breast Center, and the Sidney Kimmel Center for Prostate and Urologic Cancers. It has a top-notch program encompassing patient care, research, access to the latest treatments, and state-of-the-art facilities. It also has an outstanding education and training program given by physicians.

The following five centers offer essentially the same approach to combination standard and complementary medicine and should be among those sought out when seeking primary care or a second opinion for cancer.

◇ **M.D. Anderson Cancer Center (NCI CCC)** is a branch of the University of Texas in Houston, Texas—like Memorial Sloan-Kettering, it has an outstanding reputation for cancer care (see also References—#2 endnote in Introduction)

◇ **H. Lee Moffitt Cancer Center and Research Institute Foundation (NCI CCC)** in Tampa, Florida

◇ **Fox Chase Cancer Center (NCI CCC)** in Philadelphia, Pennsylvania

◇ **City of Hope (NCI CCC)** in Los Angeles, California

◇ **Mayo Clinic (NCI CCC)** in several locations—Rochester, Minnesota, Phoenix/Scottsdale, Arizona, and Jacksonville, Florida

The following are two examples of non-NCI CCC centers that advertise conventional and alternative medical treatments.

◇ **Cancer Treatment Centers of America.** Headquartered in Schaumberg, Illinois, with facilities in several locations throughout the United States. These centers have been subjects of some controversy over their advertising, suggesting their advertisements contain unsupported and misleading claims as to the efficacy of their cancer treatments. In 2001, the FDA issued the CTCA a Warning Letter concerning three clinical trials that were conducted in violation of FDA requirements. While being a good hospital, they may have been overzealous in their advertising, appealing to extremely sick patients with anecdotal examples of remarkable cures. Again, while their treatments may well be very significant and valid, their approach to patients is often misleading, and this causes the standard medical physician concern in referring patients.

◇ **New Hope Unlimited in Sonora, Mexico.** This center offers conventional, alternative, and holistic medicine, stressing noninvasive therapies, and their Mexico facility offers some therapies not permitted in the United States. They also include a disclaimer: "It is important to understand that as of today's standard; only conventional medicine is known to be FDA-approved. New Hope Unlimited, LLC, does not make any stated or implied claims regarding results. The extent of the response to treatment varies from patient to patient."

Again, the bias I have is probably due to a long history of the Western medicine's attitude toward certain therapy, but I also know that people in this country have grown up relying upon the Food and Drug Administration to protect everyone (warranted or unwarranted) from ineffective or dangerous therapies.

### Clinical Trials

Clinical trials are human research studies designed to test new ways to prevent, detect, diagnose, or treat diseases such as cancer. A clinical trial may be local or national in scope and involves having what is called a *protocol* that states what will be done, how it will be done, the risks, the ethical implications, and the endpoint of the study. Coverage for clinical trials is often underwritten by insurance companies or the businesses supplying the therapeutic agent involved. It should be noted here that the most trustworthy trials are those done by unaffiliated outside groups with no financial stake in the outcome.

Clinical trials are important because they examine the use of new modalities in thousands of individuals to determine whether there is acceptable success using a particular therapeutic method. One of the problems conventional Western doctors have with many alternative therapies is the lack of clinical trials, which makes them skeptical of their validity. More and more herbal and other alternative treatments are undergoing clinical trials, many with great success, and this bolsters the acceptability of these treatments among the medical establishment. But what needs mentioning here is why there are so few clinical trials for natural products in the first place. It's simple. Since natural products cannot be patented, *Big Pharma* (as the drug companies are referred to in alternative circles) doesn't want to spend any money doing clinical trials on them, so they don't get done for the most part, and everyone in the natural health field knows this.

Clinical trials may involve drugs, new surgery or radiation therapy, vaccine, immunotherapy, or herbal and nonconventional therapies. Generally these studies are sponsored by governmental agencies, such as the NCI (National Cancer Institute) and other parts of the NIH (National Institutes of Health), but may be initiated by private physicians, medical centers, foundations, volunteer groups, or biotechnical and pharmaceutical companies.

Regardless of who sponsors or underwrites the trial, national and international policies and regulations have been instituted to assure that strict scientific and ethical principles are followed. These trials may be done in doctors' offices, cancer centers, hospitals, and clinics. The safety and efficacy of the studies are under the watchful eye of Institutional Review Boards (IRBs) and are reviewed on a regular basis.

There exist strict rules as to who is eligible to run or participate in these trials, and results must be published or generally made available so participants, as well as other healthcare practitioners, can be made aware of the results. Statistical evaluations should be done to show whether or not the positive or negative findings truly have significance.

In what is known as informed consent, any patients participating in clinical trials must be informed of the important facts about the trial so they can intelligently decide if they want to participate, and they need to be continually updated in case there's any new information or data that may affect them. Part of a clinical trial may involve dividing the participants into two groups, where one receives the new medicine or modality and the other receives a placebo (i.e., instead of a new chemotherapeutic agent, they would receive a sugar pill). This is called a double-blind study. Some patients will not participate in a clinical trial unless they know they are receiving the new agent or modality. In some cases of terminal cancer, or at the special request of the oncologist, patients are given this information, but these cases would not be included in the case studies.

The benefits of participating in a clinical trial include having access to new interventions that may be more effective than anything else, having more frequent checkups with physicians, and knowing that their participation is altruistic in that it is helping others who have the same disease and is advancing the progress of science. The disadvantages are that the therapy may not work, or may have deleterious side effects, that there may need to be more doctor visits than are desired, and that there may, in some instances, be costs not covered by insurance. Medicare does reimburse participants in clinical trials for cancer, and TRICARE participants are reimbursed for NCI-sponsored phase II and III trials.

## NATIONAL INSTITUTES OF HEALTH (NIH)

As part of a discussion of cancer diagnosis and therapy, it's important to mention the National Institutes of Health, the largest and most comprehensive healthcare biomedical research institution program in the world. The NIH consists of 27 separate institutes, 1,200 principal investigators, and over 4,000 postdoctoral fellows doing basic and clinical research. Their research is carefully reviewed by outside scientists, and funding is given only to the most valid projects. Their research is responsible for many advances in medicine, including lithium for bipolar disease, fluorination of water preventing tooth decay, and numerous vaccines and treatments. The NIH has their own laboratories and also supports many outside research facilities in medical schools, universities, hospitals, and research institutions throughout the United States. Among the twenty-seven NIH institutes are the following.

**NCI.** National Cancer Institute, focusing primarily on cancer research;

**NLM.** National Library of Medicine;

**NIAID.** National Institute of Allergy and Infectious Diseases (infectious, allergic, and immunologic diseases);

**NIGMS.** National Institute of General Medical Sciences (genes, proteins, and cells, etc.);

**NIEHS.** National Institute of Environmental Health Sciences (environmental exposure, genetic susceptibility, and age-related issues);

**NIAMS.** National Institute of Arthritis and Musculoskeletal and Skin Diseases;

**NHGRI.** National Human Genome Research Institute.

Phase Trials for cancer are the step-by-step processes of evaluating a new drug for cancer treatment.

◈ **PHASE 0** refers to the earliest step or microdosing studies. A very small dose of the new drug is given to ten to fifteen people to gather preliminary information; these test subjects usually have an advanced form of the disease where effective treatment options are no longer available.

◈ **PHASE I (1).** Maximum tolerated dose trial to evaluate safety and maximum dosage; also given to twenty or more of the sickest patients with no other available therapy.

◈ **PHASE II (2).** This tests the effectiveness of the drug on specific cancers in 50–300 individuals who may or may not have received standard therapy; there are also continuing safety studies (throughout the trials, whenever any safety issues arise, such as allergic or other untoward side effects, the study may have to be altered, abridged, or stopped).

◈ **PHASE III (3).** This compares a new drug with an existing drug and compares side effects with the existing drug. It involves a control group (receiving the placebo) and an experimental group (getting the new drug), and one hundred to several thousand people are randomly assigned to one or another of the groups.

◈ **PHASE IV (4).** Several hundred to several thousand people are tested to determine the drug's effectiveness and long-term safety; this is usually done after approval by the Federal Drug Administration (FDA), and the trials are usually sponsored by drug companies.

When the clinical trial has ended, the results are usually published in scientific journals and are reviewed by experts in the field to determine whether the drug's use should be considered the standard of care.

## SURGICAL TREATMENT—SURGICAL ONCOLOGY

Surgical oncology is the application of surgical principles to the management of cancer. The surgeon has completed four years of medical school, five years of residency training, and sometimes additional training in surgical oncology. He is board certified by the American Board of Surgery and in many instances will have FACS after his name (Fellow of the American College of Surgeons). For many malignancies, the surgeon works closely with the medical oncologist and radiation therapist in designing the appropriate treatment for the patient with cancer.

For diagnostic purposes, the surgeon is asked to do invasive biopsies or excisions. In many instances, diagnostic open biopsies have been avoided by the development of highly trained invasive radiologists who can perform percutaneous (needle through the skin) biopsies of palpable and radiological identified masses. This has become the standard with many malignancies, such as those in the breast, or tumors that are either superficial or deep in the body, thus avoiding open procedures. However, in some cases, open biopsies will be necessary where there are bleeding tendencies or critical structures near the tumor that might risk being injured by a needle biopsy.

Lymph nodes often need to be biopsied and the mode of biopsy will vary with the disease. For certain solid tumors, carcinomas, many head and neck cancers, lung, liver, and intra-abdominal tumors, biopsies are now done with a fine needle or larger needles (called core biopsy needles). In suspected lymphoma, the surgeon needs to do an open biopsy and remove an entire lymph node because the needle biopsy will not supply sufficient information for treatment. Other biopsies are performed by other specialists—gastroenterologists perform endoscopic biopsies of the stomach, intestine, colon, and even the pancreas; pulmonologists biopsy the bronchi; and dermatologists biopsy (and sometimes completely remove) skin cancers.

Once the specimen is removed, it is sent to the pathologist to confirm the diagnosis and several tests will be done to determine certain characteristics of the cancer. After a diagnosis has been made, a course of treatment is designed, which may be a decision to remove the cancer, to do debulking (the surgical removal of part of a malignant tumor that cannot be completely excised), or palliation (easing symptoms without curing the underlying disease). If surgery is decided upon, the patient must have a complete medical workup to determine whether it will be tolerated. The old saying, "The surgery was a success, but the patient died," is a sad truism that must be avoided if possible.

Resection is the surgical removal of tissue, and it can be performed for cure, debulking (removing a large portion of a cancer), or palliation (removing cancer to make the patient's remaining life more pleasant). The expression *wide excision* means taking out the tumor plus some normal tissue around the edges to be sure it is all removed. It has been a general principle to handle the actual cancer or cancer-bearing tissue as little as possible, to prevent shedding or spreading tumor cells during the resection. New techniques, such as a laparoscopy for removing cancer with smaller skin incisions, and newer robotic techniques are being developed. The robotics are used primarily in prostate and gynecologic procedures but may prove useful in a whole host of procedures. Various surgical techniques will be discussed under each of the specific cancers, including sentinel-node biopsies and lumpectomies for breast surgery, newer modifications to older techniques, as with head, neck, and colon surgery, or a lymphadenectomy (removal of lymph nodes).

On many occasions, the surgeon will be called on to perform palliative surgery to alleviate situations where curative surgery is not possible or would not be tolerated because of other underlying conditions, such as severe heart or lung disease. The patients and family play a major part in this type of surgery because the patient understands that the disease is not curable and may want to resort to other modes of therapy. These individuals have to be very careful to avoid charlatans who prey on dying cancer patients, often presenting them with expensive, useless treatments.

Surgeons are called upon to do diverting procedures in patients with extensive colon or ovarian cancer who present with intestinal obstructions and require an ileostomy or a colostomy (bringing a loop of intestine to the surface of the abdomen and allowing its contents to drain into a bag) to alleviate the pain of the obstruction. In some instances, incurable cancers just below the level of the skin may present with impending ulceration through the skin, resulting in infection, pain, and hemorrhaging, and these may need removal to ease any complications caused by further growth of the cancer. Some palliative procedures for incurable brain or spinal-cord cancers may alleviate neurological deficits, pain, or cognitive problems for a period of time. The object of this surgery is to make the person as comfortable as possible. And with the rapid advancement of new therapies, new treatments and even cures may arise to completely eradicate the cancer in the months or years following such surgeries.

Another issue the cancer surgeon must face in severe cases is the question of resuscitation where the quality of life is such that life-preserving procedures, simple or complex, might not add any quality time to the patient's existence and would probably cause more pain and suffering. The surgeon must discuss these principles with the family, and sometimes the patient may not be coherent enough to participate in the discussion. The humanitarian approach to surgery is always foremost in the cancer surgeon's arsenal, recalling the old adage, "Physician do no harm."

## COMPLEMENTARY MEDICINE

Complementary integrative medicine is the combination of traditional alternative medicine with standard establishment medical and surgical care. It is at once the enlightened approach to a coordinated effort by two schools of thought to reach the best outcome for the patient in terms of prevention, treatment, and palliation of cancer patients. There is a wealth of information available to the lay public, much of it of historical validity. Because of my mainstream medical background, I tend to gravitate to the word complementary rather than alternative, but these therapies are often bundled under the term CAM (complementary and alternative medicine) and generally encompass a group of healing philosophies, diagnostic methods, and therapies that are not in the conventional medical armamentarium.

Included in this group is holistic medicine, naturopathic medicine, Ayurvedic and Chinese herbal medicine, folkloric, non-Western, unorthodox, herbal therapies, among others. These are generally not taught in conventional Western medical schools and are not usually available in conventional hospital settings. They are, and have been for centuries, very popular throughout the world and can include nutritional/dietary programs, spiritual approaches, vitamin/mineral supplements, herbal productions, mind-body therapies, manipulative therapies, bioelectromagnetics and other energy approaches, and a whole host of other therapies. In the last decades, there have been more scientific examinations of many of these treatments, but many have used flawed methods to determine the validity of this or that method. This is a well-known fact in the alternative world. Study after study ballyhooed as showing faults with this or that alternative method have been improperly set up, often due to the incomplete knowledge of the researchers.

Complementary medicine has been the source of continual debate, and dietary supplements, safety, and claims are a continual source of controversy since a given drug may be legal in the United States, but the herbal source of the same drug is banned. There is the continual problem of regulation and insurance coverage for complementary medicine that won't be resolved until a better understanding develops between the two groups of practitioners. If mainstream medicine persists in labeling all alternative and complementary medicine as snake-oil science, then no progress can be made. Complementary and alternative medicine providers are in agreement that health fraud occurs in both systems and both groups feel this fraud should be investigated and dealt with appropriately, but this attitude should not be extended to all aspects of this type of approach to patient care.

There are many legitimate healthcare products advocated by those who practice alternative and complementary medicine. It behooves those who practice Western mainstream medicine to open their minds to the possibility that many of the ancient, truly traditional, practices that have come down through the centuries and the millennia may have significant value. Because Western medical practitioners do not understand the basis for Chinese traditional and Ayurvedic practice, or other philosophies, that should not hinder their desire and ability to educate themselves about it. When the editor in chief of the prestigious *New England Journal of Medicine* comes out with the statement, "There is really no such thing as alternative medicine—only medicine that has been proved to work and medicine that has not," and another editor of the same journal states, "It's a new name for snake oil," then all possibility for evaluation and judgment is thrown to the wind. A website called *Quackwatch* professes to enlighten the public to much of the quackery and health fraud, promoting what they say are intelligent decisions. After reviewing many of their articles, however, it becomes apparent that many of the authors are so closed-minded against any form of alternative therapy, that they are contentious, and in many areas seem to show contempt prior to investigation, making blanket statements where focal and limited criticism might (or might not) be indicated.

The bias of one group of practitioners against the other has only slowed the acceptance of many modalities that although used successfully for centuries, are scoffed at by conventional Western medical practitioners. It's time to open people's eyes and ears to the wisdom of four thousand years of medical practice. Without being blind to possible fraud and charlatanism, it's important to examine the validity of treatments that have been effective in alleviating the suffering of many, whatever the mechanism. In line with this, in 1992, the U.S. Congress set up the Office of Alternative Medicine, a part of the National Institutes of Health, to establish guidelines for testing the complementary methods. Since it is estimated that almost 80 percent of those with cancer use CAM therapies, it behooves the conventional practitioner to determine what therapies are valid and useful.

Many complementary therapies have been shown to have definite, clinically proven validity and are coming into use in some oncology practices, among them maitake mushrooms, phytoestrogens in other than breast-cancer patients, and a shark cartilage derivative AE941 for kidney and lung cancer.

As a practicing surgeon, I am aware of the bias of many Western practitioners against complementary, Ayurvedic, Chinese, and holistic medicine and hope this book might spur some enlightenment in these closed minds through the impact that intelligent, well-informed patients can have on their physicians.

There are many beneficial complementary treatments in supportive-care therapy for treating nausea, cachexia, chemotherapy toxicity, side effects from radiotherapy, and constipation, as well as for general well-being. In addition, there are therapies used for cancer prevention that have validity and warrant further examination. Among these are aloe, cranberry, eucalyptus oil, grapeseed extract, green tea, lactobacillus acidophilus, lycopene, oleander, omega-3 fatty acids, psyllium, selenium, vitamins A, C, and E, and others.

Of particular interest is the long history of the effects of alkalinization on the human body. In the beginning of the twentieth century, several distinguished researchers emphasized the theory that cancer cannot exist in an alkaline milieu. Dr. Linus Pauling, the Nobel Prize winner, asserted this theory and maintained its validity throughout his scientific career. Today, there are several companies involved in manufacturing machines that alkalinize water, with the findings that individuals who maintain an alkaline body milieu are much less susceptible to developing malignancies. In fact, one in five families in Japan shares this point of view and the popularity of the alkaline-water hypothesis has grown in the United States as well, with the introduction of Kangen water. While everyone acknowledges the importance of clean water, most Americans don't realize that tapwater is acidic until it's neutralized by lye to make it a pH of 7.0, and most of the bottled designer water is strongly acidic.

The findings of numerous clinical studies in Japan and the United States bear witness to the health advantages of maintaining an alkaline body fluid to help prevent many nonmalignant as well as malignant diseases. This is one area that will be expanding as the public is made more aware of the advantages of this alternative approach to cancer prevention and treatment, and it should be examined by anyone interested in finding alternative routes to maintaining a healthy body.

## A Brief Compendium of Complementary and Alternative Treatment for Cancer

This section will serve as an example of the more popular therapies advocated by complementary medicine for the prevention or treatment of cancer. It includes herbal medicine, nutrition, dietary supplements, energy medicine, mind-body medicine, biology-based practices, manipulative therapy, and acupuncture. The beneficial results will be discussed under each individual cancer, but here I wanted to just give a list of the more commonly used therapies.

The complementary practitioner should be involved from the beginning, and the patient should be made aware of how the ensuing benefits will complement the person's treatments. The range of therapies are what this book is about, and I have been trying to meld this total view of patient health in order to encourage the family physician, oncologist, surgeon, and other medical personnel to work together with the alternative practitioner.

### *Herbal and Dietary Treatments and Remedies*

These are perhaps the most widely accepted and used aspects of complementary medicine. The use of herbal combinations for prevention and remedies dates back thousands of years, and the success of many over the centuries must be evaluated. The therapeutic effect of many proposed anticancer herbs is through inhibiting cancer-activating enzymes, stimulating DNA repair, enhancing the immune system, and promoting antioxidant activity. Certain herbs also affect hormones and enzymes, and others help during chemotherapy by reducing nausea and other toxic side effects of standard therapy. More than three hundred actively used anticancer herbs have been studied, and among them are the following.

* African willow tree *(Combretum caffrum)*, with combretastatin, a small organic molecule found in the bark of this tree, inhibits the blood supply to tumors. It will only affect blood vessels that supply cancer cells.

- Aloe vera activates macrophages.

- Astragalus and ligusticum (Chinese herbs) have anticancer effects. Astragalus has proven efficacious as an adjunct cancer therapy. Ligusticum, and its active components, have been investigated for enhancement of the immune system, treatment of ischemic disorders, and as an anti-inflammatory.[8]

- Betulin (*Betula utilis*) inhibits the growth of melanomas, and lung and liver cancer.

- Bioflavonoids, particularly quercetin, citrin, flavones, and anthrocyanins, can reputedly inhibit cancer growth and convert cancer cells to normal cells.

- Bromelain (*Ananas comosus*), from pineapple, enhances cytotoxic activities.

- Camptothecin (*Quinolone*) is an antileukemia, anticancer agent. This class of compounds has been demonstrated to be effective against a broad spectrum of tumors.[9]

- Cat's Claw (*Uncaria tomentosa*) contains the antioxidant compounds polyphenols, stigmasterol, and beta-sitosterol used for treating brain cancer.

- Carotenoids (carrots, kale, beets, tomatoes, squash, etc.) are reputed to reduce the risks of cancer.

- Ellipticine (*Pyrido carbozoles*) has potent anticancer properties and is used for breast and kidney cancer.

- Essiac, an herbal tea from Canada, is purported to enhance activity of immune cells and reduce toxic side effects of chemotherapy—used to treat melanoma, lymphoma, and many cancers.

- Flaxseed and flaxseed oil are said to reduce the growth of cancer cells in colon and breast cancer, and another component of flaxseed called *lignans* is believed to help prevent these cancers.

- Garlic (*Allium sativum*) restores killer-cell activity in AIDS patients and inhibits cancer in lab animals and humans (as per example Allium sativum in Chinese herbal medicine).

- *Ginseng* is believed to inhibit cancer growth.

- Green tea (*Camellia sinensis*) is known to inhibit urokinase and slow or stop the spread of cancer—prevents covalent bonding of carcinogens to DNA, and users have a lower incidence of stomach cancer.

- Himalayan May apple (*Podophyllum hexandrum*) and American May apple (*Podophyllum peltatum*) contain podophyllum that affects dividing cancer cells—podophyllotoxin is used in treatment of several cancers, including Hodgkin's and non-Hodgkin's lymphoma.

- Hoxsey herbal formula (*Arctium lappa, Berberis vulgaris, Glycyrrhiza glabra, Larrea tridentate, Picramnia antidesma*, et al.) contains anti-cancer abilities.

- Iscador–Mistletoe (*Viscum album*) has been used in advanced cases of breast cancer and has increased survival in other cancers. Iscador treatment can achieve a clinically relevant prolongation of survival time of cancer patients.[10]

- Kombu (*Laminaria japonica*) is a seaweed (kelp) containing significant amounts of glutamic acid and reputed to reduce the risk for breast cancer.

- Larch arabinogalactan (*Echinacea angustifolia*) is effectively used for metastatic esophageal and colon cancer.[11]

- Larix (*Larix ocidentalis*) enhances the cytotoxicity of natural killer cells.

- Macrobiotic diet (near-vegetarian) consisting of beans, miso soup, nuts, seaweed, seeds, vegetables, whole grains, and herbal teas is useful in reducing the risk for cancer.

- Madagascar periwinkle, rosy periwinkle (*Catharanthus roseus*). The experimentation with this folkloric hypoglycemic drug led to the development of alkaloids like vinblastine, vincristine, and other pharmaceutical drugs used for leukemias, lymphomas, and other cancers.

- Maitake (*Gyrphora esculenta*) is a mushroom that inhibits cancer by enhancing natural killer cells.

- Milk thistle (*Silybum marianum*) protects against cancer by helping with the regrowth of liver cells.

- Multivitamins, vitamins B, C, thiamine, $B_{12}$, folic acid, and the mineral zinc have anticancer functions.

- Pau d'arco bark (*Tabebuia impetiginosa*), as lapachol, is used for tea and has anticancer results, prolonging survival of patients with leukemia.

- Periwinkle plants (*Vinca rosea*) were the first alkaloids used to treat cancer.

- Selenium and calcium are considered anticancer supplements.

- Soy-based diets (*Isoflavones*) are believed to reduce risks of breast and prostate cancer.

- Taxanes–Pacific yew tree (*Taxus brevifolia*) is used pharmaceutically as anticancer drugs paclitaxel (Taxol) and docetaxel (Taxotere).

- Turmeric (*Curcuma longa*) is effective in all phases of cancer development, initiation, promotion, and progression. It enhances natural antioxidant functions and is used for squamous skin cancer and oral cancers.

- Valerian (*Valeriana officinalis*) is an herb used to defray anxiety during treatments for cancer.

These are only a few of the preparations used extensively in China and India for the treatment of cancer. They are slowly being investigated by American drug companies, and many have already been used in formulating chemotherapeutic agents. There is great probability that many have value, although it may take a while before they are accepted by the American Food and Drug administration. They are, however, currently in use as herbs and supplements by alternative practitioners.

A few others used by American herbalists include azovin, blue tonic, chaga mushroom (*Tsi-ahga*), chicory root, custom elixir RAD, gingerroot oil, klivina trem, Murill mushroom (*Agaricus blazei*), organic black cumin, organic clary sage oil, organic lemon oil, organic peppermint oil, quanzor, reishi mushroom (*Ganodermum lucidum*), tovil, and wild juniper berry—the list goes on and on.

It is interesting to note that, according to researcher Kaushal Chovatiya, only "5–15 percent of approximately 250,000 higher plants have ever been investigated for bioactive compounds."[12]

### Indian Ayurveda

Ayurvedic medicine has been practiced in India for over five thousand years. Ayurvedic means science of life and focuses on the mind, body, and spirit to restore normal harmony and homeostasis to the human body. In this manner, it is similar to Chinese medicine, which utilizes *qigong* (*qi* is vital energy that flows along invisible pathways in the body called meridians), as well as acupuncture and herbs.

Ayurvedic medicine bases diagnoses on three metabolic body types called *doshas,* and everyone has one predominant type. Your own dosha is determined by which group you predominately fall into.

1. **Vata.** Thin with cool dry skin, dry curly hair, vivacious and imaginative personality, easily fatigued, quick to learn, prominent joints and veins, and prone to constipation, PMS, anxiety, insomnia. (It is characterized by *changeable.*)

2. **Pitta.** Medium build, articulate, strong with endurance, thin fine hair, ruddy, freckled complexion, dislikes sleep, moderately sound sleeper, perspires heavily, often thirsty, medium mental capacity, irritated under stress, prone to acne, hemorrhoids, ulcers, and other stomach ailments. (It is characterized by *predictable.*)

3. **Kapha.** Solid, heavy, curvy, and strong, procrastinators, slow in everything, obstinate, dark full hair, oily smooth skin, dislikes damp and cold, compassionate, good memory, relaxed under stress, prone to high cholesterol, allergies, and sinus problems. (It is characterized by *relaxed.*)

Ayurvedic medicine uses pulse and tongue diagnosis and also evaluates the eyes and nails. Of interest is that, in ancient times, Ayurvedic doctors were only paid when the patient was well; when you got sick, payments stopped. The focus was on preventive medicine, utilizing spiritual healing and mental hygiene, cleansing and detoxifying, palliation and rejuvenation.

The Ayurvedic doctor has to complete five years of training in India (there are no U.S. schools) and receives a BAMS degree (Bachelor of Ayurvedic Medicine and Surgery) but is not licensed in the United States. However, there are some dual Western and Indian physicians who promote and treat using both philosophies. The treatment utilizes herbal therapy, meditation, purification, and yoga, and each cancer diagnosis will discuss this.

### *Traditional Chinese Medicine*

Traditional Chinese medicine (TCM) is basically a philosophy of looking at the body in a different way. Codified over 2,500 years ago, TCM is truly the forerunner of holistic health care. The direction is partly through preventing disease by paying attention to, or altering, the environment, diet, lifestyle, and emotional state of the person. It is all about the *qi* or energy system in the body. Chinese medicine seeks to strengthen *qi* with a tapestry of therapies, including acupuncture, dietary and lifestyle changes, exercises with breathing movements, such as tai chi, herbs, and even using lovemaking techniques to enhance all aspects of life.

The ears are considered a microsystem of the body, and massaging the ears is thought to enhance the flow of *qi* through the entire body. With centuries of history and documentation and the experience of three billion Chinese, many practitioners state that Chinese medicine can help heal cancer, as well as arthritis, fatigue, gastrointestinal disorders, heart disease, nausea, pain, respiratory conditions, and sexual dysfunctions. Even the diagnostic terms are different from Western medicine. In addition to the term *qi*, you will hear such terms as yin and yang, which refer to the opposite qualities in life, male and female, hot and cold, light and dark, wet and dry. Deficiencies in yin or yang call for specific approaches, using the modalities of Chinese medicine, including herbal, acupuncture, and *qi* manipulations. This is a far fly from Western medicine and it is not surprising that most Western surgeons and oncologists look upon this therapy with doubt and hesitation. With increasing interaction and knowledge, perhaps the American patient will be able to benefit from both philosophies. I say this knowing that, to some extent, there is a growing knowledge of these modalities. I also know that many of my patients are not aware of them, and are excited and interested to hear about alternative therapies. And many physicians are not aware of many of these alternative treatments either, so this book by a fellow physician can serve as an introduction for them as well.

## Selection of Ayurvedic or Chinese Practitioners.

Just as it is important to select a qualified surgeon or oncologist in Western medicine, it behooves the patient to seek out highly qualified practitioners of both Ayurvedic and Chinese medicine. With regard to

Indian Ayurvedic medicine, be sure the doctor has a BAMS degree. The Chinese practitioner should be certified an O.M.D. (Oriental Medical Doctor) or D.O.M. (Doctor of Oriental Medicine) by the National Certification Commission for Acupuncture and Oriental Medicine (NCCAOM), and practitioners of acupuncture should have L.Ac. (Licensed Acupuncturist) or C.A. (Certified Acupuncturist) after their names.

This book aims to clarify and integrate these two forms of medicine into the care of cancer patients as each individual cancer will be examined in the ensuing chapters.

## Chinese Herbal Medicine

The following herbal medicines are used in China today and many have been tested by Chinese research agencies and found effective in the treatment of cancers.

◇ Amygdalin (*Laetrile*), used in China for over three thousand years, contains nitrilosides (benzaldehyde and cyanide), and, while supposedly efficacious in treating cancer, can also be deadly when used in incorrect dosages

◇ Angelica sinensis (*Dong quia*) for cancer of the cervix—by stimulating interferon production

◇ Astragalus membranaceus (*Huang qi*) for advanced liver cancer

◇ Fu Zhen (combination of six herbs—*astragalus, atractylode, ganoderma, ginseng,* and *ligustrium*) strengthens the body defenses against cancer

◇ Ginkgo biloba protects DNA from radiation effects and inhibits cancer growth

◇ Glycine max (soybean) has a concentrated extract Haelan851, rich in selenium, multiple vitamins, zinc, isoflavone, and protease inhibitors, causes conversion of cancerous cells to normal cells

◇ Goldenseal hydrastis Canadensis (*Berberine*) treats bone-marrow depression

◇ Panax ginseng (*Ren Shen/ginseng*), used for more than two thousand years, inhibits killer cells

◇ Polyporus umbellatus (*Zhu Ling*) increases cancer-patient life span by enhancing immune system cells

◇ Rabdosia rubescens (*Dong ling cao*) for esophageal cancer

A combination of ingredients called Cancer Soup is often used. It contains angelica root, dandelion root, garlic, ginger, ginseng, hawthorn fruit, leeks, lentil beans, mung beans, olives, onions, parsley, red date licorice, scallions, senegal root, sesame seeds, shiitake mushrooms, and soybeans.

### Kampo—Japanese Herbal Medicine

◇ Juzen-taiho-to (angelica, astragalus, cinnamomum, ginseng, glycyrrhiza, et al.) enhances natural killer cells.

◇ Sho-saiko-to (bupleurum pinellia, ginseng, scutellaria, ziziphus jujube, et al.) enhances macrophages fighting cancer.

### Nutrition

Nutrition plays a major part in maintaining health both in the conventional and alternative modalities. The term RDA (Recommended Daily Allowance) indicates the daily dietary intake of a certain nutrient sufficient to meet a person's daily needs.

The American Cancer Society and the American Institute for Cancer Research both have guidelines that may help prevent cancer, and these are similar to those advocated by all alternative therapies. They include the five points below.[13]

1. Eat less meat and food low in fat and salt.

2. Limit alcohol intake.

3. Eliminate tobacco.

4. Eat a diet that includes grain products, fruits, and vegetables.

5. Maintain a healthy weight.

Some cancers make substances that alter the way your body uses certain nutrients, and nutritional therapy is aimed at supplementing and improving absorption and utilization of the carbohydrates, fats, and proteins that are lacking.

Nutrition is a key factor in maintaining a healthy immune system, rebuilding body tissue, decreasing the risk for infection, recuperating faster from cancer treatment, increasing energy, and improving the quality of life in general. Supplementary vitamins and minerals often provide nutrients not in your diet.

Similarly, most of the alternative and complementary systems advocate diets rich in fiber, antioxidants, micronutrients, and amino acids. They stress avoidance of red meats. Co-enzyme $Q_{10}$, found in grape-seeds, pistachios, soybeans, spinach, and walnuts, is said to prevent cancer and cause a regression of advanced breast cancer. Omega-3 fatty acids, found in fish, plant oils, such as corn, flax, pumpkin, and safflower, are anticancer agents. Vitamin A is an antioxidant and strengthens the immune system, vitamin D promotes the absorption of calcium and phosphorus and is felt to prevent certain cancers, vitamin $B_6$ helps the immune system, and vitamin C (ascorbic acid) promotes healing. Vitamins C, D, and E are believed to prevent cancer. Several other dietary supplements are recommended to ward off or treat cancer—calcium, copper, germanium, iodine, magnesium, manganese, potassium, selenium, and zinc. Natural estrogens found in legumes (diadzein and genistein) inhibit hormone-dependent cancers by blocking estrogen. Lactobacilli are anticancer agents because they detoxify chemical carcinogens. Many other nutritional supplements are used, including ginger, green tea, maitake (*grifola frondosa*), soy products, and turmeric.

Avoid animal fat and animal-based protein, eat food low in cholesterol, avoid gluten, and focus more on a plant-based diet.

## Energetics

Years ago, work on energetically enhancing the body's ability to fight disease and improve health was in its infancy. As a consequence, improving health energetically seemed something useful to do, but not vital. But once quantum physics had proved that everything was essentially energy, that led visionary health professionals to talk about how, in the future, energetic medicine would be the strongest form of healing. With the development and release of a series of powerful frequency enhanced elixirs, using energetic frequencies to improve health and fight disease is now possible. They include a group of therapies that are listed here.

◇ Corvix, made from three oils, angelica root, chamomile, and sage, greatly increases the ability of every cell in your body to produce more energy, enabling them to function more effectively and detoxify more efficiently.

◇ Elixir waters. A whole series of crystal elixers exist to support detoxification. One stimulates and improves the function of the kidneys, liver, and other detoxification organs. Excess toxins are an underlying major cause of cancer. You may have been further poisoned by chemotherapy. Your body needs to get rid of those toxins, and your liver needs support. Dead cancer cells are toxic, and the liver can easily get overwhelmed. In fact, an overwhelmed liver leaving behind a large amount of toxins in the body can lead to death.

◇ Koch's homeopathic energy remedies. Cancer cells are geared up to replicate rapidly, many times faster than normal cells, but Koch Energy turns off the replication of cancer cells and initiates the repair of respiratory enzymes in the cells, stopping the spread of cancer and helping to slow down the growth of, or even kill, cancer cells.

◇ Quantum Variable Field Technology. Removing blocks so the energy can flow. According to practitioner Garland Landrith, Ph.D., in his website (www.theuniverselieswithin.com/DVD.aspx) today's science explains that our whole physical system is governed by the flow of electrical energy within our bodies. According to acupuncture theory, he says, when there is a block in the energy flow, it creates a corresponding effect in our bodies that, in turn, creates disease or pain. In theory this makes a lot of sense because scientists today are finding all sorts of mind-body connections that seem to indicate how negative emotions can actually cause all kinds of physical problems. In essence what is being proposed here is that there are mind, emotional, and body connections that can be healed simply by getting rid of the blocks to the flow of energy in our bodies.[14]

◇ QuZu increases the production of endorphins and glutathione and enables your immune system to function better.

◇ Quantum X uses subtle vibrations and energy to encourage cells to release their toxins and establish a new pattern of repair. This supports wellness at all levels.

◇ Zernix is a powerful immune-system booster composed of essential oils—cedarwood oil, Douglas fir needle oil, frankincense oil, pine oil, spruce oil, thuja oil, yarrow oil—and a blend of trace amounts of the minerals copper, gold, magnesium, sodium, and strontium (2 oz.).

## Acupuncture and Acupressure

While having a role in other diseases, and in relieving stress and pains, and even their use as anesthesia, these modalities do not play an active role in cancer care in the Western sense. They are, however, extremely effective in their ability to relax patients and ease the pain and suffering of both the cancer itself, and the side effects of chemotherapy that include abdominal pain, constipation, diarrhea, loss of hair, nausea, and vomiting.[15]

## Chiropractic

Chiropractic is a form of alternative medicine that deals with the philosophy of disease being related to mechanical disorders of the human spine. These physicians perform spinal adjustments to alleviate back pain, neck pain, and headaches, as well as many general medical disorders, assuming that vertebral subluxation (*see* glossary) interferes with the body's intelligence causing these abnormalities. The main treatment involves manual therapy that many individuals swear by, claiming their back and neck pain has been alleviated by the treatments. They also advocate diet, exercises, and lifestyle counseling.

The practice originated in the late nineteenth and early twentieth century with D. D. Palmer and his son B. J. Palmer and has grown to be the third most popular medical specialty after conventional medicine and dentistry. With its usual benighted outlook, the very establishment American Medical Association has called chiropractic an "unscientific cult," and most mainstream physicians look with extreme skepticism on its principles and practice. The original practitioners claimed to have cured hearing loss and many general medical conditions with this therapy, but there have been no supportive clinical trials or data to confirm that this treatment does anything at all to alleviate symptoms.

Contrary to the clear prejudice demonstrated in this assessment, chiropractic *does* have benefits for people with cancer. Chiropractic adjustments increase certain immune cells, as well as tone down the stress hormones, the fight-or-flight mechanisms. Since the stress hormones tend to weaken the body's immune system, toning them down increases the immune system's ability to fight the abnormal cancer cells.[16]

The mother of a chiropractor named Dan Murphy had lung cancer and was given six months to live. She rejected standard medical treatment in favor of chiropractic, and thanks to her son's regular chiropractic work on her, she lived for twenty-four more years before finally succumbing to her cancer.[17]

The chiropractic philosophy includes:

◇ Holism, the belief that health is affected by everything in the environment including the spiritual;

◇ Reductionism that reduces all causes and cures to vertebral subluxation;

◇ Conservatism that emphasizes noninvasive treatment, avoiding medication and surgery; and

◇ Homeostasis that emphasizes the body's inherent ability to heal itself.

### Manipulative Therapies

Manipulative therapies, including chiropractic, while seeming foreign and ineffective to too many unenlightened conventional Western physicians, have been used worldwide for centuries, with much success and popularity. "Most conventional Western practitioners tend to think of the body as a series of segmented carapaces, each unrelated to the other, whereas the holistic alternative practitioner views the body as one complete, interrelated unit, with every part of it connected to, and impacting, every other part of this whole—this is a key difference between the two systems."[18]

Hopefully, establishment medicine will learn this core concept of alternative medicine and will integrate it into the care of cancer patients. It may be a difficult nut to crack, but it is being done slowly and surely throughout the world because patients are demanding it.

### Reiki

According to William Lee Rand, "Reiki energy is very flexible and creative, treating each unique situation with a unique response and working freely with all other forms of healing"[19]

Reiki, a Japanese word meaning universal life energy, is a form of energy medicine that has no side effects and can do no harm. It is applied to the patient through the hands of a Reiki practitioner. Some schools of Reiki teach a gentle, hands-on approach, while others teach a hands-off approach where the hands hover gently above the body.

Reiki was discovered by Mikau Usui in March 1922 while he was on a Buddhist retreat on Mt. Kurama. He was searching for solutions to his life's problems on this retreat, and, as part of the practice, he sat under a waterfall that was known for its healing properties. Indeed, he had a sudden insight into his solutions and raced down the hill to share his discovery. Along the way, he stubbed his toe. He instinctively reached out to his injured foot with his hands, and, as soon as he touched his toe, the injury healed instantly, and he discovered that, in addition to his insights, he had gained a healing ability as well.

A Reiki practitioner is able to direct *Rei-Ki* (Universal Healing Light Energy) through the hands as a method to improve body and spirit. Much like a sourdough starter, a Reiki Master must open the natural healing channels in the practitioner through a process called attunement that takes several minutes in a Reiki class. Without the attunement, Reiki energy will not flow.

Reiki healing is unique among all other kinds of energy healing in that it does not deplete the healer. In fact a small amount of healing is absorbed by the healer while working on the patient.

The benefit of Reiki in cancer treatment is that it promotes relaxation. Randomized double-blind studies support this benefit. Many cancer centers have departments of integrative medicine where Reiki is provided to hospital patients free-of-charge by volunteers. Outpatients may access Reiki at reduced rates at an integrative medical center or at nearby affiliated Reiki practitioners.

Many patients with cancer and other chronic diseases opt to learn Reiki themselves in order to self-treat. This adds a layer of care that is comforting to many who respond well to Reiki treatment.

Usui-Sensei advised a daily meditation on these five precepts:

1. Just for today, do not anger.

2. Just for today, do not complain.

3. Just for today, express gratitude.

**4** Just for today, do your work honestly.

**5** Just for today, be kind to others.

"Reiki is not a religion. It is a noninvasive form of healing that aligns the body's own natural healing ability with a higher source of energy that exists from the universe. Spirituality is often associated with Reiki practice, but there is no link to any formal religion of any kind with its use." —Carla St. Laurent, Reiki Master-Teacher, Karuma Reiki-Master-Teacher[20,21,22]

## Holistic and Other Organizations

In Ayurvedic Indian medicine, the practitioner receives his training and has documentation of his expertise in this tradition. The training in India requires at least five years and graduates receive a BAMS (Bachelor of Ayurvedic Medicine), or a DAMS (Doctor of Ayurvedic Medicine and Surgery). The United States has no standard for training or certifying Ayurvedic medicine, although some states have recognized Ayurvedic schools as educational institutions. So it is difficult for an American to know for sure the qualifications of this type of practitioner and must rely on the ability to discover the validity of the practitioner's training and expertise. Concurrently, Ayurvedic medications are regulated as dietary supplements and are not required to meet the safety and efficacy standards for conventional medicine.

Chinese Medicine is divided between Western-type medicine, following the British system, and is overseen by the Chinese Medical Association and the Chinese Academy of Medical Science, with strict requirements for licensure and practice. Chinese traditional medicine (TCM), based on *qi*, acupuncture, and a whole different approach to body homeostasis, presents a different model. One group, now based in the Beijing Institute of Traditional Chinese Medicine, provides training in this ancient art that covers a whole host of traditions and requires many years to become an expert. Unfortunately, there is no set standard for qualification in the United States and determining who is qualified to practice this ancient art is problematic. Many major American medical schools are beginning to incorporate aspects of TCM, but as yet there is no certifying board or way to accurately evaluate the qualifications of a practitioner. Currently the

# NATIONAL CENTER FOR COMPLEMENTARY AND ALTERNATIVE MEDICINE (NCCAM)

The National Institutes of Health (NIH) funds several centers, and included among them, since 1992, is the NCCAM (National Center for Complementary and Alternative Medicine). This group explores these medical practices with rigorous scientific programs to determine which ones meet standards for valid and provable additions to the standard medical regimen. Typically, this program has met with much criticism from establishment medicine, and several prominent individuals want the center closed for lack of finding any value in complementary or alternative medical programs. This is the extreme position and many scientists feel that these nonconventional programs should be examined and that information on them should be disseminated. Several researchers feel that the NCCAM facilitates the infiltration of nonscientific and non-evidence-based treatments and want the program eliminated from the NIH. It is, however, better to have these programs under some observation and evaluation than none. The problem may lie in trying to evaluate a nonstandard medical regimen, such as Chinese medicine, Ayurveda, or spiritual or herbal therapies, using conventional Western medical methods. Plus, the bias against complementary medicine is so strong among Western physicians that evaluations are often doomed before they begin.

While complementary and alternative approaches need to be critically evaluated, it is also important not to eliminate the fact that many of these methods contribute a positive asset. Improving diet and making individuals more aware of their environment, their weight, and the toxic nature of many foods and additives, is all encompassed in the alternative medical focus, and these programs should not be dismissed. In this text I present some aspects of complementary medicine, keeping in mind that traditional Newtonian physics has taken a great step forward only because scientists have been willing to look at the world through different glasses, as with quantum mechanics and string theory, which almost approach the spiritual.

gold standard in acupuncturists is those who have had lengthy training in China (Beijing).

Naturopathic and holistic medicine have schools in the United States with varying years of training. Many (though not all) states have licensing procedures for these specialties. There is an accrediting agency for naturopathic medicine, the North American Board of Naturopathic Examiners that oversees the Council on Naturopathic Medical Education, and national and/or state licensure examinations must be passed in order to practice the specialty. Similarly, there is an American Board of Integrative Holistic Medicine (ABIHM) that regulates and licenses these practitioners. Individuals wanting care from these healthcare providers should look for qualifications from these boards.

PART 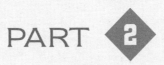 2

# THE DISEASES

# THE CANCERS

CANCER IS NOT A SINGLE DISEASE. So talking about cancer, its etiology (cause), progression, cure, or treatment, is in effect a discussion of many different diseases that have been lumped together by their natural propensity to grow indiscriminately and eventually lead to the destruction of tissue and death. Malignant tumors can, in fact, be found in all forms of higher organisms, including plants.

Concerning the staging system, most tumors in this book use the TNM system. T stands for tumor size, N for node, and M for metastasis. Surgical and oncological treatment depends on the staging of the disease. T0 means no tumor found, Tis is DCIS, T1—tumor size to 2cm, T2—2–5cm, T3—greater than 5cm, No—No nodes, N1 cancer in moveable nodes, N2—matted nodes, N3—spread to inside chest nodes.

> Each specific organ system will include advice on prevention and complementary methods, including diet and natural substances, along with medical and surgical management.

# ADRENAL CANCERS

Cancers of the adrenal gland are rare, highly malignant tumors. They are divided between the two parts of the adrenal gland—the cortex (the outer part) and the medulla (the inner part) of the gland. The cortex produces steroids (mineralocorticoids—aldosterone, glucocorticoids, cortisol, much like cortisone) and sex steroids (estrone and testosterone). The medulla produces catecholamines (dopamine, epinephrine, and norepinephrine) and can further synthesize a wide variety of other substances, such as histamine, rennin, serotonin, and others. Cancer of the adrenal gland may produce an excess of the hormone or substance from the particular part of the adrenal where it arises. There are no known causes for adrenal cancers.

## ADRENAL CORTEX CANCER

Tumors of the adrenal cortex, being very deep in the retroperitoneum on the top of the kidney, are often not diagnosed until they have grown fairly large. By this time, they have invaded large vessels, such as the kidney and vena cava arteries, and often have spread into adjacent lymph nodes or lungs. Symptoms may include abdominal mass, abdominal pain, fever, and weight loss.

If a cancer of the adrenal cortex produces cortisol, it may produce Cushing's syndrome, which is characterized by abdominal stretch marks, high blood pressure, hirsutism (excess hairiness), osteoporosis, severe acne, slow growth rate in children, and weakness.

If the cancer produces aldosterone, then it may bring about Conn's syndrome, characterized by excessive thirst, frequent urination, high blood pressure, and low potassium levels. Aside from blood and studies, the diagnosis and staging can be completed using MRI (magnetic resonance imaging), a CT scan (computerized axial tomography), and nuclear-medicine scanning using MIBG (metaiodobenzylguanidine) and PET (positron emission tomography) scan.

### ■ *Diagnosis and Treatment*

When diagnosed early, the best therapy is surgery. Advanced cancer may also be surgically treated, and, if not completely removed, debulking may decrease the symptoms and provide longer survival. These are also treated with chemotherapy, radiation, and hormonal therapy.

## Staging

The staging is according to the T.N.M. system. T=Tumor, N=Lymph nodes, M=Metastases.

- T1 tumor < 5 cm, no invasion—N0–No lymph node involvement

- T2 tumor > 5 cm, no invasion—N1–Lymph node involvement

- T3 tumor outside adrenal in fat—M0–No metastases

- T4 tumor invading adjacent organs—M1–Distant metastases

- Stage I—T1 N0 M0

- Stage II—T2 N0 M0

- Stage III—T1 2 N1 M0; T3 N0 M0

- Stage IV—any T any N M1; T3, T4

Surgery to remove the gland is called adrenalectomy and can be done through an incision in the back or through the front of the abdomen. Laparoscopic procedures are also possible if the tumor is not too large. A newer technique called robotic surgery is also available. Radiation is often used after surgery to kill remaining cells, but the adrenal cancer is not very sensitive to radiation therapy.

Chemotherapy does not work well for adrenal cortical cancer. Mitotane is used and is effective in blocking hormone production in 80 percent of the people, and stemming the growth of the cancer in 30 percent of them. Other chemotherapeutic agents are aminoglutethamide, etoposide (VP-16), 5-fluorouracil (5-FU), ketoconazole, metyrapone, paclitaxel (Taxol), and vincristine (Oncovin). Unfortunately, the side effects for these are hair loss, hand and foot rashes, loss of appetite, low blood counts, mouth sores, nausea, and vomiting. They have a tendency to lead to anemia, bleeding and bruising, and an increased risk for infections. Most of the side effects disappear after the cessation of therapy, and there are many standard and complementary regimens for control of the major side effects.

■ *Complementary and Alternative Treatment*

Among the complementary methods are acupuncture, aromatherapy, biofeedback to relieve pain, hypnosis, massage, meditation to reduce stress, music therapy, peppermint tea to relieve nausea, and yoga to relieve stress. No complementary treatments can cure adrenal cancer, and conventional allopathic medicine believes that all alternative medicine should only be used in conjunction with standard Western oncological care.

The best approach is to understand that there are no known preventives or lifestyle changes for adrenal cancer although adherence to a good diet and avoiding tobacco are certainly important. Individuals with a family history of adrenal cancer or with the unusual syndromes listed below are at increased risk for adrenal cancer and should have genetic testing and the diagnostic studies described above.[1,2]

## ADRENAL MEDULLA CANCER

Tumors of the medulla are predominately neuroblastomas (from precursors of nerve cells) and pheochromocytoma, which produce adrenaline compounds and can present with very high blood pressure, heart arrhythmias, headaches, anxiety attacks, sweating, and weight loss. The symptoms are treated medically, and when stable these tumors can be removed surgically.

## MEDICAL SYNDROMES WITH INCREASED RISK FOR ADRENAL CANCER

◇ Beckwith-Wiedemann syndrome

◇ Li-Fraumeni syndrome

◇ Multiple endocrine neoplasia type 2

◇ Neurofibromatosis type 1 (von Recklinghausen's disease)

◇ Paraganglioma syndrome

◇ Von Hippel–Lindau syndrome

### ■ *Diagnosis and Treatment*

The radiological workup is the same as adrenal cortical tumors; the blood and urine tests focus on the by-products of the substances produced by the cancer (fractionated plasma metanephrines, urinary catecholamines, and urine metanephrines). Surgery to remove the tumor and the adrenal gland is performed after medication has stabilized the blood pressure or other extreme symptoms.

Chemotherapy includes streptozosin, and occasionally with cyclophosphamide, vincristine, dacarbazine, doxorubicin and epirubicin.

### ■ *Complementary and Alternative Treatment*

The complementary treatments and cautions are the same as with the adrenal cortex cancers.

## METASTATIC CANCER TO ADRENAL GLAND

In conclusion, you should be aware that the most common cancers of the adrenal gland are the metastases from another cancer in another part of the body. These include kidney cancer, melanoma, lung cancer, colorectal cancer, breast cancer, and lymphoma. The treatment is adrenalectomy, and the drugs used are those prescribed for the primary tumor. Radiation will be used for these types of metastases.

## AIDS AND CANCER

Human immunodeficiency virus (HIV) is the cause of AIDS. The incidence of cancer in those with AIDS (acquired immunodeficiency syndrome) hovers at 40–45 percent and increases as the survival of the person infected with HIV improves with therapy. AIDS-related cancers include Kaposi's sarcoma, non-Hodgkin's lymphoma, and cancer of the anus and cervix.

Kaposi's sarcoma, described by Morris Kaposi in 1872, was once a very rare disease until the rising incidence of it seen with AIDS patients. Kaposi's sarcoma is a cancer involving the lining of blood vessels and the form of the tumor seen in this group is much more highly malignant in its behavior. With the HIV epidemic, it became a more common entity because HIV destroys the immune cells that normally defend the body against certain infections and against cancer development.

In 1995, with the inception of HAART (highly active antiretroviral therapy), there was a marked decrease in the deaths from AIDS and initially a marked decrease in the occurrence of AIDS-related malignancies. However, while there has never been a cure for HIV infection, the long-term survival has increased and the total number of those with the disease has increased. Therefore, there is a larger group at risk for developing these malignancies over their prolonged lives.

## ■ Diagnosis and Treatment

Kaposi's sarcoma in AIDS may present as a series of bulky tumors of the legs, with swelling and pain, or may present with enlarged lymph nodes, liver, and spleen. The HAART therapy is the main therapy directed toward AIDS, and local treatments may involve cryotherapy, intralesional injections, photodynamic therapy, radiation therapy, and topical application of drugs. In addition to HAART, commonly used systemic therapies include ABV (adriamycin, bleomycin, daunorubicin, doxorubicin, interferon-a, paclitaxel, vinca alkaloids), and, more recently, imatinib (Gleevac) and thalidomide.

AIDS-associated lymphoma is a highly malignant disease arriving predominately from B-lymphocytes, and it often involves bone marrow, the central nervous system, and the liver. Treatment includes chemotherapy, the HAART protocol, and a number of new agents, including CHOP (cyclophosphamide-Cytoxan, doxorubicin, etoposide, prednisone, rituximab, and vincristine).

Women with HIV have twice the incidence of developing cervical cancer, and the nature of this cancer is usually more vigorous and is discovered at a later stage than in women who are not HIV-positive. Because of the immune suppression, the incidence of oral cancers is also higher in individuals with HIV.

## ■ Complementary and Alternative Treatment

There are several alternative therapies recommended as complementary therapies for individuals with HIV and HIV malignancies. Herbs, including aloe vera, echinacea, ginseng, and licorice, have been used extensively to improve the immune response and reduce the symptoms of AIDS and the incidence of related malignancies. St. John's Wort, however, is not recommended, even though it has many positive effects on other cancers, because it can significantly reduce the effect of standard HAART therapy.

Chinese herbal medicine, Indian Ayurvedic therapy, and Native American medical practices are used to treat HIV and AIDS, along with standard therapy. These include acupuncture, herbal formulas, massage techniques, and meditation.. Diet and nutrition, dietary supplements, and mind-body therapies, which are often foreign to Western physicians, have a significant effect on improving the quality of life of patients with HIV and related malignancies. In my opinion, these therapies should be used in an integrative fashion, in tandem with standard oncologic medical management.

Supplements that may be helpful are coenzyme $Q_{10}$, fish oil, garlic, and whey protein, which tend to boost the immune system and counteract the side effects of anti-HIV drugs.

## ANAL CANCER

The anus or anal canal consists of the final 3–4 cm of the gastrointestinal tract, extending from the rectum to the skin around the anus. There are four different areas in this short segment of the intestine, each with its own lining cells and epithelium, and cancer is treated differently here than rectal and colon cancer. The outer area looks like skin with the same hair and glandular bearing tissue; slightly more inward, the anus is lined with modified squamous epithelium; a little farther up, in an area called anal valves and the dentate or pectinate line, the lining is made up of a combination of squamous and transitional epithelium that has rectum, squamous, and urinary-tract features. A little higher up, the mucosa blends with that of the lower rectum.

This cancer is more common in men and usually occurs between fifty and sixty years of age. There is a strong connection between immuno-suppression diseases, tobacco smoking, and human papilloma virus (HPV). Among unmarried men, a two-times higher incidence may be related to homosexuality and the incidence of anal intercourse.

### ■ *Diagnosis and Treatment*

The signs and symptoms of this disease—bleeding, pain, recurrent anal infection, and sensations of a mass—are so similar to many common benign conditions that diagnosis is often delayed. Diagnosis is usually made with a rectal examination and by endoscopic ano-rectal examination. Because of pain, a careful exam and biopsy may require general anesthesia. A chest x-ray, liver function tests, and a pelvic PET (positron emission tomography) scan are necessary.

Although most of these cancers are classified as squamous-cell carcinomas, there are a few rare neoplasms, such as adenocarcinoma, melanoma, and small-cell carcinoma.

### Staging

The staging is by the TNM (T=Tumor, N=Node, M=Metastasis) system but is divided between anal canal carcinomas (with a grading system to help the oncologist in treatment) and anal margin cancers that behave more like skin cancers and are thereby staged like skin cancers.

- Tis carcinoma in situ—Grade 1–well differentiated (almost normal)
- T1 tumor < 2 cm—Grade 2–moderately differentiated
- T2 tumor > 2 cm but < 5 cm Grade 3–poorly differentiated
- T3 tumor > 5 cm—Grade 4–undifferentiated (looks nothing like anal cells)
- T4 tumor—any size—but invades adjacent organs (bladder, urethra, and vagina)
- N0—No nodes with cancer
- N1—Spread to perirectal lymph node
- N2—Unilateral inguinal or iliac node
- N3—Perirectal and inguinal nodes bilateral
- M0—No metastases
- M1—Distant metastases
- Stage 0—Tis–N0 M0
- Stage I—T1–N0 M0

- Stage II—T2–3 N0 M0
- Stage IIIA—T1–3 N1 M0
- T4—N0 M0
- Stage IIIB—T4–N1 M0
- Any T N2—3 M0
- Stage IV—Any T–Any N M1

**Anal Margin Cancers**

- Tis Carcinoma in situ—N0–No nodes
- T1 Tumor 2 cm or less—N–Positive nodes
- T2 Tumor > 2 cm but < 5 cm
- T3 Tumor > 5 cm—M0–No metastases
- T4—Invades deep tissue (bone, muscle, etc.); M1–Distant metastases
- Stage 0—Tis N0 M0
- Stage I—T1 N0 M0
- Stage II—T2–3 N0 M0
- Stage III—T4–N0 M0
- Any T—N1–M0
- Stage IV—Any T–Any N M1

With small T1 anal-canal tumors, local excision is adequate for cure, often giving postoperative radiation to prevent recurrence. Whereas, in the past, a radical removal of the ano-rectum and a colostomy (abdominal-perineal resection) was performed, much lesser surgical procedures can be done with the introduction of chemotherapy and radiation therapy. Combined modality therapy for Stages I–III has been used for several years and involved upward of 3000cGy of radiation over three weeks, along with a regimen of chemotherapy, which includes several drugs, among them cisplatin, fluorouracil, and mitomycin.

The anal-margin cancers are treated like skin cancers with wide local excision. This therapy may be augmented with radiation and, in some cases, chemotherapy, depending on the stage.

### ■ *Complementary and Alternative Treatment*

Complementary and alternative therapies are not specific for anal cancers and are primarily based on good colon and ano-rectal health. Avoid tobacco, know your family genetic history, and be sure to use a condom if you participate in anal sex to prevent both HPV and HIV viral infection. The Mayo Clinic states that alternative treatments can't cure anal cancer but that several alternative medicine treatments may help you cope with the side effects of cancer treatment. Among those noted are: hypnosis, massages, meditation, music therapy; exercise and relaxation techniques for anxiety, and gentle exercise and tai chi for fatigue; acupuncture, hypnosis, or music therapy for nausea and pain; and relaxation techniques and yoga for sleep problems.

## BONE CANCER

There are 206 bones in the human body and most of them are subject to involvement with cancer of one form or another. The subjects here are the primary cancers that originate in the bones and surrounding tissues. Elsewhere, the book has discussed the various metastatic cancers that have spread to the bone from their origins in other organs, the most common being breast, kidney, lung, prostate, and thyroid.

Below are several types of primary bone cancers depending on the cell types and their location of origin.

1. Osteosarcoma—osteogenic sarcoma, originating from the bony substance of long bones

2. Chondrosarcoma—arising from cartilage

3. Ewing's sarcoma—from immature nerve tissue in bones

4. Fibrosarcoma—from connective tissue in bones

5. Malignant giant cell tumor—connective tissue of bone marrow

There is no known specific etiology (cause) for bone cancers, but a few predisposing factors have been identified, among them the presence of other cancers or cancer syndromes—adrenal and brain tumors, breast cancer, leukemia, and Li-Fraumeni syndrome—or previous chemotherapy and radiation therapy. Although there has been some suggestion that trauma and orthopedic implants may play a role, there is no definitive proof of any relationship.

Osteosarcoma is the most common primary bone cancer, more frequent in men than women, and usually occurring during the second and third decades of life. It often presents as a swelling around the knee or shoulder and may also present as a pathological fracture, a broken bone caused in part by deformity and weakness due to the growth of the cancer. Diagnosis of the tumor is by biopsy, bone scan, CT scan, and x-ray.

Chondrosarcoma is the second most common bone cancer and occurs between the ages of forty to sixty and may affect bones in the femur, humerus, pelvis, ribs, and scapula. Chondrosarcoma cancers are categorized as low-grade (slow growing) and high-grade (rapidly growing) tumors and may involve adjacent tissue causing pain and, when involving the spine, neurological symptoms and a collapse of vertebrae. As with osteosarcoma, diagnosis is made with CT, open or needle biopsies, PET scans, and x-rays.

The third most common primary bone cancer, Ewing's sarcoma, occurs in the long bones of children, usually white; it is rare in Asians and African Americans.

Fibrosarcomas arise from bone and surrounding soft tissue and are most common in men from ages thirty to forty, in the arms, hips, legs, and pelvis. They cause bone destruction and metastasize, via lymph channels, to adjacent nodes and the lungs. They are diagnosed by biopsy, CT, and x-rays.

Malignant giant cell tumors are more common in women between thirty and fifty. Arising in the ends of long bones, they present as painful swellings near the joints, and occasionally as pathological fractures. They spread to adjacent tissue and metastasize to the lungs.

### ■ Diagnosis and Treatment

In all these tumors, common symptoms are pain and a lump, in some cases, pathologic fractures. After a complete workup to determine the size and extent of the cancer, staging is completed and helps the oncology team decide on the appropriate type and timing of therapy. These cancers may affect blood chemistries of alkaline phosphatase, the blood-phosphorus level, calcium, and the parathyroid hormone.

**Staging**

- IA—Low-grade tumor localized to the bone

- IB—Low-grade tumor extending outside bone (extra-compart-mental)

- IIA—High-grade tumor localized to bone

- IIB—High-grade tumor extra-compartmental

- III—High-grade tumor occurring in two or more places on the same bone

- IV—Any grade at any site with metastases, often to brain, liver, or lungs

The first choice for treatment is complete surgical excision, removing segments of bone and replacing with bone grafts or prostheses. For high-grade tumors, chemotherapy or neoadjuvant radiation may be indicated. Only in extreme cases are amputations necessary. Surgical resection is often accompanied by chemotherapy and radiation therapy. Some patients who develop solitary, or even several, lung metastases are candidates for surgical removal of the metastases (metastasectomy).

The drugs used are cisplatin, dacarbazine, doxorubicin, etoposide, ifosfamide, mesna, and methotrexate, often in combinations.

## ▣ *Complementary and Alternative Treatment*

The specific causes of bone cancer are unknown and there are no specific dietary guidelines except as offered by the National Cancer Institute.[3]

There are several recommendations regarding complementary treatment of bone cancer in conjunction with standard medical and surgical practice. These include herbal medicine and nutritional therapy—foods rich in omega-3 fatty acids, fruits, and vegetables—and some physicians recommend green tea, turmeric, art therapy, and mind-body medicine that includes imagery, meditation, music therapy, prayer, and visualization to ameliorate the symptoms of the disease and the side effects of the chemo- and radiation therapy. Selenium in vivo and in-vitro studies have shown an inhibition of osteosarcoma.[4]

Double-blind Chinese herbal medicines have been tested in China and have shown to be of help in alleviating the pain, nausea, and vomiting associated with bone cancer and its treatment. In addition to alleviating pain, Chinese herbs have been shown to prolong life for people with this cancer. Genistein can cause the death of sarcoma cells but is contraindicated in breast, ovarian, and prostate hormone-dependent tumors.[5]

Some Chinese doctors recommend herbs to also diminish swelling, increase appetite, and reduce the size of the tumor. Other Chinese and Ayurvedic practitioners have a large compendium of useful therapies.

## BRAIN AND CENTRAL NERVOUS SYSTEM CANCER

Brain cancer may be either primary (beginning in the brain) or metastatic (beginning in other parts of the body and spreading to the brain). Because of the confined space defined by the hard skull, any tumors in the brain, even the nonmalignant ones, have a dangerous ability to cause serious damage because there is no allowance for expansion of normal tissue around the growing tumor. Whereas benign tumors, such as meningiomas, can cause critical mental and physical changes only relieved by removal of the mass, a malignant tumor is doubly serious because of its dual pressure and its infiltrative capacities.

The cause of primary brain tumors is essentially unknown. A few people (5 percent) may have genetic factors that may be associated with inherited diseases, such as Li-Fraumeni syndrome, multiple endocrine neoplasia, neurofibromatosis, tuberous sclerosis, Turcot syndrome, von Hippel–Lindau, and a family history of brain tumors. There are probably mutations and deletions of tumor-suppressor genes as well. There is an association between brain cancer and prior radiation therapy to the brain, and possibly chemical exposure at work (vinyl chloride), but there is no definite relationship to alcohol, cellphone use, obesity or smoking. There are a few genetic markers, such as MGMT—methylguanine-DNA methyltransferase—that may predict survival in gliomas, but in general there are few genetic or other consistent markers for primary brain cancer.

The pathology of brain tumors depends on the site from which the cancer arises. Gliomas or astrocytomas arise from astrocytes and are graded I–III by the pathologist. Other cancers are ependymoblastoma, germ-cell tumor, medulloblastoma, neuroblastoma, oligodendroglioma, pineoblastoma, naming the origin of the cancer and adding blastoma in most cases. The most common metastatic brain cancers come from breast, colon, kidney, lung, and melanoma.

The symptoms associated with brain cancer may be from the tumor growing and destroying certain portions of the brain, or from the effects of pressure exerted on certain brain-function areas. These may include headaches of a new and different type, migraine headaches, nausea and vomiting, or stiffness of the neck. As well there can be hearing problems, loss of motion or sensation in an arm or leg, personality and behavior changes (confusion, and seizures), speech problems, and visual problems (blurring, difficulty with balance, double vision, loss of peripheral vision). Irritation from any tumor can cause fatigue, tremors, and seizures.

Many of these can be attributed to an increase in intracranial pressure when a tumor expands against a brain in a fixed (skull) environment. This intracranial pressure causes edema (swelling) and more pressure, which causes headaches, nausea and vomiting, and can lead to a coma. Examination of the eyes may show papilledema (changes in the back of the eye), anisocoria (one pupil larger than the other) and, in severe cases, the pressure can push the brainstem downward, leading to severe neurological dysfunction and death. The specific dysfunctions (hearing loss, speech problems, weakness) are related to that portion of the brain responsible for those functions being invaded or destroyed by the cancer. These symptoms apply not only to primary but also to secondary (metastatic) brain cancers.

## ■ *Diagnosis and Treatment*

Years ago, the diagnosis and location of brain cancer was accomplished by a detailed history and neurological examinations, calling for the most acute and scholarly intellectual findings. Today, in addition to the physical examination and EEG (electroencephalogram to pick up abnormal electrical waves in brain function), definitive location and size can be determined by CT scans (computerized axial tomography) and MRIs (magnetic resonance imaging). Once a tumor is found, examination of the rest of the body is necessary to determine whether there is a primary cancer somewhere else in the body (i.e., breast or colon). The final diagnosis, however, rests upon the pathologist examining tissue under a microscope. The tissue may be obtained by needle biopsy or, at the time of definitive excision of the cancer, by a neurosurgeon (brain surgeon).

As opposed to most other malignancies, there is no formal staging for brain cancer because these malignancies are locally invasive and never metastasize to lymph nodes or outside the brain. All metastatic brain cancers are, of course, stage IV by definition.

The treatment of brain cancer depends on the type, location, size, and symptomatology. Decisions about therapy are usually determined by committees of physicians, or at a tumor conference where all aspects of the disease are considered. The optimum therapy would be to remove the entire cancer, but this might not be possible without causing unacceptable damage to the brain, or risking terrible dysfunction or death. So the decision may be made to remove an entire tumor if possible, or just do a biopsy, or remove a portion of the tumor and utilize another modality to get rid of most or all of the remaining cancer. This decision is made not only with the professional staff but also with the understanding and consent of the patient.

Other modalities include chemotherapy (intravenous, oral with pills, or intraoperative with a wafer containing chemotherapy placed in the tumor bed by the surgeon), and radiation therapy or radiosurgery (cyber-knife, gamma-knife, Novalis Tx radiosurgery—stereotactic radiation using multiple beams to a small area).

A minimal amount of response and success has been found in treating malignant gliomas with hydroxyurea, imatinib (Gleevac), procarbazine (Matulane), and tomozolomide (Temodar). Anti-angiogenic agents are being tested (bevacizumab-Avastin and thalidomide) with moderate response rates. Chemotherapy has no role in the treatment of astrocytomas. Procarbazine, iomustine (CeeNu), and vincristine (PCV) produced 70–90 percent response rates for oligodendrogliomas. Capecitabine (Xeloda) is effective in treating brain metastases from breast cancer, and temozolomide has been effective against brain metastases from melanoma and non-small-cell lung cancers.

Treatment is also aimed at controlling the swelling caused by the cancer, and corticosteroids are given liberally throughout the therapy. Seizures, which occur in up to 30 percent of patients, is controlled with phenobarbitol, phenytoin, tegretol, or valproic acid. Newer medications include levetiracetam (Keppra), lamotrigine (Lamictal), andtopiromate (Topamax).

There is a large volume of ongoing experimentation with various agents, but no encouraging positive and definitive results have been forthcoming.

### ■ Complementary and Alternative Treatment

In addition to the side effects of the tumor itself, most patients have the added burden of side effects from the chemotherapy and radiation therapy. The therapies of complementary medicine have been most helpful with cancers in the brain, not just in offsetting the side effects, but in some cases augmenting the effects of the standard therapies, and even acting on the tumor itself. Most major medical centers have begun to focus on time-tested alternative herbals and therapies with great success, and these non-Western approaches are rapidly becoming part of the oncologist's armamentarium.

Fish oils, omega-3 fatty acids, soy lecithin, and vitamin D are helpful for various anticancer and supportive functions. Coenzyme $Q_{10}$ helps mitochondria function properly, and curcumin and echinacea stimulate the immune system.

Several Chinese herbs have been tested and found effective in brain cancer treatment. Dang gui (*Angelica sinensis*) slows and/or reverses development of glioblastoma multiforme, gardenia fruits (*Shan zhi zi*) reported a measurable inhibition of glioma tumor cells and induced apoptosis and/or arrest growth. Exercise is helpful, as it reduces excess fat, and sunshine acts on cholesterol to produce vitamin D, a powerful cancer preventive.

Other suggestions for therapy include Resveratrol, pine bark, and grapeseed extracts, and eating more greens. When used in conjunction with standard therapy, several Swiss clinics have reported mistletoe, under the name of *iscador*, to be successful against brain tumors. A ketogenic diet low in carbohydrates that become glucose in the body is felt to be antitumor, with the belief that brain cancers use glucose and normal cells can use ketones. This is under study in several laboratories.

Preliminary reports show concern about exposure to several possible contributing factors for brain cancer, including regular use of cell phones.[6] And there is the ongoing controversy about the use of aspartame (Nutrasweet and Equal), pesticides, high-voltage power lines, and possible child exposure to electromagnetic fields. [7,8,9,10,11,12]

## BREAST CANCER

One out of every eight women in the United States will develop breast cancer during her lifetime.

Fifty years ago most women who presented to their physicians with breast cancer had a large mass, and the disease was diagnosed at a later stage, with a relatively poorer prognosis. As I explained in my book, *Comprehensive Breast Care and Surviving Breast Cancer,* the attitude toward breast disease has changed significantly. "Breast disease has come out of the closet of embarrassment and negative stigma, and with this public recognition comes earlier diagnosis, less radical treatment, and better prognosis and cosmetic outcomes." Centers for Breast Care have arisen, focusing on breast health, and awareness of the causes and diverse treatments of the disease have led to a steady improvement in the outcomes and survival.

Up to the mid-1800s, most women died from their breast cancer. With the development of the Halsted radical mastectomy in the late 1800s the mortality dropped to 30 percent, and, throughout the twentieth century, doctors have been able to make earlier diagnosis of smaller cancers and develop less radical deforming treatments.

But first, a brief discussion of the anatomy of the breast and a description of the types of cancer are indicated.

The female breast or mammary gland is, strictly speaking, a modified sweat gland whose primary function is the nourishment of the infant. Today, of course, breasts play an important psychosexual role so surgeons have learned to preserve as much of the gland as possible while attempting to eradicate disease. The breast consists of fifteen to twenty segments, or lobes, arranged in a circular (radial) fashion around the nipple and each lobe has its own tube or duct ending and exiting at the nipple. The area around the nipple is called the areola. Underlying the breast are the pectoral muscles, and lymph nodes that drain lymph and waste from the breast are in the armpit (axilla). In the breast and axilla are several tiny sensory nerves that supply the breast tissue and skin, and these are frequently disturbed during breast surgery. These usually regenerate over time. There are two motor nerves (nerves that innervate muscles) in the axilla that surgeons must preserve to prevent weakness of the chest wall and back muscles.

The female breast is affected by hormones. Natural estrogen in the female at the time of puberty causes the deposition of fat in the breasts and, along with progesterone, causes the development of various other areas of the breast, such as the lobules and ducts.

The College of American Pathologists has developed a chart to indicate the risks for certain types of abnormalities that could develop into invasive breast cancer. I will list them so that when you are given a diagnosis by a physician you can understand their relative risk.

### No Increased Risk

◇ Apocrine metaplasia, duct ectasia, fibroadenoma without complex features, fibrosis, mastitis, mild hyperplasia without atypia, ordinary cysts, sclerosing adenosis, and squamous metaplasia

### Slightly Increased Risk (1.5–2.0 times)

◇ Fibroadenoma with complex features, moderate or florid hyperplasia without atypia; sclerosing adenosis when present, with atypical ductal hyperplasia; solitary papilloma with co-existent atypical ductal hyperplasia

### Moderately Increased Risk (4–5 times)

◇ Atypical ductal hyperplasia, atypical lobular hyperplasia

### Markedly Increased Risk (8–10 times)

◇ Ductal carcinoma in situ (this is actually stage 0 cancer)

◇ Lobular carcinoma in situ

### The Cancer Itself

The earliest form of true cancer is called ductal carcinoma in situ, DCIS, or Stage 0 cancer, where the cancer is confined to the duct and apparently does not have the ability to spread or metastasize. This form of cancer is essentially 99.5 percent curable. The next group begins what is referred to as invasive cancers. Invasive cancers increase in stage by their size, by the presence or absence of cancer in the lymph nodes, and by the presence of metastasis, where the cancer has spread beyond the breast and axilla to other parts of the body.

## ▪ *Diagnosis and Treatment*

- Stage 0 is DCIS—Tis N0 M0
- Stage 1—T1 N0 M0
- Stage 2A—T0 N1 M0; T1 N0 M0; T2 N0 M0
- Stage 2B—T2 N1 M0; T3 N0 M0
- Stage 3A—T0 N2 M0; T1 N2 M0; T2 N2 M0; T3 N2 M0
- Stage 3B—T4, Any N M0; Any T N3
- Stage 4—Any T; Any N M1

Why is this important? Because the surgeon and oncologist will base therapy on the staging of the cancer and can give a general idea of prognosis, cure rates, and survival depending on the staging. The lower the stage, the better the prognosis, so early diagnosis and treatment is best.

There are several types of breast cancer relating to the location (ductal, lobular, tubular) or type (inflammatory, invasive, in situ).

It is recommended that women over forty years of age have mammograms every two years. Hopefully, using this method, and possibly augmenting this with MRIs (magnetic resonance imaging), breast cancer can be detected long before a palpable nodule develops. The earlier the diagnosis and the smaller the tumor, often the better the prognosis and possibility for complete cure of the disease. Of course it is important for every woman (and man) to take enough interest in her or his own body to manually self-examine every few months. But more important is to discover an abnormality even before it has developed to the point where it can be felt by the fingers. As a surgeon, I am now seeing more and more patients with the earliest stage of breast cancer and can offer them the least cosmetically disturbing surgery.

When a woman has a mammogram, she should understand there is a 10–15 percent false-negative error in diagnosis; in other words 15 percent of cancers may not be seen because they are too small, or because the breast tissue is very dense (as in pregnancy or young women). In women who have a strong family history of breast cancer, or who have certain genetic predispositions to cancer (certain genes called BRCA1 or BRCA2), a more sensitive test, an MRI, might be indicated, in addition to the mammogram and ultrasound. When a radiologist reports a suspicious area on a mammogram or MRI, a biopsy must be performed. Today we recommend needle, or core, biopsies done by the radiologist, instead of open breast biopsies. Surgical open biopsies may be indicated when there is not adequate tissue, or when a definite diagnosis cannot be made by a needle biopsy, but this is a rare occurrence today. Usually after a core needle biopsy, the radiologist leaves a tiny titanium clip to identify the site of the biopsy; later, at the time of the lumpectomy, the patient returns to the radiologist prior to surgery and a fine wire is placed in the breast, with its curled tip at the site of the clip so the surgeon can identify the site during his lumpectomy. This is called needle localization.

Once a pathologist has examined the biopsy and given a diagnosis, the surgeon and oncologist can design a course of treatment. For large cancers, the oncologist may recommend treating the patient with chemotherapy and radiation before surgery to decrease the tumor size and make a cosmetic surgical approach more feasible. The surgery of choice for small cancers is usually a lumpectomy (removing the cancer), being sure to allow for extra normal tissue around the tumor (free margin). Today a sentinel-node biopsy is also performed, which means taking out the first one or two lymph nodes, and draining the breast; these are located in the axilla and are identified by two methods, blue dye or radionucleotide, which a surgeon will explain to the patient. If the sentinel node does not have cancer, no further node removal is necessary. If the sentinel node has cancer, many oncologists and surgeons are recommending removal of many of the lymph nodes in the axilla. It is important to note there is a difference of opinion about the management of the lymph nodes, and each surgeon will have to discuss this with the patient and explain why he or she chooses one particular pathway. The major complication of removing a large amount of lymph nodes in the axilla is the 15–20-percent chance of developing lymphedema, a swelling of the arm that can be treated by therapy and sleeve application.

The lumpectomy procedure is the preferred method of surgical treatment for many cancers. It is sufficient for DCIS, but when invasive cancer is present (Stage I–IV), the surgery must be followed up with some type of radiation therapy to the involved breast because, in cases where a lumpectomy alone has been done rather than a mastectomy, the local recurrence rate of cancer is 25 percent. So, as far as results are concerned, a lumpectomy and radiation equals a mastectomy for invasive cancers. Today, breast surgeons use what are called oncoplastic techniques to remove portions of the breast and accomplish cosmetically pleasing results by mobilizing remaining tissue employing plastic surgical techniques.

A mastectomy may be indicated in cases where a cancer is very large, or multifocal (in several areas of the breast), and in situations where previous resection margins cannot be cleared of cancer, also sometimes during pregnancy. The radical mastectomy originally done over one hundred years ago, with complete removal of the breast, the underlying muscles, and the axillary lymph nodes, is rarely necessary anymore. Today, a mastectomy implies only the removal of the breast and is often accompanied by a reconstruction performed by a plastic surgeon at the time of the initial surgery. The plastic surgeon usually puts in a synthetic expanding silicone or saline-filled prosthesis in a procedure that may require one or two more reconstructive surgeries.

After breast surgery, the surgeon may insert temporary drains to remove any subsequent blood or serum collections and these drains are usually removed in a few days. Most breast surgery is outpatient, or sometimes an overnight stay is needed. Complications are not common and can include bleeding, infection, or the development of a fluid collection (seroma or hematoma) that may require placement of a drain several days after surgery. With extensive surgery, there is the remote possibility of skin loss requiring further procedures, and even skin grafting.

Most major medical centers have boards for breast tumors where a collection of physicians and nurses meet to discuss each case of breast cancer. The committees consist of medical oncologists, radiologists, surgeons, radiation therapists, plastic surgeons, nurses, and social workers. After the presentation of each case, a discussion ensues and a concerted plan of action is decided for each patient. Decisions are made as to whether or not the patient needs radiation therapy and also what types of medical therapy should be instituted, such as hormone therapy, preoperative chemotherapy (neoadjuvant), and postsurgical chemotherapy (adjuvant). These can include a whole host of agents— CMF (cytoxan, methotrexate, 5-fluorouracil), Herceptin (for patients with an overexpression of the gene Her2/neu, TAC (taxotere, adriamycin, cyclophosphamide), FAC (5-FU, adriamycin, cyclophosphamide), trastuzumab (a so-called monoclonal antibody medication), and many other combinations of drugs. There are endocrine therapies, including tamoxifen and aromatase inhibitors, biphosphonates for treating bone metastases, and special regimens of high-dose chemotherapy for advanced disease. The uses and side effects of these medications need to be explained to the patient by the oncologist—the tumor board is, in effect, a second opinion for the patient.

And lastly, in terms of treatment, what is the value of a bilateral mastectomy, a very radical approach to the problem? There is no doubt that removing all the breast tissue will prevent the development of breast cancer. But it should be understood that the breast, unlike some organs, such as the liver, lung, or testicles, does not have distinct boundaries. Even the woman who has a mastectomy probably has some residual breast tissue left after her surgery, thereby retaining a small risk for cancer development. However, in certain cases, where there is bilateral extensive cancer, where there is a very strong history of familial breast cancer, or where the woman has an inordinate fear of developing breast cancer, bilateral mastectomies may be indicated, often with immediate reconstruction.

### ■ Complementary and Alternative Treatment

Consider what a woman can do to prevent breast cancer or at least lower her chances of getting breast cancer. It is known that breast cancer is much less common in Japan, but when a Japanese woman moves to the United States, her incidence of cancer becomes the same as an American woman within a few years, so diet and environment play a significant role in cancer prevention. Estrogen supplements increase risks, and obesity and a sedentary lifestyle also increase the risk. Other preventive actions include decreasing the fat intake, increasing fiber by incorporating whole grains, legumes, fresh fruit, and vegetables, and avoiding excess alcohol.

Several scientists have determined that fruits and vegetables are beneficial because they are low in fat and high in fiber, high in antioxidants and vitamins, and lower in calories. Among the powerful cancer-fighting groups are phytochemicals, or plant chemicals, such as carotenoids (carrots, kale, tomatoes), flavonoids ( leafy green vegetables), indole-3 carbinols (broccoli, Brussels sprouts, cabbage, cauliflower, mustard seeds, radishes, and others), and many fruits, such as apples, grapefruit, and oranges, that are high in D-glucaric acid. These foods have substances that affect the growth cycle of the cancer cell, or prevent the development of cancer by protecting against damage caused by oxygen free–radicals.

Eating organic foods free from pesticides is considered advantageous in preventing breast cancer. Man-made or trans-fats should be avoided, as well as excessive IGF (insulin-like growth factors that are used to promote increased milk development in American milk cattle). It's a good idea to avoid large amounts of *unbalanced* omega-6 fatty acids, such as those found in commercial salad dressing, corn oil, cottonseed oil, margarine, mayonnaise, peanut oil, safflower oil, and soybean oil (a balanced intake of omega-3s and omega-6s is normally optimal). Several foods are considered anticancer, including garlic, ginseng, green tea, maitake mushrooms, red clover, seaweed, turmeric, and possibly even coffee. There are many who advocate vitamin therapies and a whole group called antioxidants. Foods it's best to decrease in your diet include animal protein, saturated animal fats, and red meat. There are many dietary do's and don'ts that are readily accessible to readers.

Other recommendations are aerobic exercise and programs that help a person cope with stress (Ayurvedic routines, breathing routines, and meditation). Greek women who derive 40 percent of their calories from fat, mostly olive oil, have reduced rates of breast cancer, but reports also state that an increased intake of starch may increase the risk of breast cancer, and selenium and zinc supplements may be helpful. Some physicians feel that grief and depression suppress immunity, giving malignant cells the chance to grow into perceptible tumors. While others have suggested there is a relationship between prayer and healing, skeptical Dr. Larry Dossey has compiled an impressive catalog of saints who have died of cancer (in fact cancer almost seems to be an occupational hazard of sainthood). Yet there are many dramatic instances of spontaneous remissions of cancer, some under the aegis of Zen Buddhist practitioners and other spiritual guides. One naturopathic doctor states that four hours of exercise a week can reduce the risks of breast cancer by 50 percent.

I mention all these alternative medical therapies because, although there are few clinical trials, there is ample historical evidence that these modalities do have a place in augmenting the standard treatment therapies. I emphasize the difference between pure alternative medicine, which recommends sole treatment with nonconventional methods, and complementary medicine, which recommends alternative medicine in conjunction with conventional Western medical practice.

There is no question in my mind that many of the holistic approaches to the treatment of disease may work in conjunction with standard mainstream medical and surgical care, even if they only ease the patient's anxiety and create peace of mind. Among these approaches are the following.

◇ Acupuncture                    ◇ Meditation

◇ Biofeedback                     ◇ Music therapy

◇ Chiropractic                    ◇ Self-help groups

◇ Herbal therapy                  ◇ Stress management

◇ Homeopathy                      ◇ Yoga

◇ Massage

Frequently, I have women come to my office with varying stages of breast cancer. I discuss their cases, explaining the disease and the therapy. I always recommend getting a second opinion before undergoing a major surgical or medical treatment. I recommend major medical centers, teaching-university settings, and physicians prominent in the management of breast cancer. I advise against radical nonconventional approaches to breast-cancer management while encouraging their full utilization of complementary medical adjuncts. I know that, when faced with the diagnosis of cancer, most women retain very little of what I have told them in the office and, for that reason, I give them a copy of my book *Comprehensive Breast Care and Surviving Breast Cancer.* I have found there is too much inexpert *expert* advice on the Internet and women can be led down dangerous paths through their own investigations into therapy and prevention.

I also strongly suggest that all women with breast cancer join support groups for breast cancer, where they can discuss their questions, anxieties, and doubts with women who have undergone similar treatment and who have answers to many of their most gripping questions and doubts.

In the above book of mine that was published more than ten years ago, I took unwarranted pride in stating that several alternative therapies were unproven and probably of no value in the treatment of cancer. However, having recently begun to look into alternative and complementary medicine from a more open and broad-minded point of view, I am learning it was truly my bias as a conventional surgeon that was the basis for my thinking. Among those I listed negatively then was a collection from A-Z that included the following.

- Aromatherapy
- Bach's flower remedy
- Chiro-crystal healing
- Dousing
- Electro acupuncture
- Faith healing
- Gerson therapy
- Horsley regimen
- Iridology
- Iscador
- Johnson's remedy radionics
- Krebiozen
- Laetrile moxibustion
- Negative ionizers
- Orgone accumulators
- Pyramidology
- Quinine
- Simonton's cure
- Trepanation
- Urine therapy
- Vrillium tubes
- Water remedy
- Xanthine remedy
- Yoga
- Zebethium

Although my personal bias was probably based on a rigid adherance to the scientific method, I had to reevaluate my thinking in view of the broad acceptance and success of many of these regimens.

I also noted that the National Cancer Institute had examined several of the complementary approaches in regard to breast cancer and, in their studies, they claimed that vitamins $B_6$, $B_{12}$, E, and C, beta carotene, folic acid, and selenium had not been shown to lower the risk of breast cancer. Another study by the Agency for Healthcare Research and Quality alleged that no convincing evidence existed that antioxidant supplements, vitamins C and E, and $CoQ_{10}$ had any cancer-preventive benefits. And another study of 1.6 million participants found "insufficient and conflicting evidence" regarding an association between green-tea consumption and cancer prevention.

In more carefully examining these studies, I found a remarkable bias against complementary care and research in the face of overwhelming support in alternative American, Chinese, Indian, and other literature. Perhaps the arrogance and stalwart refusal of established Western medicine to honestly evaluate these methods has led to a lot of confusion, animosity, and perhaps incorrect conclusions. While some therapies may be of little value, most others are being adopted by major medical centers and warrant attention. The person with cancer, as well as the physician and any interested, healthy individual, needs to look more intelligently into these modalities, demanding excellence, professionalism, and an open-minded, unbiased approach toward evaluation. As Hamlet said to his super-rational friend, "There are more things in heaven and earth, Horatio, than are dreamed of in your philosophy." (Hamlet Act 1, scene V.)

## CANCER OF THE PENIS

Cancer of the penis is a relatively rare malignancy in the United States. However, it is a major health problem in South America, Asia, and Africa, comprising almost 8–10 percent of cancers in those regions. Usually seen in men older than sixty, it is seen to be associated with poor hygiene and phimosis (a condition of the penis where the foreskin is so tight it cannot be drawn back over the head of the penis). This condition leads to the accumulation of infected cells called smegma under the foreskin, which has been postulated as a cause for cancer. In cultures (as in the Jewish population) where there is neonatal (at birth) circumcision, the incidence of penile cancer is practically percent. Interestingly, delaying circumcision until later in life does not seem to increase the incidence of cancer seen when the procedure is carried out in the newborn. HPV (human papilloma virus) also plays a role in the development of this cancer, as well as tobacco, which tends to promote cancerous growth in the presence of the other factors.

The symptoms are usually abnormal skin changes, infections, along with the development of a mass that may even be ulcerated and bleeding at intervals. As the cancer progresses, there may be pain, fistulas, and foul-smelling infections. Most of the cancers are squamous cell, and most of the remaining ones may be AIDS-related Kaposi sarcomas.

### ■ Diagnosis and Treatment

The diagnosis is made by biopsy, and, depending on the size and histologic characteristics, further radiological studies, including MRIs (magnetic resonance imaging) and CT scanning (computer axial tomography) may be indicated, as well as a CT-guided biopsy of lymph nodes in the groin to determine the staging.

## Staging

The staging is according to the TNM system. T=Tumor, N=Node, M=Metastasis.

- Stage 0—T in situ cancer; N0–no nodes involved; M0–no metastases (superficial lesion called Erythroplasia of Querat)
- Stage I—T1 N0–N0 nodes M0
- Stage II—T1 N1 M0
- T2—N0 M0
- T2—N2 M0
- T2—N2 M0
- Stage III
- T3—N0 M0
- T1–3—N1 M0
- T1–3—N2 M0
- Stage IV—T4–Any N M0
- Any T N3 M0
- Any T Any N M1–Distant metastases

Stage 0 cancers may be treated with topical creams, such as 5-FU cream, but excellent results have also been achieved with carbon dioxide and Nd:YAG laser therapy. In addition, Mohs micrographic surgery is an alternative with less cosmetic distortion, as is local radiation therapy.

Stage I cancers and beyond are treated surgically if there is a significant chance for cure. If the cancer is in the distal end or distal half of the penis, the organ can be saved, but proximal cancers at the base of the shaft may require complete removal and reconstructive surgery. When lymph nodes are involved, varying degrees of lymph-node dissection are indicated, along with radiation therapy. Because of the paucity of cases in the United States, there are few clinical trials to rely upon, and the use and success rate of chemotherapeutic drugs is still under investigation. At present, combinations of bleomycin, methotrexate, and vincristine have been used with response rates of 50–60 percent.

### ▩ Complementary and Alternative Treatment

Penile cancer is preventable by adhering to good hygiene principles, avoiding HPV infection, and not smoking tobacco.[13]

## CARCINOID TUMORS

Carcinoid tumors are relatively uncommon cancers and can occur anywhere in the intestinal tract, as well as the lung and pancreas. The most common site is actually in the appendix where it presents as acute appendicitis and is therefore diagnosed and treated very early, with a high cure rate. When it occurs elsewhere, the diagnosis usually comes later in the progression of the cancer and is more difficult to manage. There are many variations in the type of cells found, and they generally fall under the heading of neuroendocrine or APUD tumors (amine precursor uptake and decarboxylation); they may produce various substances, depending on their origin and extent of growth. (There are over fifty named substances produced by carcinoid tumors, including catecholamines, dopamine, gastrin, histamine, insulin, and serotonin.)

The etiology (origin) of the cancer is not known. The risk factors include family history, older age, and smoking tobacco. The cancer is more common in women.

Tumors less than 1 cm do not metastasize, but a significant number of those above 2 cm do metastasize, and some develop what is called the carcinoid syndrome, which is triggered by the tumor, producing catecholamines, along with the individual's drinking alcohol and having emotional stress. The symptoms can be abdominal cramping, bronchospasm and wheezing (due to histamine production), decreased blood pressure and fainting, diarrhea, flushing, intestinal obstruction, rectal bleeding, recurrent pneumonia, swelling of the arms and legs (edema), and valvular heart disease.

## ▓ *Diagnosis and Treatment*

The diagnosis is made with CT and MRI studies, as well as urine collection for a metabolic product of serotonin produced by the tumor called 5-HIAA (5-hydroxyindoleacetic acid). A nuclear medicine scan is also helpful in determining cancer spread and a blood test for the tumor marker chromogranin A (CgA) is sometimes positive with carcinoid cancers. Tissue diagnosis is obtained by needle biopsy of the primary or metastatic tumor; there are no staging criteria for this disease and the tumors are usually characterized as local, extensive local, or metastatic.

The treatment and management of carcinoid tumors depends on the size and extent of disease. Carcinoids of the appendix found incidentally are usually cured by an appendectomy if less than 1–2 cm. Large tumors should have a right hemicolectomy (removal of the appendix along with half the colon), along with lymph nodes. Other intestinal areas need to have wide excisions of the involved bowel. When there is liver involvement, debulking of the tumor surgically, using radiofrequency ablation, or hepatic artery embolization is indicated. In those cases where there is no demonstrable disease outside the liver, a liver transplant may be recommended.

The tumor is radiosensitive and often well palliated with local therapy. For the most part, the cancer is not responsive to chemotherapy, although new anti-angiogenic approaches using bevacizumab and temozolomide with FOLFOX (a combination chemotherapy), and several other drugs in clinical trials, such as sunitinib, temsirolimus, thalidomide, and vatalanib. Another study is using interferon alfa-2b and octreotide.

Palliation of symptoms is achieved using alpha and beta adrenergic blockers, lanreotide (Somatuline Depot), octreotide, steroids, and thorazine.

## ▓ *Complementary and Alternative Treatment*

The alternative methods of treatment include massage, meditation, relaxation techniques, tai chi, and yoga. Multiple recommendations are listed for alternative treatments, food supplements, antioxidants, and Chinese herbal recipes.

# CANCERS OF CHILDHOOD

Cancer in children is relatively rare, but, after accidents, it is the major cause of death in children from one to fourteen. Childhood cancers differ from adult cancers in their growth pattern, their response to treatment, and the problems encountered. The emotional impact on both the physician and the family is often devastating and care must be taken to assure that only the best therapies are offered. Whereas the adult may select from a panoply of choices, it behooves the physician and the parents to opt for only the most accepted standard approaches for the child.

The most common cancers in children are leukemia (acute lympho-cytic, granulocytic, and lymphoblastic) and brain tumors (astrocy-tomas, ependymomas, gliomas, and medulloblastomas). Certain cancers are more common in children than adults—bone tumors (Ewing's sarcoma, osteogenic sarcoma), an eye tumor (retinoblastoma), a kidney cancer called Wilm's tumor, a liver tumor (hepatoblastoma), a muscle cancer (rhabdomyosarcoma), and a nervous-system tumor called neuroblastoma. Children may also get Hodgkin's lymphoma and non-Hodgkin's lymphoma.

The etiology of cancer in children is more of a puzzle than that of adults, since there has been no prolonged exposure to alcohol, tobacco, obesity, and the environmental toxins that are associated with adult cancers. So, many of these cancers are assumed to have a congenital or genetic basis. Of course, children exposed to radiation, such as in Hiroshima and Chernobyl, were apparently more sensitive and suscep-tible to the dosages received and had a significantly higher rate of can-cers than adults.

Certain other diseases appear to predispose to higher risk for cancer, including Down syndrome, Fanconi's Syndrome, and several rare hereditary syndromes, including Ataxia-telangiectasia, Beckwith-Wiedeman, Bloom's, Gorlin's, Li-Fraumeni, and Rothmun-Thomson syndromes. It is beyond the scope of this book to do more than name these entities, only to know that genetic abnormalities have predis-posed these children to develop rare cancers, posing severe manage-ment and therapy problems.

These children appear to have inappropriately activated oncogenes, abnormal genes, and inactivation of tumor-suppressor genes (genes that prevent cancer). Of course, some children have such severe genetic abnormalities that they do not survive to birth and die in utero or early infancy. In many, the developmental stages are normal, but shortly after birth, genetic abnormalities activate tumor oncogenes, causing cancer cells to germinate and grow.

## ■ Diagnosis and Treatment

The staging and treatment of this multitude of rare childhood cancers is too complex to describe here. However, in many cases, the cancers are more responsive to radiation and chemotherapy than in an adult with the same or a similar disease.

Although alternative and complementary therapies may one day be among the first-line treatments, at this time the focus should be on standard Western oncological care in comprehensive pediatric medical centers where many of the nonstandard therapies dealing with pain and nutrition are carefully examined and utilized when indicated.

The treatment of childhood cancers is surgery, chemotherapy, and radiation therapy, a team approach that includes medical experts in pediatric oncology, pediatric oncology nurses, social services, physical and occupational therapy, educational, and other special child services. Generally, cancer in children should be managed at dedicated children's hospitals where a multidisciplinary approach can be accomplished at a center of excellence, and where tumor boards discuss each case and make recommendations.

Children can be enrolled in clinical trials and have access to the most innovative and progressive investigational treatments, and they are sometimes treated with bone-marrow transplantation. Dealing with childhood cancer is often a question of placing optimism before pessimism for both the patient and the family. Children usually have recurrent admissions to the hospital, side effects from their therapy they don't understand (hair loss, nausea, sores, ulcers, and vomiting), allergic reactions, and of course the complete change in their growth and development in school, outside activities, and planning for the future.

The focus has to be that each child can be cured, regardless of whether the therapy is weeks, months, or years, giving hope and encouragement to both patient and family, while supporting the family in those instances when they recognize that the child will not survive.

■ *Complementary and Alternative Treatment*

This is such a broad and highly specialized area that I do not feel it would be appropriate for me to offer advice or information. While I am sure there are many alternative treatments, most children's hospitals offer comprehensive programs that include standard, alternative, and numerous other therapies. A local children's hospital or cancer center would be the best place to start.

## COLON AND RECTAL CANCER

Cancer of the colon and rectum is the third most common malignancy after prostate and lung in men and lung and breast in women. In the last few years, because of the attention brought by public figures, more attention, and therefore more information on the subject, has been brought to the public eye. The lifetime risk for Americans is about 7 percent. Like alcoholism, homosexuality, and breast cancer thirty years ago, this disease has come *out of the closet,* and we are seeing more public and media information about prevention, early diagnosis, and treatment. Unfortunately, Western medicine has lagged behind in recognizing the dietary causes of this disease, allowing a whole host of pseudo-professional information to seep into the public coffers of information.

Cancer of the colon and rectum are malignant tumors that arise in the colon (ascending, cecum, descending, sigmoid, and transverse), the appendix, and the rectum (that extends to about 15–20 cm above the anus—the anus has a different cancer and different treatment recommendations). Most cancers develop as small growths on the inner lining or mucosa of the colon, often benign, and called polyps or adenomas. Given enough time, these small growths may develop into cancer. This is the reason why most physicians recommend a complete evaluation of the colon on a regular basis (every five years) after age fifty. Removal of polyps and adenomas endoscopically (through the scope) under sedation will prevent the development of cancer, and finding small cancers at an early stage can lead to 100 percent cure.

The genetic changes found in cells with colon cancer have to do with the loss of certain cancer-suppressor (cancer-preventing) genes and the presence of oncogenes (cancer-causing) that require several steps before a cancer develops. Certain syndromes appear to shorten the multistage concept of colon cancer's development, and dietary considerations play a significant role in the prevention, diminution of risk, and survival of people with this disease. The most commonly mutated gene in colon cancer is the APC gene that normally protects against cancer by diminishing the protein Beta-catenin that causes DNA changes and can lead to a malignant change. This is called the Wnt-APC-beta-catenin signaling pathway that, along with other mutations, may cause a cell to become cancerous. The process is complex and beyond our scope here. Also, mutations in the p53 protein (produced by the TP53 gene that normally monitors cell division) prevent it from protecting the cell against malignant change. Other proteins that lead to normal cell apoptosis (death) are deactivated by other genes (DCC, TGF-beta), and many oncogenes are developed by creating overexpression of normal growth-stimulating genes, such as P13K, KRAS and RAF; several different mutations or changes in the cell affect the DNA and lead to changes in cellular function that cause it to multiply out of normal control or not destroy itself when it becomes very abnormal. The normal controls of the body have broken down.

Cancer of the colon has several hereditary syndromes that increase the risks for developing the disease. Certainly a family history of colon cancer increases a person's risk of having the disease, although this may be partly related to dietary, environmental, and lifestyle considerations. Among the definitive syndromes you can look up are Cowden's disease, familial adenomatous polyposis, Gardner's syndrome, Peutz-Jegher's syndrome, and Turcot's syndrome, all of which have been determined to have genetic abnormalities. Those with Crohn's disease and ulcerative colitis have a higher incidence of developing colon cancer and must be monitored more carefully. Genetic counseling is indicated in many instances.

Other factors increasing the risk include obesity, diet with red meats and char-broiled foods, too few fruits and vegetables, cigarettes, and alcohol. Low levels of selenium, certain viruses, and environmental factors have also been implicated.

Increased consumption of fruits and vegetables and daily exercise appear to decrease the risk. Diets with increased fiber, supplements such as calcium, fish oil, or omega-3 with DHA (docosahexaenoic acid) and EPA (eicosapentaenoic acid), flaxseed, folic acid, and vitamin $B_6$ have been recommended for preventing colon cancer. Use of low-dose aspirin, anti-inflammatory drugs, supplemental vitamin D, and hormone replacement in women may be protective.

## ▪ Diagnosis and Treatment

One function of the colon is to remove water from the stool as it passes through to the anus. Therefore, on the right side of the colon and in the cecum and ascending colon, the stool is watery and loose, whereas in the descending colon and rectum it has become more formed and solid. Cancers developing on the left side will develop symptoms of constipation and obstruction earlier than those on the right, which will obstruct later in their development and bleed earlier on. Early signs may be bleeding, a change in bowel habits, cramping, flatulence, and vague pain. Left-side cancers may have constipation, diarrhea, nausea, pain, and vomiting. Right-side ones may have abdominal pain or aching, and bleeding, or just anemia from blood loss, causing lethargy, weakness, and weight loss. The most important sign and symptom is *no sign or symptom*. The cancer may develop without being recognized, and this is the reason a regular examination is recommended. A rectal exam will identify a rectal tumor and a colonoscopy will find precancerous, early, and late cancers. The earlier the diagnosis, the better the prognosis.

Screening can include testing for blood in the stool, proctosigmoidoscopy, a virtual colonoscopy using CT scans, and the older method, a barium enema. Lesions found should be biopsied and examined by a pathologist.

### Staging

Colon cancer is staged depending on its location, the presence of nodes with cancer, and the presence of metastatic disease. T=Tumor size, N=Nodes, M=Metastasis.

Primary tumor—Lymph node tumor–Distant metastasis

- Stage 0—Tis (in situ carcinoma) N0 M0

- Stage I—T1 (tumor invades submucosa) N0 M0–T2 (tumor invades muscularis) N0 M0

- Stage IIA—T3 (tumor invades pericolic tissue) N0 M0

- Stage IIB—T4 (tumor directly invades other structures) N0 M0

- Stage IIIA—T1–2–NI (1–3 nodes) M0
- Stage IIIB—T3–4–NI M0
- Stage IIIC—Any T N2 (4 or more nodes) M0
- Stage IV—Any T–Any NMI

A less complicated old classification method called the Duke's System is:

- Tumor confined to the intestinal wall
- Tumor invading through the intestinal wall
- With lymph node involvement
- With distant metastasis

The pathologist may also grade a tumor according to its appearance under the microscope. Well-differentiated means the cancer approaches a normal cell appearance whereas poorly differentiated means it looks unlike its original cell of origin. There are different gradings.

◇ **Grade 1.** Well differentiated

◇ **Grade 2.** Moderately differentiated

◇ **Grade 3.** Poorly differentiated

◇ **Grade 4.** Undifferentiated (totally unlike cell of origin)

The pathologist will also note whether there are lymphatic channels with cancer, a blood-vessel invasion, as well as the histologic type, such as medullary, mucinous, signet ring, or small cell.

The grading, microscopic findings, histologic type along with the stage determine the treatment of colon cancer. Like other cancers, these findings are usually discussed at a tumor conference to obtain several opinions and develop a plan of treatment.

After a diagnosis, several options exist. If the cancer in the rectum is large, but not obstructing, the recommendation may be for presurgical treatment with chemotherapy and radiation (neoadjuvant treatment) to shrink the cancer and allow for a better surgical resection. If a cancer is very low and close to the end of the rectum near the anus, a more radical removal of the lower colon and rectum may be needed to achieve a complete removal of the cancer. This may involve removing the rectal/anal muscles and necessitating a permanent diversion of the stool called a colostomy (abdomino-perineal resection). If radiation and chemotherapy can sufficiently diminish the size of the cancer, the surgeon may be able to get around the cancer, preserving the lower musculature and eliminating the need for a permanent colostomy.

Part of the preoperative evaluation may be further studies to determine the presence or absence of tumor spread. This might include colonic endoscopic ultrasound (done at a few institutions) to determine the extent of a local spread in designing surgery, a CT scan of the abdomen, pelvis, and chest, and a PET scan (positron emission tomography) looking for a metastasis to the liver or lung. If there are neurological symptoms, such as a headache, a mental change, or vision changes, then a CT or an MRI of the brain may be indicated. It's important to get as much information as possible before starting the treatment.

**Surgery**

There are three indications for urgent surgery with colon cancer.

1. When a cancer grows through the colon call and perforates into the abdominal cavity, causing infection and sepsis
2. Uncontrollable bleeding
3. Obstruction of the colon or ureter

Surgery can be curative or palliative. This is usually decided before the procedure. Hopefully the entire cancer and the adjacent lymph nodes can be removed in an attempt to cure the patient. But in cases where there are extensive metastases, a palliative procedure may be indicated where removal of the cancer may still be recommended because of bleeding or obstruction. Or in cases where a resection of the cancer is not possible because of the extent of the cancer invading surrounding tissues, a diverting colostomy or a fecal-stream diversion might offer temporary relief of pain and suffering from the obstruction.

The surgical approach depends on the location of the cancer. Generally, the recommended procedure is to remove the cancer-bearing segment of colon with the lymph node draining tissues for that area, and allowing wide margins on either side of the cancer. When this segment is removed, the colon is put back together. Surgery today may be per-formed by open surgery where the abdomen is opened with a large incision, laparoscopic-assisted surgery (smaller openings), or the newest, robotic surgery (small openings). The efficacy of the latter is still under investigation since the surgeon wants to insure the best can-cer operation without compromising because of the size of the inci-sion. Cosmetic appearance has to play a secondary role when dealing with cancer. It may sound nice to advertise performing cancer surgery through a keyhole-sized incision, but this might not entail complete removal of all cancer-bearing tissues. Time will tell.

Technically, the surgeon uses automatic stapling devices to divide and connect the bowel, uses staplers to control bleeding along with electrocautery and other devices, and the old suture techniques. Skin can be closed with sutures, staples, or a special glue. The surgeon may put rubber or plastic drains in place to drain off blood or infection, and these are removed several days after the surgery.

To prepare for this type of surgery, a patient will need to have a bowel-cleansing that can involve swallowing pills, liquid preparations, or rectal enemas. Before surgery, laboratory studies and nothing to eat after midnight the night before will be required. When a person is older than forty years of age, additional groundwork may include blood and urine studies, a chest x-ray, and an EKG. CEA (carcino-embry-onic-antigen) is a protein found in a blood sample that measures colon cancer. It can be followed in the postoperative period. The value may be elevated before surgery, go down after the cancer is removed, and then followed after surgery, using blood tests—if it rises, this can indi-cate a recurrence of the cancer.

At the start of a surgical procedure, an IV is started in the pre-op room, and the patient is usually given an intravenous, relaxing sedative medication before being wheeled into the operating room. The surgery can take anywhere from an hour to many hours, depending on the can-cer location, skill of the surgeon, and difficulty of the surgery. In cases where cancer is found in the liver or other areas (usually recognized and diagnosed preoperatively), attempts may be made to remove the metastasis or metastases during this first surgery.

When a cancer recurs, or when metastatic disease is found in the lungs or liver, further surgery may be indicated. Only recently, the pres-ence of liver or lung metastasis was usually an indication of incurability. However, more vigorous approaches to removing segments of the lung or liver have been advocated and have resulted in many cases of cure, even after metastasis. This is called metastasectomy and is becoming part of the cancer surgeon's arsenal. In addition to this therapy for metastatic disease, other modalities, including radio-frequency ablation and chemo-embolization, are being used.

Complications of surgery include bleeding, dehiscence of the skin (splitting open along the wound), infection (wound or deep infection), or fascial closure, hernia, injury to other organs (bladder, intestine, spleen, ureters), leakage from the new colon connection (anastomosis), abscess, fistulas, infections, and peritonitis, all of which could require a re-operation. In addition, there are always risks for heart and lung problems. Surgeons are careful to watch for, and try to prevent, pulmonary emboli (blood clots to the lung) that can be fatal; surgeons use special leg wraps and, in many cases, low-dose anticoagulants (Lovenox) to prevent blood clots in idle legs or in pelvic or abdominal veins. Surgery is not like changing a muffler, and with anatomical differences and cancer abnormalities, complications can occur. Batting .500 percent is excellent for a baseball player; batting less than 100 percent is unacceptable for a surgeon yet rarely attainable. Depending on the procedure, patients are usually in the hospital from two to ten days and may have pain and tiredness for several weeks.

### Oncological Treatment

Treatments recommended by oncologists can be divided into three categories: neoadjuvant (before surgery), adjuvant (after surgery), and palliative.

**The neoadjuvant regimen,** predominately for low rectal cancers, consists of combination radiation therapy and chemotherapy, usually intravenous or oral 5-FU (5-fluorouracil), but may also be in combination with oxaliplatin (Eloxatin) and leucovorin (LV, folinic acid), FOLFOX regimen, or capecytabine (oral Xeloda). Radiation therapy for colon and rectal cancer is usually given as neoadjuvant to shrink the tumor and clear away lymph nodes prior to surgery, or at any time for pain relief or relief of symptoms due to the tumor invading other organs.

**Adjuvant chemotherapy** involves the same chemotherapeutic agents.

**Palliative treatment.** When a cancer has progressed beyond the ability to completely eradicate or cure it, then palliative treatment is instituted to make the patient more comfortable, extend life, and limit disability.

Metastatic disease poses a more difficult problem and the oncologist will start with the above regimens and may add combinations of the following drugs.

◇ Bevacizumab (Avastin)

◇ Capecytabine (Xeloda)

◇ Cetuximab (Erbitux)

◇ 5-fluorouracil (5-FU)

◇ Gemcitabine (Gemzar)

◇ Irinotecan (Camptosar)

◇ Leucovorin (LV, folinic acid)

◇ Oxaliplatin (Eloxatin)

◇ Panitumumab (Vectibix)

◇ UFT, Tegafur-uracil

◇ Newer experimental drugs include bortezomib (Velcade), gefitinib (Tarceva), and topotecan (Hycamtrim)

◇ Immunotherapy using Bacillus Calmette-Guerin (BCG) is still in the investigative stage, as is Vax, a cancer vaccine.

| TABLE 5.1. SURVIVAL RATES FOR COLON CANCER BY STAGE | |
|---|---|
| STAGE | FIVE YEAR SURVIVAL RATE[17] |
| I | 74 percent |
| IIA | 67 percent |
| IIB | 59 percent |
| IIIA | 73 percent |
| IIIB | 46 percent |
| IIIC | 28 percent |
| IV | 6 percent |

The prognosis for colon and rectal cancer varies with the stage and also changes each year with new and more promising therapies. As of now, the statistics on Table 5.1 (p. 125) are given, but many very recent studies are now showing higher survival rates for Stages III and IV with newer drugs and with new and more promising complementary therapies each year.

## ◼ *Complementary and Alternative Treatment*

Complications and side effects of chemotherapeutic agents are of concern. Among them are diarrhea, fever, hand-foot syndrome (pain, redness, and rash of hands and feet), malaise, nausea, vomiting, and suppression of bone marrow, anemia, decreased appetite, depression, and weight loss. There are also changes in, or absence of, the menstrual cycle, changes in taste, hair loss, lymphedema (swelling of arms or legs), mouth sores, skin reactions, and cardiac toxicity. Many of these are managed with other drugs, but this is an area where alternative and complementary treatment may be of significant help.

Here are some of the complementary methods for preventing cancer or for dealing with cancer or the side effects of standard therapy.

Vegan diets are recommended for cancer patients, along with diets containing fruits and vegetables, plus the additives of vitamins and minerals.

Supplements often recommended to prevent cancer include calcium, $CoQ_{10}$, omega-3 fatty acids, quercetin, resveratrol, selenium, and vitamins B, C, D, and E.

Herbs that are recommended to alleviate the side effects of chemotherapy, including depression and nausea, are: cinnamon, fenugreek, ginger, kava, peppermint, St. John's wort, and valerian. Bromelain is said to increase the effectiveness of 5-FU, and combination therapies containing anticancer combinations include Gerson therapy and Hoxsey therapy. Alternative therapies that help relieve stress include art therapy, dance or movement therapy, exercise, meditation, music therapy, and relaxation exercises that may direct the patient's thoughts away from their fears.

Many Chinese herbal remedies are recommended to augment conventional treatments. Zuo gui wan/you gui yin formulas work by augmenting your immune system and reducing the side effects of chemotherapy and radiation; the marrow plus formula used by the Quan Yin Herbal program in San Francisco is believed to decrease bone-marrow suppression due to chemotherapy and radiation. Because gaining expertise in Chinese herbal medicine or Indian Ayurveda requires many years of study, it will be difficult for people to try and learn the appropriate path to follow on their own, and finding a reputable guide in any alternative or complementary therapy whose credentials are carefully researched, just as you would a Western mainstream doctor, is recommended. This can help to avoid any potential mistreatment and lead to successful outcomes.

Treatments that can be examined for therapy and can alleviate the side effects of chemotherapy are as follows:

◆ Adjunctive—Chelation, DMSO, hyperthermia, oxygen

◆ Aromatherapy

◆ Biological. Antineoplastins, hydrazine sulfate, Revici therapy

◆ Energy Medicine. Acupuncture, Ayurveda, bioelectric, Chinese

◆ Immune. Immuno-augmentive therapy (IAT)

◆ Metabolic. Gerson therapy, Kelley's nutritional therapy

◆ Mind-Body. Meditation and relaxation

◆ Nutritional. Macrobiotics, wheatgrass

◆ Spiritual Healing and healing retreats

◆ Yoga and tai chi

In all of this, do your homework—be proactive and be careful.

Once colon cancer has appeared, it is a surgical and medical disease to be addressed immediately by standard Western medicine. While complementary medicine can play a significant role in the prevention of cancer and the alleviation of symptoms, and may alleviate the side effects of chemotherapy and radiation as well, using this modality as the primary therapy for cancer may delay proper standard therapy for so long that the window of opportunity for a complete cure may pass.

## ESOPHAGUS CANCER

The esophagus is essentially a tube that extends from the back of the throat or pharynx down to the stomach at the GE (gastroesophageal) junction. The inner lining or mucosa is made up predominately of tissue called squamous cells (the same sort found in the skin), so it is not surprising that 95 percent of esophageal cancers are of the squamous-cell variety. The remaining cancers are mostly adenocarcinomas (arising from glands) and are usually at the junction between the esophagus and the stomach. There are a few rare tumors of the esophagus—melanomas, lymphomas, and sarcomas.

Esophageal cancer is seven times more common in men than women, more common in blacks than whites, and the median age at diagnosis is around seventy years. The incidence of the disease is 20–30 times higher in China and the Middle East and most patients present with advanced disease.

The early cancers are often not diagnosed because of the paucity of symptoms. When the cancer becomes larger, the primary symptoms are dysphagia (difficulty swallowing) and odontophagia (painful swallowing). Initially these patients avoid swallowing bulky foods because of severe heartburn and then progress to tolerating mostly liquids. Because of the diet change they often lose weight even though the cancer has not spread beyond the esophagus. Occasionally there may be hematemesis (vomiting up blood). More advanced disease may have hoarseness from involvement of the recurrent laryngeal nerves (to voice box), coughing due to extension to the throat, or development of a fistula (tract) between the esophagus and the trachea. When the cancer becomes metastatic, there may be ascites (fluid in the abdomen) or bone pain.

There are several risk factors for esophagus cancer. The two most prominent are alcohol and tobacco acting together (90 percent), followed by high-fat, low-protein diets with exposure to nitrosamines. Individuals whose close relatives have cancer experience a higher incidence of the disease. As well, GERD (gastroesophageal reflux disease) that leads to Barrett's esophagus (chronic irritation of the lining of the esophagus) can lead to cancer (usually adenocarcinoma). Other contributing factors include burns on the esophagus due to drinking hot liquids, celiac disease, obesity (probably due to increased reflux), HPV (human papilloma virus), injury to the esophagus from strong acid or lye, radiation therapy to the chest, and several congenital syndromes (Howel-Evans syndrome, hereditary thickening of the skin of the palms and soles, and Plummer-Vinson syndrome, with webs in the esophagus and anemia).

Surprisingly, individuals using daily aspirin and NSAIDs (non-steroidal anti-inflammatory medication) have a lower risk. Also, there is a lower incidence stemming from diets with fruits, green and yellow vegetables, cruciferous vegetables (broccoli, cabbage, and cauliflower), and moderate coffee intake.

### ■ Diagnosis and Treatment

The diagnosis is often made with either a barium swallow or EGD (esophago-gastro-duodenoscopy—a fiberoptic lighted tube) where biopsies of a suspected lesion can be done. After the diagnosis has been confirmed, other studies are performed to evaluate the extent and operability of the disease. These include CT (computerized tomography) of the abdomen, chest, and pelvis, and PET (positron emission tomography) scans. Frequently EUS (esophageal endoscopic ultrasound) can be used to determine the level of tumor invasion.

If the tumor is so large that swallowing is impossible for the patient, a metal stent can be placed through the obstructing tumor to allow continuation of eating; if this is not possible, a feeding tube can be placed in the stomach (through the abdominal wall) to improve the nutrition of the patient during therapy or prior to definitive surgery. Often the patient is treated with preoperative chemotherapy (neoadjuvant) and tube feedings or total parenteral nutrition (intravenous feeding) to improve the general health and decrease the risks of surgery.

### Staging

The esophagus has four layers from inside to outside: mucosa, submucosa, muscularis, adventitia that are important in staging.

The TNM system is used. T=Tumor, N=Nodes, M=Metastases.

- Tis—Carcinoma in situ–in mucosa–N0=No nodes with cancer–M0=no metastases

- T1—Invades submucosa

- T1—Regional nodes with cancer–M1=metastases

- T2—Invades muscularis

- T3—Invades adventitia

- T4—Invades adjacent structures

*Staging—5-year survival*

- Stage 0—Tis N0 M0 > 90 percent
- Stage I—T1 N0 M > 70 percent
- Stage IIA—T2–3 N0 M0–00 percent
- Stage IIB—T1–2 N1 M0–00 percent
- Stage III—T3 N1 M0 <10 percent
- T4—Any N M0

## Surgery

The surgical approach depends on the stage of the cancer and the condition of the patient. Very early stage I disease can sometimes be treated with endoscopic resection of the mucosa or mucosal ablation with a laser (Nd-YAG or argon plasma laser). Lasers use high-intensity light to destroy tumor cells. Another type of laser PDT (photodynamic therapy) involves the use of drugs that are absorbed by cancer cells, making the cells very sensitive to destruction when exposed to special light.

Stage 0 and Stage I cancers are treated with surgery; IIA and IIB with surgery, chemo, radiation, or a combination; Stage III with chemo, radiation, and palliative resection; and Stage IV with palliation, intubation, and possibly chemotherapy and radiation. The extent of the surgery depends on the location, pathology, and stage of the disease. When indicated for a cure, many surgeons recommend complete removal of the esophagus (total esophagectomy), while others may recommend lesser procedures, especially for cancers in the area of the esophago-gastric junction. The surgery can be done through the abdomen or chest, or a combination of the two. To reestablish intestinal continuity, either the stomach has to be brought up into the chest, or a loop of colon needs to be interposed to function as a new esophagus. In addition, several surgical centers recommend extensive removal of lymph nodes. The surgery is complex and has much potential for complications and side effects, including leakage at the anastomosis (connections), bleeding, heart attack, infection, lung collapse, pulmonary embolus, stenosis, and stroke, along with the usual postoperative problems of nausea, pain, and the need for continual breathing assistance on a ventilator.

## Chemotherapy

Chemotherapeutic agents used alone, or in combination, are bleomycin, cisplatin, docetaxel, 5-FU, gemcitabine, leucovorin, oxyplatin, paclitaxel, and vindesine, as well as capecytabine, erlotinib, flavopiridol, and gefitonib. The side effects include anemia, anorexia, fatigue, hand-foot syndrome, fever, lethargy, nausea and vomiting, and neutropenia (decreased white blood cells).

## ■ *Complementary and Alternative Treatment*

Alternative and complementary medicine will not cure esophageal cancer but can play an important part in relieving the symptoms, both of the cancer itself and the side effects of chemotherapy and radiation therapy. Hypnosis, massage, meditation, and relaxation techniques are helpful in allaying anxiety, fatigue, and stress; acupuncture, aromatherapy, hypnosis, and music therapy can be very effective against nausea and vomiting, as well as pain management. Exercise, relaxation techniques, tai chi, and yoga are beneficial for sleep problems.

Chinese medicine offers several herbal approaches to therapy, and many are aimed directly at the cancer. The Ayurvedic approaches to therapy are also directed toward alleviating symptoms of the disease as well as diminishing the side effects of standard therapy. Several alternative and complementary clinics offer consultation and therapies including:

◇ **Abhayanga.** Harmonizing, synchronous herbal oil massage

◇ **Shirodhara.** Oil applied to the forehead for harmonization of vegetative system

◇ **Svedana.** Herbal steam bath with medicinal plants

◇ **Padabhyanga.** Harmonizing Ayurvedic foot reflex zone massage

◇ **Shiroabhyanga.** Invigorating massage of head, neck, and shoulders with herbs

The regimens of Chinese, Ayurvedic, and other alternative and complementary systems occupy thousands of pages and hundreds of years experience. Many of these appear obscure and foreign to the Western physician's approach to cancer management, so it is recommended that patients with esophageal cancer seek out qualified practitioners, listen to their recommendations, discuss the therapy with their oncologist, and then make a decision as to its efficacy, considering outcome, cost, and time required. Because of the ominous nature of esophageal cancer, early evaluation and treatment along standard Western medicine lines are recommended, with alternative and complementary therapies used in tandem. In my experience with patients with advanced stage cancer, seeking alternative therapy is recommended, but judgment and common sense should always prevail.

Acceptance is an important aspect of dealing with any cancer. Don't close the door on any potential reasonable therapy, but make sure that wisdom and caution also enter into the equation. Unfortunately, many Western physicians are averse to complementary and alternative approaches, and this is wrong. Hopefully when dealing with esophageal cancer, an aggressive disease with difficult management, the diagnosis, treatment, and support can be a coordinated effort between the two, often divergent, approaches to management.

## EYE CANCER

Cancers in the eye may be either primary (originating in the eye) or metastatic (originating in another organ and spreading to the eye).

The most common cancer in the area of the eye is the basal-cell carcinoma affecting the eyelid. Other cancers of this area are melanoma, sebaceous carcinoma, and squamous cell. Because of the location and local irritation, all these cancers are usually diagnosed early and can be removed surgically without risk of them spreading.

In children, the most common intraocular tumor is the retinoblastoma that has a cure rate over 95 percent when diagnosed early. The earliest findings are blurred vision, crossed eyes (strabismus), red and painful eye, and a whitish or yellowish glow to the examined eye.

The second most common childhood eye cancer is the meduloblastoma affecting the ciliary body and uvea (the middle layer of the eye), which is also highly curable when diagnosed early.

In adults the most common intraocular tumor is the melanoma, which may initially be symptomatic and only diagnosed early by a routine eye exam. As the tumor grows, it will appear as an enlarging black spot, with blurring of vision, double vision, and eventual blindness. Pain may also be a symptom.

Primary intraocular lymphoma is the second most frequent adult ocular malignancy.

Metastatic cancers to the eye can come from cancer of the breast, lung, and, rarely, from the colon, kidney, prostate, skin, and thyroid.

The treatment of intraocular cancers is widely variable, depending on the specific location in the eye, the size, and the danger of spread. The objective is to leave the patient with a cure if possible, followed by vision, and an acceptable cosmetic appearance.

## ◼ *Diagnosis and Treatment*

After consultation and workup, including an ophthalmologic exam and x-rays of the skull and soft tissues around the orbit, a multidisciplinary approach to therapy will be reached. This may include one or a combination of the following treatments.

### Chemotherapy

◇ Enucleation. Removal of the eye, leaving muscles and eyelid

◇ Evisceration. Removing the inside of the eye leaving the white part (sclera)

◇ Exenteration. Removal of the entire contents of the orbit—eye, eyelid, and muscles

◇ Laser treatment

◇ Local excision

◇ Radiation therapy

◇ Surgical removal. Either portions (iridectomy, choroidectomy), or the entire eye and surrounding tissue

Radical treatments are followed by replacement of the eyeball with matching prostheses and appropriate plastic reconstruction (often appearing so natural that only family members are aware of the prosthesis).

Radiation treatment, in an attempt to salvage the eye, may involve external beam or internal radiation brachytherapy with the insertion of radioactive discs. These therapies, however, may result in cataracts, loss of eyelashes, and dry eye, or, in rare cases, retinopathy (abnormal blood-vessel development in the eye), or optic nerve damage (optic neuropathy) that may result in loss of vision in that eye.

### ■ *Complementary and Alternative Treatment*

With eye cancer, alternative treatments are only recommended to manage the side effects of chemotherapy and radiation therapy, and to alleviate the stress and anxiety involved with the symptoms and, later, with the possible loss of the eye.

## GALLBLADDER AND BILE-DUCT CANCER

The gallbladder, situated under the right lobe of the liver, is a globular saclike organ that stores and concentrates bile, the green liquid that is produced in the liver. It flows through the liver's bile ducts, or tubules, into a main hepatic (liver) bile duct toward the gallbladder or the intestine. When it joins up with the cystic duct (the tube from the gallbladder), it is called the common bile duct, and this leads to, and connects to, the duodenum, the first part of the small intestine after the stomach. When a person eats certain foods, especially fatty or spicy foods, the gallbladder contracts, sending bile into the intestine to help digest the foods and vitamins A, D, E, and K. When there are dysfunctions of the gallbladder, or when it concentrates the bile too much, stones form, and these can cause pain, nausea, and vomiting. This is called acute or chronic cholecystitis and often results in surgical removal of the gallbladder in a procedure called a cholecystectomy (either laparoscopic, using four tiny openings and a fiberoptic scope, or open, through a large incision).

Cancer can occur in the gallbladder itself or in any of the ducts. When it arises in the gallbladder, usually from the innermost lining, or mucosa, it is called an adenocarcinoma. When cancer forms in the bile ducts, it is called a cholangiocarcinoma and may affect ducts in the liver (intrahepatic) or outside the liver (extrahepatic).

Gallbladder cancer is two times more common in women, Mexican Americans, some South Americans, and Native American, usually more than seventy years old. Although the incidence of gallstones and cholecystitis is very high, only a few people develop this cancer. However, in most individuals with gallbladder cancer, stones *are* found in the organ. So among the risk factors for developing gallbladder cancer are gallstones and cholecystitis, as well as typhoid fever (the bacteria settles in the gallbladder), obesity, family history, and a condition known as porcelain gallbladder, where so much calcium is deposited in the gallbladder wall that the organ becomes a solid porcelain-like receptacle. Cancer of the bile ducts, cholangiocarcinoma, is felt to be more common in individuals with small stones in these ducts, as well as those with chronic infections in other areas of the body, or harmful habits. Among these chronic conditions are diabetes mellitus, hepatitis C, smoking, ulcerative colitis, and parasites seen in other areas of the world and uncommon in the United States. Some abnormalities in bile-duct development (choledochal cysts) predispose an individual to bile duct cancer.

In its early stages, gallbladder cancer does not cause symptoms, and, as an unfortunate result, most of these cancers are not identified until the disease has spread and become difficult to treat. Because the gallbladder is directly adjacent to the undersurface of the liver, there is a propensity for it to spread directly into the liver, as well as the lymph nodes and adjacent structures (bile ducts, colon, intestines, stomach). The symptoms usually parallel those of cholecystitis and gallstones, namely pain, nausea, fever, and a sense of bloating. But when the cancer starts to obstruct the flow of bile from the liver, jaundice (yellow skin and eyes due to a buildup of a substance called bilirubin) will develop, along with late stages of weight loss, fatigue, and even the development of a mass.

Cancer of the bile ducts may present earlier, with blockage of the bile ducts causing jaundice. Intrahepatic disease is more ominous because of the early involvement of the surrounding liver, while extra-hepatic bile-duct cancer may present early enough to allow surgical removal and possible cure.

### ■ Diagnosis and Treatment

Most gallbladder cancer is diagnosed incidentally at the time of removing the gallbladder (a cholecystectomy); bile-duct cancer presents as jaundice. In cases of cancer of the distal common bile duct, there may be a backup of bile into the gallbladder, causing massive distention of the structure. This is called Courvoisier's sign and is often characteristic of bile-duct cancer. Blood tests for gallbladder or bile-duct cancer are unfortunately not very diagnostic, often suggesting a benign disease, such as cholecystitis, or gallstones. Among these test results are the elevation of bilirubin, or such liver function tests as SGOT, SGPT, and alkaline phosphatase. The tumor markers

CA19–9 and CEA may be elevated but are so nonspecific that they are of little help.

Once cancer of the gallbladder or bile ducts is suspected or diagnosed, further studies will be performed to evaluate the stage and plan for treatment. These include CT (computerized tomography), ultrasound, MRCP (magnetic resonance cholangiopancreatography), or PET scan (positron emission tomography) to identify metastases. If a tissue diagnosis is needed, a needle biopsy can be done through the skin by a radiologist, by a gastroenterologist through endoscopy (looking down the esophagus past the stomach into the first part of the duodenum and up into the bile duct), ERCP (endoscopic retrograde cholangiopancreatography) by the surgeon, using laparoscopy (placing a fiberoptic scope into the abdomen under anesthesia), or through open surgery.

### Staging

The staging of these diseases will help to determine how they should be handled medically and surgically. Although the TNM (T=Tumor size, N=Lymph node involvement, M=Metastasis) system is used for gallbladder cancer, there are only three stages to be discussed—localized disease that is completely removable, localized disease that is not removable because of its extent and the involvement of liver and other adjacent structures, and advanced metastatic disease.

Similarly, cancer of the intra- and extrahepatic bile ducts has a complex T, N, M staging. The only important determination is whether the involvement, location, and extent of the disease allows it to be resected (surgically removed) or not.

### Surgery

Gallbladder cancer is often found at the time of a cholecystectomy, and often the surgeon may not even know about it until several days later when the pathologist calls him or her after completing the studies. In the rare cases where the tumor is small, where there is only a small involvement of the adjacent liver, or when the cancer has been detected before the cholecystectomy, an open operation must be performed. This includes the removal of the gallbladder, if not already done, as well as removal of the portion of the liver adjacent to the gallbladder (the gallbladder bed of the liver). Usually, upon exploration, the cancer

has been found to have spread beyond the point where a curative operation can be performed.

Bile-duct surgery may be very complex. If the cancer is in an intrahepatic bile duct, a partial hepatectomy (liver resection) may be possible. If it occurs at the junction of the right and left hepatic ducts as
they exit the liver to form the common hepatic duct (Klatskin tumor),
the surgery is very difficult and requires reconstructing the bile ducts
using the intestine. If the cancer is in a distal extrahepatic bile duct, a
Whipple procedure is sometimes possible (removing the gallbladder,
bile ducts, head of the pancreas, part of the stomach, and local lymph
nodes).

In most instances, only palliative procedures can be done, and these
involve bypassing the obstructed area using a loop of intestine. Sometimes a gastroenterologist can relieve blockage of a duct by passing a
stent or tube through the obstructed area.

In cases where there is severe pain, a radiologist or a specialist in
pain management can do a nerve block (neurolysis) of the celiac nerve
plexus and eliminate or lessen the pain.

### Chemotherapy

Chemotherapy is not curative but can sometimes shrink the gallbladder or bile-duct tumor and extend the life of these patients. The usual
regimen includes gemcitabine plus platinum-based drugs, and a new
trial drug call sorafenib. Direct infusion of drugs into the hepatic artery
has been shown to extend survival, as has adiation therapy, alone or
with chemotherapy, or a radio-sensitizing drug (a drug that makes the
cancer more sensitive to radiation).

### ■ *Complementary and Alternative Treatment*

Because gallbladder and biliary-tract cancers are often rapid growing
and can spread very quickly, alternative measures cannot usually shrink
the tumor fast enough to relieve obstruction. However, following several complementary regimens may help in slowing its growth, or even
preventing its metastasis. Standard Western medical and surgical therapy is recommended, along with such alternative therapies as vitamin
$B_{17}$ (laetrile) or the Cellect-Budwig diet, basically vegetable juicing
(with carrots as the primary element), cottage cheese, and flaxseed oil,
that may be of help and that are not harmful to other therapies.

Ayurvedic herbal medicines are replete with many treatments that reduce swelling and alleviate jaundice, as well as many of the side effects of radiation and chemotherapy, such as decreased appetite, nausea, vomiting, weakness, and weight loss. Some even state they can slow down or prevent metastasis, thereby prolonging and improving the quality of life.

The Gerson diet is considered especially advantageous for gallbladder and bile-duct (and liver) cancers because its focus is on eliminating toxins that are processed in the liver. The regimen also includes enemas, a variety of minerals and vitamins, fruit juices, and vegetarian diets. As with many holistic therapies, the addition of beta-carotene, vitamins C and E, and selenium are recommended, along with acupuncture.

NCCAM (National Center for Complementary and Alternative Medicine) has several recommendations.

◇ Dandelion (*Taraxacum officinale*), also called lion's tooth or blowball, is rich in vitamin A and has been used by Native Americans as well as Ayurvedic practitioners for liver and gallbladder cancer, but not for blocked bile ducts.

◇ Licorice (sweet root, *Glycyrrhiza glabra*) is an ingredient in many Chinese herbal remedies. It has been used for centuries in China for cancer treatment and prevention by preventing DNA mutations and inhibiting cancer growth, even killing cancer cells. Laboratory studies in the West are still inconclusive.

◇ Milk thistle (*Silybum marianum*) contains a flavonoid that is believed to protect liver and gallbladder cells from damage by free radicals.

◇ Turmeric, a yellow herb often found in Indian curry dishes is used in Ayurvedic medicine for gallbladder and bile-duct cancers.

◇ A Chinese medicine, *Canelim* capsules, is the only class A medicine listed in the Chinese national Basic Insurance Catalog for promoting the killing of gallbladder and bile-duct cancer cells, boosting body immunity, alleviating pain and other symptoms, and prolonging life. It is recommended together with standard Western therapies and in terminal stage disease.

Clinical trials are being instituted in China, India, and several major American Cancer Centers to determine the effectiveness of these various remedies. But in all cases, the treatment recommended is complementary only—standard Western medicine and surgery in conjunction with alternative and complementary medicine.

## GYNECOLOGICAL CANCER— CERVICAL, UTERINE, OVARIAN

### CERVICAL CANCER

The cervix is a globular round structure serving as the mouth of the uterus projecting into the vagina. The incidence of cancer of the cervix is decreasing and primarily affects women in their thirties and forties in the lower socioeconomic class where there is poor access to adequate medical care. While this is a relatively rare disease in the United States, throughout the world it is the third leading cause of cancer deaths in women.

Invasive cervical cancer is essentially a sexually transmitted disease, not occurring in women who have never been sexually active. The etiology (origin) is felt to be the human papilloma virus (HPV) that is sexually transmitted. There are more than 200 types of HPV, of which forty infect the genital tract. Types HPV 16 and 18 account for 70 percent of the cervical cancers. Gardasil, a quadrivalent vaccine is now approved for use in women ages nine to twenty-six and is supposed to prevent upward of 70 percent of cervical cancer.

Other risk factors are cervical dysplasia (a precancerous condition of the cervix), chronic cervicitis (cervical and vaginal infections), cigarette smoking, immune-system deficiencies found with HIV disease, multiparity (many pregnancies and deliveries), and oral contraceptives. Additional risk factors are chronic chlamydia infections, early age at first intercourse and first pregnancy, family history of cervical cancer, stress-related disorders, and use of the hormonal drug diethylstilbestrol.

The symptoms of cervical carcinoma are infected, foul-smelling, vaginal discharge, metrorrhagia (persistent vaginal bleeding throughout the month), and postcoital (postintercourse) spotting (bleeding). Late symptoms are bladder infections, fistulas between the vagina and rectum, involvement of the bladder with blood in the urine, pelvic and rectal pain, and pain with intercourse. Extreme advanced disease may cause back pain from spinal-nerve involvement, impaired kidney function when the ureters are involved, and swelling of the legs from lymph-node involvement.

Prevention is through screening (Pap test), use of condoms, and vaccination. Reduction of risks is seen with the use of vitamins A, $B_{12}$, C, E, and beta-carotene.

### ■ Diagnosis and Treatment

The most widely used screening test for cervical abnormalities is the Pap test developed by George Papanicolaou in 1928, where a scraping of cells is taken from the cervix and examined by a pathologist. Early diagnosis of mild abnormalities and precancerous lesions of the cervix allow the gynecologist to treat the early disease and obviate the development of frank invasive cancer of the cervix. This simple test has saved thousands of women.

Diagnostic measures also include cervical biopsy, often done as the loop electrosurgical excision procedure (LEEP), or colposcopy, where an examination of the cervix and vagina is performed with a special scope and appropriate biopsies are taken.

There are two main types of cervical cancer, squamous (80 percent) and adenocarcinoma (20 percent).

### Staging

The International Federation of Gynecology and Obstetrics (FIGO) clinical staging, which is fairly complex, differs slightly from the standard TNM system, T=Tumor, N=Nodes, and M=Metastasis. This is an abbreviated version.

- Tis—Carcinoma in situ. N0–No nodes involved

- T1—Invasive cancer limited to the cervix. N1–Nodes involved

- T2—Cervical cancer invading beyond the uterus, but not to the pelvic wall. M0–No metastasis

- T3—Cancer extends to pelvic wall, vagina, and M1. Distant metastases and possible kidney dysfunction

- T4 tumor—Involves bladder, rectum, and pelvic wall

## FIGO Staging

- IA—Preinvasive carcinoma

- IA1—Minimal invasion

- IA2—Tumor invasion 3–7 mm

- IB—Confined to cervix

- IB1—No greater than 4 cm

- IB2—Greater than 4 cm

- II—Invades beyond uterus, but not to pelvic wall or lower third vagina

- IIA—No parametrial involvement

- IIB—Parametrial invasion

- III—Extends to pelvic wall, lower third of vagina, causes ureter obstruction

- IV—Invades bladder, rectum, and beyond

## Surgery

The generally accepted standard of care of cervical cancer is surgical removal of the cervix. Whether more extensive surgery is indicated depends on the staging. Stage 1A can be treated with a simple hysterectomy, either abdominal, vaginal, laparoscopic assisted, or robotic. If preservation of fertility is a high priority with the patient, an extensive excision of the cervix with margins free of tumor is occasionally done. For Stage IA2, IB1, and some IIA, a radical hysterectomy is recommended. This includes removal of the uterus, tubes, ovaries, pelvic lymph nodes, and some of the aortic lymph nodes. Postoperative radiation therapy may be recommended. For stages IB2 and bulky IIA disease, the recommendation is cisplatin and radiation therapy followed by a radical hysterectomy.

The management of higher stage and/or recurrent cervical cancer is tremendously variable and the object of many ongoing clinical trials. The various therapies include intracavitary brachytherapy, using cesium-137 introduced directly into the uterine cervix, and external beam radiation to the pelvic and para-aortic lymph nodes. In some cases there may be a possibility for cure with a radical surgical procedure called the pelvic exenteration, which involves removing all the pelvic organs in a long, complicated, surgical operation in the hands of specially trained gynecologic oncologists. (Intraoperative radiation may be used along with this procedure.)

### Chemotherapy

Advanced and recurrent disease states are also treated with many chemotherapeutic agents, including alkylating agents (CCNU, cyclophosphamide, iphosphamide, etc.), heavy metals (carboplatin, cisplatin), alkaloids (vincristine vindesine), antimetabolites (5-FU, methotrexate), antibiotics (doxorubicin, mitomycin), and other agents (irinotecan, paclitaxel, teniposide, etc.). Palliative radiation and chemotherapy are used for advanced disease, and, in cases of solitary lung metastases, actual removal of the metastasis may be indicated (metastasectomy).

The use of various combinations of chemotherapy and radiation therapy as salvage modalities is complex and beyond the scope of this book.

In general, the prognosis for Stage I disease is an almost 90 percent cure, with Stage II at 45–60 percent, and Stage III at 15 percent. However, with newer and combined therapies these figures have been improving steadily.

### ■ Complementary and Alternative Treatment

This disease is common in Asia and Africa, and there is a focus on complementary treatment in these areas. Ayurvedic approaches to cervical cancer are always recommended in conjunction with standard conventional treatment. There is a large armamentarium of therapies that act on the rasa, rakta, and mansa tissues of Ayurvedic medicine with names that are strange to the Western ear, including indrayav, kutki, patol, saariva, and patha, all used to curtail metastatic disease, and such medicines as ashwaghanda, shatavari, kamadudharas, and others to prevent or reduce the effects of radiation and chemotherapy, or improve the immunity of the body. Approaching Ayurvedic practitioners for complementary medicine may not be as popular in the United States because of the rarity of cervical cancer, but it is very popular in India where the incidence is significantly higher.

Chinese and other herbal therapies have been helpful in protecting against cervical cancer and in ameliorating the side effects of standard therapy. Among these therapies are garlic, goldenseal with anti-inflammatory components, Lempoyang pine ginger, natural green tea, turmeric, and zedoania). Suffice it to say that alternative therapies, including acupuncture, herbal therapy, and massage, can be of significant benefit to patients with advanced disease requiring combination therapies with many side effects.

## UTERINE CANCER

Uterine cancer (endometrial carcinoma) arises from the inner lining of the uterus and is the most common gynecological cancer in the United States. It is associated with diabetes mellitus, estrogen replacement therapy, heavy alcohol consumption, hypertension, obesity, pelvic radiation therapy, polycystic ovaries, use of oral contraceptives, and the use of Tamoxifen. Those with endometrial hyperplasia (florid growth of the lining cells), nulliparous (no children), women with late menopause, and a positive family history for this cancer are also at higher risk. A family history of breast, colon, or ovarian cancer seems to indicate a higher risk as well.

These cancers spread into the wall of the uterus and into the cervix and can eventually grow through the uterus into the surrounding tissue of the bladder and the rectum. More advanced spread comes via the lymphatic system to lymph nodes in the groin and above the clavicle (collarbone), throughout the abdomen and pelvis, and through the bloodstream to the liver, lungs, and brain.

The common signs are abnormal uterine bleeding, anemia, clear vaginal discharge in postmenopausal women, back and pelvic pain, weight loss, and weakness; 5–10 percent of women who have this cancer have no symptoms.

### ■ Diagnosis and Treatment

Diagnosis through clinical evaluation after a pelvic examination is accomplished by an endometrial biopsy or, in some cases, a D&C (dilation of the cervical opening and curettage—done under anesthesia). Hysteroscopy, the inspection of the uterus by fiberoptic scope with access through the cervix, allows direct visualization of the endometrium and a possible direct biopsy. The actual thickness of the cancer can be determined by a transvaginal ultrasound. Chest x-rays, PET/CT scans, and MRIs are used to determine the extent and operability of the cancer. The Pap test, while excellent for cervical cancer, may show some abnormal change but is not generally a good screening method for uterine cancer.

Although 80 percent of uterine cancers are adenocarcinomas, there are also several rarer cancers, such as serous carcinoma, clear-cell carcinoma, and sarcoma. The staging of uterine cancer is complex and often differentiates between medical and surgical staging with determinations made after a surgical procedure more carefully delineates the extent of the disease. However, the FIGO system is generally used.

**FIGO Staging**

- Stage IA—Tumor confined to uterus, no or $<1/2$ myometrial (muscle layer) invasion
- Stage IB—Tumor confined to uterus, $>1/2$ myometrial invasion
- Stage II—Cervical invasion but not beyond uterus
- Stage IIIA—Tumor invades serosa and adnexae (tubes and ovaries)
- Stage IIIB—Vagina or adnexae involved
- Stage IIIC1—Pelvic lymph nodes involved
- Stage IIIC2—Para-aortic lymph nodes involved
- Stage IVA—Cancer invades bladder or/and rectum
- Stage IVB—Distant metastases

**Surgery**

Treatment of uterine cancer is surgical, usually by abdominal hysterectomy (rather than vaginal hysterectomy) so that abdominal cavity washings (free cells in the abdomen for examination) can be obtained to evaluate for the presence or absence of cancer. In this radical hysterectomy procedure, the fallopian tubes and ovaries, along with abdominal lymph nodes, are removed. In stages I and II disease, chemotherapy may be offered in conjunction with the surgery. Stages III and IV usually require chemotherapy along with radiation therapy, as well as surgical intervention. Laparoscopic, as well as robotic, techniques are now being used when the surgeon is experienced in these modalities.

### Radiation and Chemotherapy

Radiation therapy techniques can include brachytherapy, which places the radiation source into the uterus, external beam radiation, and vaginal irradiation.

Chemotherapy drugs used for treatment of uterine cancer include cisplatin (Platinol), doxorubicin (Adriamycin), and paclitaxel (Taxol). Occasionally, progesterone-like drugs are used to palliate or slow down the growth of advanced tumors, and tamoxifen (Nolvadex), an antiestrogen drug has a similar effect.

### ■ Complementary and Alternative Treatment

The complementary approach to uterine cancer is predominately one of helping to promote health and wholeness and improve the quality of life. Many young women have to face the fact that they will never have children and may have significant sexual and emotional setbacks. Mind-body therapy deals with these issues through couples sessions, guided imagery, deep breathing exercises, laughter therapy, Reiki (a gentle hands-on practice) and *qigong*, an ancient Chinese healing art using soft, flowing motions to refocus the mind and body, reduce stress, build stamina, and enhance the immune system.

Ayurvedic treatment for uterine cancer is aimed at both the cancer and at preventing or reducing the amount the cancer spreads. Its many therapies have been used for centuries, and consultation with qualified practitioners may lead to the improvement of a patient's condition. Responsible Ayurvedic specialists always state that their patients should be under the care and supervision of an oncology team.

As with other cancers, there are many herbal remedies for nausea, vomiting, pain, and depression offered by complementary medicine that will not interact negatively with oncologic treatments.

Obesity and a diet high in animal fats are associated with an increased risk for many malignancies and especially endometrial (uterine) cancers. Conversely, diets high in vegetables and fruit appear to provide some protection against this malignancy.[18]

While many herbs and nutrients are used in any balanced nutritional program, in estrogen-stimulating endometrial cancer, certain substances with anti-estrogenic properties, such as soybean isoflavones and resveratrol, may be of significant value. Those herbs with estrogenic effect are contraindicated—dong quai, licorice, and red clover among them.[19,20]

## OVARIAN CANCER

The study and understanding of ovarian cancer is broad-reaching and at times complex. This disease is difficult and problematic because it is rarely diagnosed at early stages, and, by the time its symptoms become apparent, the cancer has usually progressed to stage IV. On the rare occasions it is identified early, it is highly responsive to treatment and curable. But even with the advanced disease, marked advances in treatment, both surgical and chemotherapeutic, have allowed for a notable increase in survival and palliation in the last twenty years.

This cancer occurs in women ages fifty to seventy-five and is more common in Caucasians than African Americans (17.9/100,000 vs. 11.9/100,000). The cause is unknown although there appear to be many discrete genetic defects involved in its development and there is an increased incidence in women who have the BRCA1, BRCA2, and HNPCC (hereditary nonpolyposis colorectal cancer) genes. Other risk factors include endometriosis, a family history of breast or ovarian cancer, infertility (no history of having children), and postmenopausal use of estrogen replacement therapy. Obesity, radiation, talc exposure, and, possibly, certain virus exposures are also suggested as increasing the risk for developing ovarian cancer.

Ovarian cancer is subtle in its early stages, with vague gastrointestinal symptoms—nausea, vomiting, constipation, and diarrhea—often attributable to other causes. With more advanced disease, women develop abdominal distention, ascites (accumulation of fluid in the abdomen), accompanied by bladder and/or rectal symptoms, a palpable mass, and weight loss. Once the possibility of ovarian cancer has been entertained, a workup should be undertaken that includes a pelvic examination, abdominal and transvaginal ultrasound, an abdominal CT (computerized tomography), and an MRI (magnetic resonance imaging). In advanced disease, laboratory tests include CA-125 and

CEA; in younger women, beta HCG (human chorionic gonado-trophin) and AFP (alpha fetoprotein) elevations help diagnosis germ-cell tumors.

### ■ Diagnosis and Treatment

The definitive diagnosis is made histologically (through microscopic studies) by obtaining tissue from abdominal fluid or by surgical explo-ration (exploratory laparotomy or laparoscopy). Approximately 90 per-cent of ovarian cancer is epithelial adenocarcinoma coming from the cells on the surface of the ovaries, and the pathologist will determine and grade the severity of the cancer by the degree of cellular change seen under a microscope. The remaining ovarian cancers arise from the ovarian stroma (deep tissue) or germ cells and include almost fifty dif-ferent types of cancer that often occur in younger women.

### FIGO Staging

The FIGO staging (International Federation of Gynecology and Obstetrics) is the system most used today and is abbreviated below.

- Stage I—Cancer limited to the ovaries

- Stage II—Growth involving one or both ovaries with pelvic exten-sion of disease

- Stage III—Tumor involves both ovaries, peritoneal implants, lymph node involvement and has implants on the intestine and liver

- Stage IV—Involving both ovaries with distant metastases

### Surgery

Surgical staging of the disease involves abdominal exploration (inci-sional, laparoscopic, or robotic) with a sampling of all areas for tumor cells (cytological washings), removal of ovaries, uterus, and fallopian tubes, omentectomy (removal of large fatty apron in abdomen), ran-dom biopsies of peritoneum, and diaphragm and lymph node sam-pling. This extensive procedure usually demands the expertise of a specially trained team of surgical gynecological oncologists, and women undergoing this extensive surgical procedure might want to ask for the inclusion of a gynecological oncologist on the operative team. When an expert is not present, the amount of cyto-reduction (removal of cancer tissue) is often less than adequate and long-term survival is poorer. In cases where the cancer is limited to only one ovary, it may be possible to preserve the uterus and remaining ovary in young women wishing to have children, although a discussion with the patient and her family needs to emphasize the risks involved.

**Chemotherapy and Radiation**

In addition to surgery, early stage ovarian cancer is treated with systemic chemotherapy, using such agents as carboplatin, cisplatin, doxorubicin, paclitaxel, phosphorus-32 (P-32), and topotecan. Whole abdominal radiation is also used in some cases of an early-stage cancer, but its use in late-stage disease is less successful.

For advanced disease, repeat surgery and more complex chemotherapy regimens have been used, including intraperitoneal infusion of chemotherapy and palliative radiation and chemotherapy. Studies using angiogenesis inhibitors (Avastin, Bevacizumab, ) and anti-VEGF therapy (sorafenib-Nexavar, and sunitinib-Sutent) are being undertaken and in many instances have converted ovarian cancer to a chronic disease with treatable recurrences (relapses) followed by partial or complete remissions (disappearance of cancer).

### ■ *Complementary and Alternative Treatment*

Many of the alternative CAM therapies are helpful in relieving the symptoms and improving the lives of patients with ovarian cancer by reducing the side effects of therapy and providing psychological support. Among these are mind, body, and spirit methods, including aromatherapy, art therapy, imagery, meditation, tai chi, and yoga. Other methods include acupuncture, massage therapy, and transcutaneous electrical nerve stimulation (TENS), using a portable unit that will afford considerable pain relief.

Among the herbs recommended (for example by the Johns Hopkins Cancer Center) are echinacea, which may provide immune enhancement and increase resistance to cancer ( though some studies actually indicate echinacea may suppress immune function). Kava may relieve anxiety, insomnia, nervousness, and stress, and ginkgo is used for dizziness, improved memory, motion sickness, and tinnitus (ringing in the ears). However, since ginkgo may interfere with normal clotting mechanisms, it should not be used prior to any surgery. Ginseng, promoted as a remedy for fatigue, improves concentration, and some believe it can prevent cancer. St John's Wort, used for anxiety, depression, and sleep disorders, may interfere with anesthesia, anticoagulants (coumadin), chemotherapy, and heart medicine (digoxin). Before using this herb, a consultation with an oncologist is recommended. Dietary supplements include vitamins A, C, E, folic acid, and coenzyme $Q_{10}$.

Green tea is often recommended as a preventive and to augment therapy for ovarian and other cancers.

The long-named, complex Ayurvedic therapies are successful adjuncts to the management of ovarian cancer. A consultation with a certified practitioner will introduce the patient to this form of alternative therapy. Similarly, a whole host of Chinese herbal preparations are available to counteract the complications and side effects of standard chemotherapy.

Similar to uterine cancer, a balanced diet high in vegetables appears to result in a reduced rate of ovarian cancer. Consumption of nutrients, such as curcumin, ginkgo biloba, quercetin, vitamins A,C, D, and E, are felt to inhibit ovarian cancer-cell growth. Melatonin, as well as the antioxidants beta-carotene, vitamins C, E, and $CoQ_{10}$, may increase the sensitivity of ovarian cancer cells to the chemotherapy agent cisplatin.[21,22,23]

## HEAD AND NECK CANCER

Head and neck tumors are a cluster of cancers that are grouped together because of their location and because 90 percent of them are similar in cell origin—the squamous cells that line the areas involved. Generally these cancers are more common in men (3:1), usually occur between ages fifty and seventy, and behave in an aggressive manner, with over 40 percent showing signs of lymph-node metastasis at the time of diagnosis. The areas involved are the oral cavity (mouth and lips), nasal cavity (inside nose), nasal sinuses, pharynx (swallowing area of throat), and larynx (breathing area of the throat, including the voice box and vocal cords), and the trachea.

The risk factors for head and neck cancer are tobacco (cigarettes, cigars, smokeless tobacco, and marijuana), alcohol, UV light (for lip cancer), occupational exposures (paint fumes, petroleum, nickel, or wood dust), previous radiation exposure (for thyroid and salivary glands), some viruses (HPV, the human papilloma virus; EBV, the Epstein-Barr virus), chewing betel nuts, GERD (gastroesophageal reflux disease), people who have had long-term immune suppression, such as with transplantations, poor diet, and vitamin deficiencies.

These cancers may be preceded early on by white patches in the mouth called leukoplakia. The signs and symptoms of this group of cancer are diffuse and may overlap with many other causes that are benign. This is why they are not often discovered very early and have already progressed to a more advanced stage by the time of diagnosis. The many symptoms can include the following.

◇ Bad breath

◇ Bleeding mouth

◇ Coughing up blood (hemoptysis)

◇ Difficulty in swallowing

◇ Earaches

◇ Enlarged neck glands

◇ Hoarseness

◇ Lump on lip or in mouth

◇ Mass in neck

◇ Neck pain

◇ Nosebleeds

◇ Red or white patches in mouth

◇ Sinus congestion

◇ Slurring speech

◇ Sore throat

◇ Sore tongue

A full understanding of these varied cancers requires a broad knowledge of the complex anatomy of the head and neck. Generally the neck is divided into five levels, going from the lower jaw and chin down to the clavicle, and is too detailed to explain here. The lymphatic drainage of a specific cancer is associated with a specific level, and determining the presence or absence of cancer in these draining areas assists the surgeon and oncologist in designing the appropriate therapy.

### ■ Diagnosis and Treatment

After obtaining a complete history and performing a physical exam, further evaluation is obtained by indirect (using mirrors) or direct laryngoscopy, fiberoptic endoscopy, and any of several diagnostic imaging procedures, including plain x-rays, CT (computerized tomography) scans, MRIs (magnetic resonance imaging), or PETs (positron emission tomography scans). When the tumor or abnormality has been localized, depending on the location, a punch biopsy, fine needle aspiration (FNA), core biopsy, or open biopsy may be performed.

As mentioned above, more than 90 percent of the head and neck cancers are of the squamous-cell variety, and most of these have the p53 gene mutation as one of the causative events. (HPV—human papilloma virus—causes this change in the p53 gene.) Other tumor types are exceedingly rare and include adenocarcinomas, adenoid cystic carcinomas, and mucoepidermoid carcinomas.

Most squamous-cell cancers may progress from leukoplakia (whitish patches from chronic irritation by carcinogens) to erythroplakia (reddish friable areas) to dysplasia (where the cells show marked atypical changes) to carcinoma in situ (a stage 0 cancer).

## Staging

The staging of head and neck cancers varies slightly with location, but in general the following basis applies. T=Tumor, N= Nodes, M=Metastasis. Tx—Primary tumor cannot be assessed. Nx—Nodes cannot be assessed. T0—No evidence of primary tumor. N0—No involved lymph nodes.

- Tis—Carcinoma in situ
- N1—Single node same side <3 cm
- T1—Tumor <2 cm
- N2—Nodes less than 6 cm
- T2—Tumor 2–4 cm
- N3—Nodes >6 cm
- T3—Tumor >4 cm
- T4a—Tumor invades nearby structure
- Mx—Metastasis can't be assessed but is removable surgically
- M0—No distant metastases
- T4b—Inoperable primary tumor, but M1-distant metastases treatable with radiation and chemotherapy

- Stage I—T1, N0, M0
- Stage II—T2, N0, M0
- Stage III—T3, N0, M0 or T1–3, N1, M0
- Stage IVA—T4a, N0–2, M0 or T1–3, N2, M0
- Stage IVB—T4b, any N, M0 or any T, N3, M0
- Stage IVC—Any T, any N, M1

**Surgery**

The treatment of these cancers is very complex. The object is to accomplish eradication of the tumor, but the location may make extensive surgery impossible or create living conditions unacceptable to the patient. Extensive removal of the mouth, tongue, or vocal cords may be unacceptable, considering the quality of life after treatment. Surgical treatment may also involve removal of lymph nodes, often requiring a procedure known as a radical neck dissection, with complete removal of nodes in the area of the cancer, along with other structures and muscles. This can be very disfiguring surgery and often requires plastic surgery for reconstruction.

There is combined use of surgery, radiation therapy, and chemotherapy, using different schemes and schedules for delivery of these regimens. Some patients receive treatment before surgery, others afterward.

**Chemotherapy and Radiation**

The chemotherapy combinations may include such agents as carboplatin, cetuximab, cisplatin, erbitux, erlotinib (Tarceva), 5-FU, gefitinib, methotrexate, paclitaxel, taxol, and taxotere. Amifostine is a drug administered to protect the salivary glands from the effects of radiation.

Use of photodynamic therapy for some mucosal lesions is advocated, as well as laser treatments.

The complications of treatment relate not only to the problems associated with surgery but also to the chemo-radiation. Patients may have eating problems, pain, severe inflammation of the mucous membranes in the mouth and throat (mucositis), as well as decreased-to-absent saliva, resulting in dry mouth, GERD (gastroesophageal reflux), hearing deficits, and kidney problems. Some patients can develop osteonecrosis (deterioration) of the jaw from radiation.

### ■ *Complementary and Alternative Treatment*

Because of the extensive and often disfiguring nature of the standard treatments for head and neck cancers, many patients have sought out alternative therapies. One regimen, hyperthermia, is used in conjunction with lower dose radiation, and several studies have confirmed its usefulness.

There are no herbal or other alternative treatments that can cure this kind of cancer, and immediate standard treatment, in conjunction with complementary care, is recommended. Acupuncture can be useful for treating nausea from chemotherapy and can also reduce cancer pain. One clinical trial indicated that acupuncture significantly reduced mouth pain and dry mouth in patients undergoing radiation for head and neck cancers.

Mind-body therapy, hypnotherapy, and guided imagery, along with massage therapy and spirituality, have been helpful. Energy therapies, including Reiki, have showed some positive results under the aegis of experts.

Good nutrition is important as are many herbal medicines recommended by the Ayurvedic and traditional Chinese medicine (TCM) practitioners. Use of selected vegetables and fruits, along with such supplements as coenzyme $Q_{10}$, hydrazine, melatonin, and shiitake-mushroom extract have been recommended. Several Western physicians recommend an orthomolecular approach to cancer treatment, advocating the use of megadoses of vitamins A, B, C, and D, along with niacinamide, pyridoxine, selenium, and zinc, to improve the body's immune system. Several major cancer centers are exploring these regimens. Several agents are controversial, and this makes decisions about accepting alternative therapies, such as antineoplastins, Essiac, hydrazine sulfate, laetrile, and shark cartilage, difficult to determine.

While being aware of the potential advantages of traditional Chinese medicine (TCM) and Ayurvedic medicine, the patient must be careful to find a practitioner who has documented excellent training in China or India and impeccable credentials before placing her- or himself in their hands.

As with other cancers, delay of conventional treatment, especially with squamous-cell head and neck cancer, may result in the progression of a treatable, curable cancer to a higher stage and a more extensive cancer less amenable to treatment or cure.

# HEMATOLOGIC MALIGNANCIES— LEUKEMIAS, LYMPHOMAS, AND OTHERS

This is a vast subject to cover and will be divided into several subjects: acute leukemias, chronic myeloid leukemia, chronic lymphocytic leukemia, Hodgkin's lymphoma, non-Hodgkin's lymphoma, multiple myelomas, plasma cell diseases, and myelodysplastic syndromes. The objective will be to give an overview of each cancer and a basic understanding of the standard and complementary approaches to management of these diseases.

## ACUTE LEUKEMIAS

As a surgeon, I always thought of leukemia as cancer of the blood. In reality, this is a cancer of the blood-forming organs, which include the bone marrow and the lymph system (spleen or thymus). This cancer of the blood-forming cells is known as the hemopoietic system, and these leukemic cells move into the bloodstream from their place of origin and then may spread to the liver, lymph nodes, spleen, and other organs.

The molecular genetics of the leukemias has shown more than 100 mutations responsible for these cancers, with recurring chromosomal abnormalities. A large number of studies have determined the many genetic idiosyncrasies of this cancer and have led to new and innovative treatments in the last ten years, creating lines of therapy in a once universally fatal disease. There are two basic types of this cancer: acute myelogenous leukemia (AML), occurring usually after age forty, and acute lymphocytic leukemia (ALL). Sixty percent of this cancer is seen in children up to five years, with the remaining percentage appearing after age sixty.

While the exact cause of acute leukemia is not understood, exposure to benzene and petroleum products, and ionizing radiation (atomic bomb, Chernobyl, etc.) are implicated. The incubation period between exposure and development of the disease may be as long as thirty years. There is also an apparent link to smoking, hair dyes, and nonionic radiation.

A major causative contributor to acute leukemia is exposure to cytotoxic drugs. Among these are alkylating agents used in chemotherapy

—cyclophosphamide, melphalan (Alkeran), and a group called topoisomerase inhibitors—doxorubicin, etoposide, mitoxantrone (Novantrone), taxanes, and teniposide (Vumon), used in treating breast cancer.

Individuals with Down syndrome also have a higher incidence of these acute leukemias. In some cases, there is the presence of a named *Philadelphia chromosome,* which may lead to a more specifically targeted therapy.

The disease usually presents with flulike symptoms of lethargy, weakness, fever, and bone and joint pain. There may be enlarged lymph nodes (lymphadenopathy), an enlarged liver (hepatomegaly), an enlarged spleen (splenomegaly), a tendency toward bleeding (easy bruising and bleeding from skin and mucosa), and recurrent infections. There may be a marked elevation in the WBC (white blood cell) count or a depletion and low WBC count.

## Diagnosis and Treatment

After the disease is suspected, laboratory tests strongly suggesting leukemia are CBC (complete blood count), coagulation studies, and a CAT scan of the chest and abdomen. The definitive diagnosis is made by a bone-marrow biopsy, a procedure usually done under local anesthesia with a large bore needle. The cells extracted are sent for several esoteric laboratory examinations, including cytochemistry, immunophenotyping, using monoclonal antibodies and cytogenic analyses, examining the chromosomes, oncogenes, and tumor-suppressor gene abnormalities. This helps to differentiate between the myeloid and lymphocytic forms of acute leukemia. The lymphoblastic leukemias originate from early form cells called B-cells or T-cells.

### Chemotherapy

The treatment with chemotherapy is very complex and there are many different regimens. A starting therapy is given to clear the bone marrow of the leukemia and is followed by a consolidation treatment phase, reducing the number of leukemia cells. This, in turn, is followed by maintenance chemotherapy. The very complex treatments are usually very intense and have many dangerous side effects, including anemia, infections, liver and kidney failure, coagulation abnormalities, nausea and vomiting, weight loss, and depressed appetite, in addition to psychological depression.

Among the chemotherapeutic drugs used in various combinations are:

- Adriamycin (doxorubicin)
- Imatinib (Gleevac)
- Ara-C (cytarabine)
- L-asp (L-asparaginase)
- CTX (cyclophosphamide)
- MTX (methotrexate)
- Dasatinib (Sprycel)
- Nelarabine (Arranon)
- Dex (dexamethasone)
- PSE (prednisone)
- DNR (daunorubicin)
- 6-MP (mercaptopurine)
- Dox (doxorubicin)
- 6-TG (thioguanine)
- Gemcitabine (Gemzar)
- VCR (vincristine)

And newer agents:

- Cladribine
- Temozolimide (Temodar)
- Gemtuzumab
- Tipifarnib

In some cases, an attempt is made to destroy all the leukemia cells and then repopulate the damaged bone marrow with normal cells in a procedure called a bone-marrow transplant. This procedure is carried out at major medical centers, with varying success rates.

## ■ Complementary and Alternative Treatment

There is ample opportunity to apply complementary medicine principles to the management of the disease and the side effects of the therapy, but there are no generally accepted alternative treatments that will directly affect the progression of acute leukemia. Acupuncture, aromatherapy, massage therapy, meditation, and relaxation exercises will help in dealing with the side effects of standard therapy and the side effects of the leukemia itself.

Previous exposure to chemotherapy or radiation, smoking, poor nutrition, and obesity increase the risk for hematologic cancers in adults. Because of high nitrosamines, smoked fish and meats have been suggested as being an increased risk for leukemia in children.[24]

Diets with vegetables and prudent exercise appear to have preventive effects. Among the nutrients being examined for positive antitumor effects in treating these malignancies are the amino acid L-carnitine, flavonoids (quercetin from fruit, resveratrol from red grapes, and curcumin), genistein, green tea, and mistletoe. These recommendations apply for all hematologic malignancies.[25,26,27]

## CHRONIC MYELOID LEUKEMIA

Chronic myeloid leukemia (CML) is a disorder of the primitive blood-producing stem cells (the basic cells of the blood system). It is called a clonal myeloproliferative disorder because the tumor cells originate from a single-parent precursor cell. These are the early cell forms that have the capacity to either become lymphoid or myeloid and have progressed toward the myeloid group. The etiology of this disease is unclear, although some genetic or environmental factors have been reported. Some nuclear and radiation exposures are associated, but no chemical exposures are blamed.

The disease usually occurs between the ages of thirty to fifty and is characterized by decreased appetite, fatigue, low-grade fever, night sweats, and weight loss. With an enlargement of the spleen and liver, a patient will have abdominal discomfort, and bone-marrow involvement with cancerous leukemia cells and bone pain; there will be leukostasis (overpopulation of white blood cells in the blood causing sluggish flow), there may be blurring vision, breathing distress, retinal hemorrhaging (bleeding in the back of the eyeball), stupor, and tinnitus (ringing in ears). With severe disease (accelerated phase and blast crisis), there may be bone-marrow failure, leading to bleeding and infection.

There are essentially three phases of this disease: chronic, accelerated, and blastic.

◇ In the chronic stage, patients may be asymptomatic for a while, with the disease only diagnosed when a routine blood smear is taken for some other reason. However, when a more advanced disease develops, patients present with abdominal pain from hepatosplenomegaly, fatigue, the symptoms of leukostasis mentioned above, and weight loss.

◇ The accelerated phase is transitional and is characterized by blood-cell changes diagnosed by a pathologist. This phase demands urgent chemotherapeutic attention, usually with imatinib therapy.

◇ The blastic phase resembles acute leukemia and, as the name implies, has upward of 30 percent blast (early form) cells in the blood examination. Leukemic cells may aggregate in the brain, the central nervous system, the lymph nodes, or the bones, and patients have severe bleeding problems, enlarged nodes, and tender skin lesions. The prognosis in this phase is poor.

## ■ Diagnosis and Treatment

CML is characterized by the presence of the *Philadelphia chromosome,* a complex genetic abnormality called, in correct scientific terms, "a balanced translocation between long arms of chromosomes 9 and 22." This 1960 discovery was the first time a cytogenetic marker was found consistently associated with a cancer.

This cancer is now treated primarily with an orally administered drug called imatinib with a greater than 90 percent overall survival at six years. Other drugs include bosutinib, dasatinib, and nilotinib. The objective is to eliminate the Philadelphia chromosomal changes and prevent or delay progression to the accelerated and blastic phases. When these modalities fail, another treatment is a stem-cell transplant (SCT), a procedure where high-dose chemotherapy destroys the person's cancer cells and bone marrow, and healthy bone-marrow cells are reintroduced to repopulate the hemopoietic system.

A major complication of SCT is graft-versus-host disease (GVHD), a phenomenon that occurs after transplantation of stem cells or bone marrow from another person. Immune cells from the donated stem cells or marrow recognize the recipient as *foreign* and attack the recipient's body cells. This can occur within the first 100 days of a transplant (acute or fulminant form), or after 100 days (chronic form), both of which have high associated morbidity and mortality. This disease is characterized by intestinal, liver, and skin symptoms, which are graded I–IV and require treatment with steroids and other agents to reverse the effect. The worse the GVHD, the graver the consequences. GVHD is prevented and/or treated by the administration of steroids and the use of such agents as cyclosporine, methotrexate, sirolimus (Rapamune), and tacrolimus (Prograf). For those who don't respond to those regimens, a whole host of new agents is available including daclizumab (Zenapax), etanercept (Enbrel), and pentostatin (Nipent).

## ■ Complementary and Alternative Treatment

The complementary medicine recommendations are the same as those with acute leukemia, namely alleviating the side effects of the treatment. There is ample opportunity to apply complementary medicine principles to the management of the disease and the side effects of the therapy. Acupuncture, aromatherapy, massage therapy, meditation, and relaxation exercises will help in dealing with the side effects of standard therapy and the side effects of the leukemia itself.

Previous exposure to chemotherapy or radiation, smoking, poor nutrition, and obesity increase the risk for hematologic cancers in adults. Because of high nitrosamines, smoked fish and meats have been suggested as being an increased risk for leukemia in children.[24]

Diets with vegetables and prudent exercise appear to have preventive effects. Among the nutrients being examined for positive anti-tumor effects in treating these malignancies are the amino acid L-carnitine, flavonoids (quercetin from fruit, resveratrol from red grapes, and curcumin), genistein, green tea, and mistletoe. These recommendations apply for all hematologic malignancies.[25,26,27]

## CHRONIC LYMPHOCYTIC LEUKEMIA

Chronic lymphocytic leukemia (CLL) is the lymphocyte counterpart to CML, with the clonal dominant cell being a lymphocyte precursor cell (usually what is called a B-cell lineage lymphocyte), and occurs twice as much in men as women, and more often in the sixty to seventy age group. This is the most common of the leukemias, where a large number of white blood cells are produced in the bone marrow, lymphatic, and other blood-producing organs. This disease can have a long, relatively indolent course and only occasionally progress to a more active stage. Most patients remain asymptomatic, except for some fatigue and lethargy, occasional lymph-node enlargement, and more frequent infections, including pneumonia. Other skin problems, such as herpes zoster, and more significant skin reactions to insect bites and bee stings are common.

The etiology is unclear, although there is a high familial risk for CLL and there may be an association with some T-cell lymphocytic and Epstein-Barr viruses.

## Staging

The staging is as follows:

- Stage 0—Lymphocytosis (increased white blood cell count)

- Stage 1—Lymphocytosis and lymphadenopathy (enlarged lymph nodes)

- Stage 2—Lymphocytosis and splenomegaly (enlarged spleen)

- Stage 3—Lymphocytosis and anemia (Hgb < 11.0)

- Stage 4—Lymphocytosis and thrombocytopenia (low platelet count)

Treatment for chronic myeloid leukemia has in the past been chlorambucil (Leukeran) with prednisone. More recently treatment with fludarabine has found excellent success, along with cladribine and pentostatin (Nipent). Monoclonal antibody therapy with alemtuzumab, and rituximab. In more severe cases and recurrences, stem-cell transplantation may be indicated, as well as a surgical splenectomy when there is hypersplenism and splenomegaly.

### ■ Complementary and Alternative Treatment

There are no specific alternative therapies except those that are supportive, utilizing many of the CAM therapies outlined in other chapters.

There is ample opportunity to apply complementary medicine principles to the management of the disease and the side effects of the therapy, but there are no generally accepted alternative treatments that will directly affect the progression of acute leukemia. Acupuncture, aromatherapy, massage therapy, meditation, and relaxation exercises will help in dealing with the side effects of standard therapy and the side effects of the leukemia itself.

Previous exposure to chemotherapy or radiation, smoking, poor nutrition, and obesity increase the risk for hematologic cancers in adults. Because of high nitrosamines, smoked fish and meats have been suggested as being an increased risk for leukemia in children.[24]

Diets with vegetables and prudent exercise appear to have preventive effects. Among the nutrients being examined for positive antitumor effects in treating these malignancies are the amino acid L-carnitine, flavonoids (quercetin from fruit, resveratrol from red grapes, and curcumin), genistein, green tea, and mistletoe. These recommendations apply for all hematologic malignancies.[25,26,27]

## HODGKIN'S LYMPHOMA

Hodgkin's Lymphoma, or Hodgkin's disease, first described by Thomas Hodgkin in 1832, is the most common lymphoma, usually occurring in two age groups, fifteen to thirty-five, and fifty-five to seventy years old. The disease may have an increased risk for patients with Epstein-Barr virus, mononucleosis, or of Jewish heritage, and the incidence is higher among chemists, individuals with suppressed immunity (AIDS), first-degree relatives of people with Hodgkin's, and woodworkers. The disease is basically divided into four types: lymphocyte depletion, lymphocyte predominant, mixed, and nodular sclerosing varieties.

The disease presents as a painless swelling of nodes in the neck, armpit, or groin and is associated with anemia, coughing, fatigue, fever, itching, night sweats, repeated infections, and weight loss. Rarely, there may be paralysis due to compression on the spinal cord. The disease may metastasize to bones, liver, skin, spleen, and stomach.

### ▣ *Diagnosis and Treatment*

In making the diagnosis, one of the chief cellular characteristics for the pathologist is the presence of Reed-Sternberg cells, malignant giant cells with multiple nuclei. Even I, as a surgeon, was able to identify these under the microscope during one of my many forays into the pathology department.

### Staging

* Stage I—One group of lymph nodes or one organ in the body

* Stage II—More than one group of lymph nodes either above or below the diaphragm, or one organ with nodes involved

* Stage III—Different lymph nodes above and below the diaphragm

• Stage IV—Spread to other organs—bones, bone marrow, liver, or lungs

The workup will consist of routine blood work, biopsies of bone marrow and lymph nodes, and several radiological studies, including a chest x-ray, PET (positron emission tomography), and CAT scan (computerized axial tomography). These will help in defining the extent of the disease. In the past, laparotomy for examination of the abdominal nodes, liver, and spleen was standard procedure, but with present technology this is rarely indicated.

**Chemotherapy and Radiation**

In the last thirty years, treatment has significantly evolved, with survival rates in the high 90 percent ranges, using combined chemotherapy (bleomycin, epirubicin, prednisone, and vinblastine) and radiation therapy for Stage I and II disease. Stage III and IV disease is still curable, using one of several chemotherapeutic regimens.

◇ ABVD. Adriamycin, bleomycin, vinblastine, dacarbazine

◇ MOPP. Mechlorethamine, oncovin, procarbazine, prednisone

◇ BEACOPP. Adriamycin, bleomycin, cyclophosphamide, etoposide, G-CSF, oncovin, prednisone, and procarbazine

◇ Stanford V. Doxorubicin, etoposide, mechlorethamine, prednisone, vinblastine, and vincristine

◇ Newer therapies include cytokines, gemcitabine, idarubicin, immunotoxins, the monoclonal antibody rituximab, vaccination, and vinorelbine

The toxicities of the chemotherapy include:

◇ Infertility

◇ Lung and heart problems

◇ Other malignancies

Patients who do not respond to treatment, or who have relapses, are sometimes recommended for stem-cell transplantation.

■ *Complementary and Alternative Treatment*

For the most part, these are aimed at alleviating the side effects of the therapy. Since Hodgkin's lymphoma is almost totally curable using Western medicine, most Chinese and Ayurvedic therapies are reserved for the non-Hodgkin's lymphoma that has a Western-medicine cure rate of 26–73 percent, depending on the risk factors.

There is ample opportunity to apply complementary medicine principles to the management of the disease and the side effects of the therapy. Acupuncture, aromatherapy, massage therapy, meditation, and relaxation exercises will help in dealing with the side effects of standard therapy and its side effects.

Previous exposure to chemotherapy or radiation, smoking, poor nutrition, and obesity increase the risk for hematologic cancers in adults.[24]

Diets with vegetables and prudent exercise appear to have preventive effects. Among the nutrients being examined for positive anti-tumor effects in treating these malignancies are the amino acid L-carnitine, flavonoids (curcumin, quercetin from fruit, resveratrol from red grapes), genistein, green tea, and mistletoe. These recommendations apply for all hematologic malignancies.[25,26,27]

## NON-HODGKIN'S LYMPHOMA

Non-Hodgkin's lymphoma (NHL), or just plain lymphoma, is actually a group of lymph-system cancers, more common in men than women, and categorized as low grade, intermediate grade, or high grade. The etiology stems from chromosomal translocations (a type of genetic rearrangement), environmental factors (pesticides, chemists, flour workers, meat workers, painters, and petroleum, plastic, rubber, and synthetics workers), exposure to chemicals (hair dyes, organic solvents, pesticides), radiation, and patients who receive chemotherapy and radiation therapy. ATLL, HCV, Hepatitis C, HIV, HTLV, and KSHV viruses are implicated. There is an increased incidence in patients with immunodeficiency syndromes, such as Crohn's disease or sprue (celiac disease, a condition that damages the lining of the small intestine and prevents it from absorbing parts of food important to staying healthy).

Low-grade disease is painless and slow progressing, with intermittently enlarged nodes and occasional splenomegaly, but rarely with what are called the B symptoms of fever and night sweats. Intermediate disease has more adenopathy and disease outside the lymph nodes. These may be in the GI (gastrointestinal) tract, the GU (genitourinary) tract, bone marrow, central nervous system, sinuses, skin, and thyroid. The diagnostic workup is much the same as for Hodgkin's disease.

## ■ *Diagnosis and Treatment*

The problem with discussing this collection of diseases is their large number and the complexity of their diagnosis and treatment. There are physicians who specialize only in the treatment and diagnosis of these diseases, which the WHO (World Health Organization) classifies as either B-cell neoplasms, or NK-cell and T-cell neoplasms. I will list them just to give you an idea of the variety and specificity of diagnosis and treatment they demand.

B-cells fight infection by producing antibodies that destroy foreign invading cells, whereas T-cells kill the foreign invading cells directly.

### B-cell Neoplasms

◈ B-cell chronic lymphocytic lymphoma

◈ B-cell prolymphocytic leukemia

◈ Hairy cell leukemia

◈ Lymphoplasmocytic lymphoma

◈ Mature—B-cell neoplasms

◈ Plasma cell myeloma

◈ Precursor—B lymphoblastic leukemia/lymphoma

◈ Splenic marginal zone B-cell lymphoma

### MALT Lymphoma

◈ Burkitt's lymphoma (fast growing form of this lymphoma)

◈ Diffuse large B-cell lymphoma

◈ Mantle cell lymphoma

◈ Nodal marginal-zone B-cell lymphoma

## T-cell and NK-cell Lymphomas

◇ Adult T-cell lymphoma

◇ Aggressive NK cell leukemia

◇ Anaplastic large cell lymphoma

◇ Angioimmunoblastic T-cell lymphoma

◇ Enteropathy-type T-cell lymphoma

◇ Extranodal NK/T-cell lymphoma

◇ Hepatosplenic gamma/delta T-cell lymphoma

◇ Mature T-cell neoplasms

◇ Mycosis fungoides (skin lymphomas)

◇ Peripheral T-cell lymphoma

◇ Precursor T-cell neoplasm

◇ Precursor T-lymphoblastic lymphoma

◇ Subcutaneous panniculitis–like T-cell lymphoma

◇ T-cell granular lymphocytic leukemia

◇ T-cell prolymphocytic leukemia

　. . . and many more

If this is not enough to make a grown surgeon cry, I can only add that each of these cancers has a specific staging and treatment, with varying prognostic factors, immunobiological factors, and molecular profiling. There are specific cell markers for many of these, and dozens of chemotherapeutic agents and combinations, plus, depending on the antigen involved, there are more than fifteen monoclonal antibodies used to treat the diseases.

The use of interferon and radiation, as well as radioimmunotherapy, stem-cell transplantation, and vaccines needs to be discussed with a highly specialized oncologist after extensive testing and group discussions.

### ■ Complementary and Alternative Treatment

Complementary medicine is of value, along with standard oncology, in managing the lymphomas. Chinese herbal therapy is almost as complex as the above list, with literally hundreds of regimens depending on the type and symptomatology of the disease. Practitioners of traditional Chinese medicine (TCM) do stress the importance of combining the two modalities, as long as each practitioner is in contact with the other. The general consensus among TCM practitioners is that Western medicine is too *heroic,* often damaging the patient's immune system, whereas Chinese medicine alone is too slow. The best of both worlds, therefore, is an integrated therapy designed to combine Western and Chinese treatments when chemotherapy and radiation therapy are used for treatment of lymphoma. Such words as qi vacuity, yin vacuity, and heat toxins are discussed and given as treatment to maintain a healthy body homeostasis while treating the disease itself.

The Ayurvedic approach to lymphoma is aimed at improving the immune status of the body, as well as treating the tumor. Kanchnaar and manjishtha are among the principal herbal medicines used, and they reduce the side effects of conventional treatment, improve the immune status of the body, improve the quality of life, and prolong survival. The patient must be under the care of a qualified oncology team that combines standard and Ayurvedic complementary care.

Other alternative therapies include acupuncture, holistic dietary recommendations, music therapy, and relaxation therapy. Vegetables high in flavonoids, such as broccoli, kale, and spinach, are recommended.

## MULTIPLE MYELOMA AND PLASMA CELL DISEASES

Multiple myeloma is a cancer of plasma cells in the bone marrow, the white blood cells responsible for producing antibodies, and it usually occurs above fifty years of age. The disease may be unrecognized and indolent for many years before causing anemia, bone pain, recurrent infections, such as pneumonia and pyelonephritis (kidney infection); decreased platelets (thrombocytopenia) the cells that help blood to clot; decreased white blood-cell count (leucopenia); and enlargement of the spleen and liver (splenomegaly and hepatomegaly). There may be blood in the stools (epistaxis, hematochezia, and hemoptysis) coughing up blood, and nosebleeds. Production of a substance called paraprotein (Bence-Jones protein, an abnormal protein in blood or urine) can cause kidney problems. Elevated calcium levels may cause altered states of consciousness, blurred vision, and headaches. In some instances, myeloma may present as a solitary tumor called a plasmacytoma in bone or soft tissue.

### ■ Diagnosis and Treatment

More common in men, the diagnosis can be made with blood tests (protein electrophoresis and peripheral blood smear, elevated sed rate), bone-marrow biopsy, and x-rays of the bones and skull. A study called *serum free light chain assay* is helpful for screening, diagnosis, and prognosis of plasma-cell disorders. Myelomas can produce all classes of immunoglobulins including IgG, IgA, and IgM that can be detected and measured.

### Durie-Salmon Staging System

- Stage I—Hgb > 10
- Normal Calcium
- X-rays normal or single plasmacytoma
- Serum para-protein level IgG < 5, IgA < 3
- Urinary light chain excretion < 4/24 hrs
- Stage II (becomes Stage II by exclusion of the other two)
- Stage III—Hgb < 8.5
- Calcium > 12
- Skeleton. 3 or more bone lesions
- Paraprotein > 7 IgG, >5 IgA
- Urinary light chain excretion > 12/24hrs

Although it is generally felt to be incurable, long periods of remission and stable disease are achieved with chemotherapy, melphalan, steroids, thalidomide, and stem-cell transplants. Newer drugs, such as bortezomid and lenolidomide, are often used, though there is an increased incidence of pulmonary embolism and venous thrombosis with these drugs.

Another plasma cell disorder is Waldenström's macroglobulinemia, a cancer of B-lymphocytes that has an overproduction of IgG protein. It is asymptomatic for years and eventually shows as fatigue and weakness due to anemia, also blurred vision, enlarged liver and spleen, enlarged lymph nodes, peripheral neuropathy (changes in nerves to the ears, fingers, nose, and toes), and weight loss. Diagnosis is made by laboratory tests, including electrophoresis and flow cytometry. Other symptoms include cryoglobulinemia (made worse by exposure to cold), dizziness, headaches, hyperviscosity syndrome (thickening of blood) with bleeding, kidney problems, Raynaud's phenomenon, and visual problems.

Treatment is by plasmaphoresis (a procedure where blood is pushed through a machine that removes unwanted substances), steroids, alkeran, cytoxan, and rituximab. Chemotherapy includes chlorambucil, cladribine, and fludarabine. Also Monoclonal antibody treatment with alemtuzumab (Campath) and rituximab (Rituxan), and bortexomib (Velcade), another inhibitor. An emerging treatment is stem-cell transplantation.

## MYELODYSPLASTIC SYNDROMES

Myelodysplastic syndromes are a group of diseases caused by blood cells that are dysfunctional due to bone-marrow abnormalities. They occur in people older than sixty, more frequently in men than women, and may be related to such chemicals as industrial chemicals, or exposure to lead, mercury, pesticides, tobacco smoke, or previous chemotherapy or radiation treatments. There is no cure, and treatment consists of basically preventing complications of the disease and watching for a progression to cancer. Symptoms are anemia, bleeding, and recurring infections.

### ■ *Complementary and Alternative Treatments*

There is ample opportunity to apply complementary medicine principles to the management of the disease and the side effects of the therapy, but there are no generally accepted alternative treatments that will directly affect the progression of this disease. Acupuncture, aromatherapy, massage therapy, meditation, and relaxation exercises will help in dealing with the side effects of standard therapy.

Previous exposure to chemotherapy or radiation, smoking, poor nutrition and obesity increase the risk for hematologic cancers in adults.

Diets with vegetables and prudent exercise appear to have preventive effects. Among the nutrients being examined for positive anti-tumor effects in treating these malignancies are the amino acid L-carnitine, flavonoids (curcumin, quercetin from fruit, and resveratrol from red grapes), genistein, green tea, and mistletoe. These recommendations apply for all hematologic malignancies.[25,26,27]

## KIDNEY, BLADDER, AND URETER CANCERS

### KIDNEY CANCER

The kidneys, two large bean-shaped organs lying on the left and right side of the back of the abdomen, filter blood and get rid of body wastes, excess water, and salt. Cancer of the kidney occurs in 3 percent of the population in the United States and is more frequent in men. There are three types. One, Wilm's tumor, is found predominately in children, and there are two in adults, renal cell carcinoma (hyper-nephroma, Grawitz tumor) that accounts for 90 percent of this cancer, and sarcomas, which are relatively rare.

Although no definitive etiology is known, a higher incidence of this cancer, also called renal cancer, is noted with a high animal-fat diet, obesity, renal dialysis, and tobacco smoking. Certain genetic abnormalities in chromosome 3 apparently predispose to the disease and also cause von Hippel–Lindau disease. Other risk factors include exposure to certain phenacetin-containing painkillers and occupational exposure to asbestos, cadmium, organic solvents, and petroleum products.

The classic triad of symptoms for cancer of the kidney is hematuria (bloody urine), pain, and the presence of a mass. Sadly, early-stage cancers are asymptomatic and by the time symptoms occur, the tumor has grown significantly. Anemia, fever, hypercalcemia, loss of appetite, polycythemia (too many red blood cells), and weight loss, may also be late signs of the cancer.

## ▪ *Diagnosis and Treatment*

Diagnosis is confirmed by several studies, including IVP (intravenous pyelogram), ultrasound, MRI, CAT scan, and in some cases selective renal-artery angiography. Other x-rays are needed to evaluate for distant metastases. Final diagnosis is established either by needle biopsy or by removing part or all of the involved kidney.

### Staging

The TNM system is used. T=Tumor, N=Node, M=Metastasis.

- T1—Tumor confined to kidney < 7 cm–N0–No nodes involved
- T2—Tumor confined to kidney > 7 cm–N1–Single node involved
- T3—Tumor into major veins, or adrenal gland–N2–More than one node
- T4—Tumor invades beyond investing fascia (Gerota's)–M0–No metastasis
- M1—Distant metastasis
- Stage I—T1 N0 M0
- Stage II—T2 N0 M0
- Stage III—T1 N1 M0
- T2—N1 M0
- T3 N0—1 M0
- Stage IV—T4 N0–1 M0
- Any T—N2 M0
- Any T—Any N M1

An evaluation must be undertaken to determine whether the patient will tolerate radical surgery. In some instances, because of other medical conditions, prudence dictates that lesser procedures or only palliative procedures are indicated.

When the kidney cancer is confined to the kidney capsule or enclosing tissue of the kidney in Stage I and II, the treatment is a radical nephrectomy, removal of the kidney along with the adrenal gland that is closely adherent to the upper pole of the kidney, the enclosing tissue (Gerota's fascia), the surrounding fat lymph nodes, and the ureter. Sometimes, with small tumors, a partial nephrectomy can be performed. In Stage III, a radical nephrectomy may be possible, and even in Stage IV, where a definitive cure is very doubtful, debulking the tumor mass may alleviate symptoms.

Other treatments, such as cryotherapy (freezing the tumor) or radiofrequency ablation (burning the tumor away) are used as palliative measures in situations where the tumor is too large and incurable by standard nephrectomy. These are not first-line treatments and are mostly utilized in extreme cases. When a tumor is large, another procedure, arterial embolization, involves placing a tube through a groin artery and guiding it into the kidney artery, then injecting material into this artery to shut off the blood supply to the kidney making the nephrectomy less bloody.

Metastasectomy, removal of metastases, is becoming more popular for both palliation and, in rare cases, cure. With the advent of more successful adjunctive therapies, this modality may be used more frequently.

Chemotherapy is not very effective for renal-cell cancer, although a few drugs, fluorouracil (5-FU), floxuridine (FUDR), and vinblastine (Velban) have had minimal success.

Radiation therapy for renal cancer is predominately palliative . Metastatic cancer has also been treated with immunotherapy, such as Interleukin-2, with response and palliation averaging four to five years. Angiogenesis inhibitors, such as bevacizumab (Avastin) and certain biological therapies (treatments that use natural substances from the body), may be helpful in late-stage disease. Among these are everolimus (Rad001), sorafenib (Nexavar), sunitinib (Sutent), temsirolimus (Torisel), which are being studied in clinical trials.

## ■ Complementary and Alternative Treatment

Alternative medicine has been directed toward improvement of the immune system and several herbal remedies are recommended. Among these is astragalus, used by Chinese herbalists for centuries and supported by the Sloan-Kettering Cancer Center for having renal-protective powers. Cat's claw, a common medicinal herb from Peru, has been used as a kidney purifier and immune booster and is supported by the American Cancer Society. Studies conducted in Germany show that Siberian ginseng has been helpful with the side effects of radiation and chemotherapy and helps increase interferon (an immune-boosting chemical) synthesis in the body. Melatonin is recommended to offset some of the side effects of interleukin therapy.

As with other cancers, the Mayo Clinic advocates a number of complementary treatments to offset the depression, stress, and side effects of standard anticancer therapy. Among these are acupressure, acupuncture, art and dance movement therapy, meditation, music therapy, and relaxation exercises.

◆ Dietary considerations are oriented toward avoiding high blood pressure and diabetes mellitus, both of which damage the kidney cells. Obesity is a leading cause of both these diseases and a sensible, balanced diet is obviously important. Exposure to environmental toxins (pesticides, solvents, soot, vinyl chloride, to name a few) should be avoided. Vitamins A, D, E, ginseng, green tea, L-carnitine, and melatonin have been put forward for inhibition of kidney cancer-cell growth.[28,29]

◆ Use of melatonin should be limited; prolonged use can negate the body's own production of this hormone.

## BLADDER, URETER, AND KIDNEY PELVIS CANCERS

Cancer in these three anatomical areas are lumped together and called urothelial cancers. The urothelial tract extends from the collecting pelvis of the kidney down the ureters (the tubes connecting the kidney to the bladder) to the urinary bladder. The lining of these structures are composed of transitional cells (cells lining the urinary tract) and 90–95 percent of the cancers are transitional-cell cancers, with the remaining being squamous-cell cancers.

The risk factors for developing urothelial cancer are urinary tract infections, smoking, industrial toxins (aromatic amines used in the dye industry), chemicals used in printing, leather, textile, and paint products. There is an increased risk in individuals who abuse analgesic compounds, such as phenacetin. The disease is more common among Caucasians than African Americans, more common in men, and it usually occurs in the sixty-five to seventy-five age group. This cancer can spread or seed cells throughout the urinary tract and therefore the cancers may be multifocal.

The symptoms are hematuria (bloody urine), painful urination, and increased frequency of urination, all symptoms that more commonly occur with noncancerous conditions, such as infections, prostate disease, stones, and trauma. With advanced disease there may be a swelling of the legs from lymphatic obstruction.

### ■ *Diagnosis and Treatment*

Diagnosis may be suggested by urinalysis, blood count, chemistry to evaluate kidney function, and occasionally microscopic examination of the urine for cancer cells. Imaging studies include IVP (intravenous pyelogram), CAT scan, and MRI. Chest x-rays and a bone scan are used to find metastatic disease.

### Staging

The TNM system is used. T=Tumor, N=Nodes, M=Metastasis.

- Ta—Noninvasive papillary tumor–N0–No nodes involved
- Tis—Carcinoma in situ. N1–single node < 2 cm
- T1—Cancer invades below the mucosa. N2–node > 2 < 5 cm (subepithelial layer)–N3 nodes > 5 cm
- T2—Tumor invades muscle. M0–No metastasis
- T3—Tumor invades outside the bladder or ureter. M1–distant metastasis
- T4—Tumor invades prostate, vagina, uterus, abdominal wall
- Stage I—T1 N0 M0
- Stage II—T2 N0 M0
- Stage III—T3 N0 M0
- Stage IV–Any T N1–N3 M0
- Any T Any N M1

## BLADDER CANCER

Treatment of bladder cancer depends on the staging. For superficial cancers where there are no muscle invasions, treatments include excising (resection), burning out (fulguration), or intrabladder (intravesical) placement of drugs. Intravesical immunotherapy is done with BCG (Bacille-Calumet-Guerin), and chemotherapy with mitomycin (Mutomycin), doxorubicin (Adriamycin), epirubicin (Ellence), and thiotepa is recommended. Localized, superficial cancer can be treated by transurethral resection (TUR), using a special operating scope through the urethra into the bladder, laser treatment (Nd: YAG-neodymium: yttrium-aluminum-garnet laser), partial cystectomy (when TUR can't be done), and radical cystectomy (removal of the bladder), though this latter technique is usually not needed for superficial cancers.

Radical cystectomy is usually reserved for cancer not amenable to TUR, multiple cancers, high-grade cancers, tumors not responsive to the above-mentioned lesser procedures. For invasive cancers (stage II and higher), the radical cystectomy is recommended. This includes removal of lymph nodes, prostate, and seminal vesicles in men, and removal of bladder, ovaries, tubes, urethra, uterus, and partial vaginal wall in women.

After surgery, urinary reconstruction may be done by using segments of the intestine for a new bladder, or by diverting the urine outside the body in a cutaneous diversion opening onto the skin (like a small colostomy) called a Koch or Indiana pouch.

## URETER AND KIDNEY PELVIS TUMORS

For ureter and kidney pelvis tumors, partial or complete removal is indicated. If the tumor is in the distal ureter, it can sometimes be removed and the proximal ureter can be reimplanted into the bladder. For proximal ureter and/or renal pelvis tumor, the kidney and ureter on that side must be removed (nephroureterectomy).

Complex combinations of radiation and chemotherapy are recommended for different stages and locations of urothelial cancer. The combinations include:

◇ PCG—Paclitaxel, Carboplatin, Gemcitabine

◇ Paclitaxel/cisplatin

◇ M-VAC-Methotrexate, Vinblastine Doxorubicin, Cisplatin

◇ Gemcitabine/Cisplatin

◇ Paclitaxel/Carboplatin

◇ TCG–Taxol, cisplatin, gemcitabine

◇ New agents. Docetaxel (Taxotere), ifosfamide (Ifex), pemetrexed (Almita), and vinflunine.

When indicated, radiation therapy is also offered, alone or in conjunction with the chemotherapy, for both cure and palliation.

## ▪ Complementary and Alternative Treatment

Many of the standard treatments for these and other cancers cause nausea, vomiting, and decreased appetite with weight loss. These can be significantly ameliorated using alternative approaches, including acupuncture, herbal products, massage therapy, meditation, spiritual healing, visualization, vitamins, and special diets. Fruits and vegetables are a good way to get vitamins, and according to the Mayo Clinic, some research indicates that larger doses of vitamin E may reduce the risk of bladder cancer. Many studies are underway to ascertain the effectiveness of green tea for bladder-cancer therapy.

When used in combination with standard Western medical care, the herb astragalus activates the p53 gene that stops defective cells from multiplying. Cat's claw is another herb with a long history of use as an immune stimulant, raising white blood cell counts that have fallen because of chemotherapy. Garlic is another immune stimulant and can complement immunotherapy. Maitake mushrooms are beneficial after bladder-cancer surgery to help decrease the risk of recurrence. Siberian ginseng and Essiac tea also stimulate the immune system. All these therapies should be discussed with your nutritionally aware physician, and consultation can be obtained from herbalists with appropriate advanced degrees in herbal, Ayurvedic, Chinese, or naturopathic studies.

## LIVER CANCER

As I described in my book, *Understanding Surgery,* the liver "is a brownish-red, partially rounded, huge blob sitting in the right upper aspect of the abdomen. It has a right and left lobe, a large blood supply and a bile drainage system."

"The liver helps metabolize, break down and use proteins, carbohydrates, and fats, and produces bile, which flows down the bile ducts and helps digest food and absorb vitamins A, D, E, and K. It produces many substances needed for blood clotting, detoxifies many substances, and has Kupffer's cells which devour waste products."

There are two basic kinds of liver cancer, primary liver cancer that arises in the liver, and metastatic liver cancer that arises in another organ and metastasizes to the liver.

There are several primary liver cancers, but more than 90 percent are hepatocellular carcinomas (sometimes given the misnomer hepatoma, incorrectly implying a benign disease). This tumor arises from the parenchymal cells (basic liver cells); other, much rarer, cancers are the cholangiocarcinoma that arises from the bile ducts, the angiosarcomas and hemangioendotheliomas from vascular (blood-vessel) tissue, and the hepatoblastoma from primary embryonic germ layers (early cells in liver development). The focus will be on the hepatocellular carcinoma.

Liver cancer is often called the most common cancer in the world. There is a very high incidence of it in Asia, but it represents less than 2 percent of the cancers in the United States. Worldwide, the ratio of men to women who have this cancer is 5:1, and in the United States it's 2:1. The disease increases with age; in the United States, the mean age is sixty-five years and is more common among Asian immigrants and blacks than whites. The etiology of these differences is based on the prevalence of the contributing factors to the disease.

The risk factors for this cancer are aflatoxin $B_1$ (a toxic chemical product from the aspergillis flavus mold that causes mutations in the p53 gene), alcoholism or excessive alcohol intake, hepatitis B, hepatitis C, and an l-carnitine deficiency. Also implicated are anabolic steroids used by bodybuilders, estrogens, thorotrast (a contrast substance once used by radiologists), vinyl chloride (used in the plastics industry), and the presence of cirrhosis, diabetes mellitus, obesity, and certain rare congenital diseases.

The signs and symptoms of hepatocellular liver cancer are abdominal mass, abdominal pain, anemia, ascites (fluid collection in the abdomen), back pain, jaundice, itching (from the jaundice), nausea and vomiting, and weight loss. On rare occasions a patient will present with excruciating abdominal pain caused by rupture and bleeding from a liver cancer. In areas where the incidence is very high, or in high-risk patients, screening tests will find early tumors that provide a better opportunity for curative therapy before any signs or symptoms present themselves.

So the general approach to preventing this cancer includes preventing hepatitis B and C (childhood vaccination against hepatitis B is being done now), avoiding obesity and the aforementioned high-risk substances, and attempting to treat alcoholism.

## ■ Diagnosis and Treatment

Blood tests are not used to diagnose liver cancer as there is no reliable screening test for the disease. Individuals with hepatic cancer may have elevated alpha-fetoprotein (a protein normally made by immature liver cells) or an enzyme called DCP (des-gamma carboxyprothrombin), but these are only suggestive and nondiagnostic. When several signs and symptoms of the disease are present, the physician will order an ultrasound of the liver to see whether there is an abnormality; this noninvasive and relatively inexpensive study can identify tumors as small as 1 cm.

If a mass suggesting cancer is found, further studies will be indicated, including CT scan (computerized tomography), MRI (magnetic resonance imaging), and PET scan (positron emission tomography). The final pathologic diagnosis rests on actually taking a biopsy of the mass. This can be done by fine needle or core needle biopsy of the liver tumor. However, in many cases, the diagnosis is so strongly suggested by the appearance of the radiological findings that the surgeon or oncologist does not want to risk spreading cancer with the biopsy, or run the risk of bleeding (coming from the cancer). Diagnostic laparoscopy may be indicated to evaluate the extent of the cancer, to rule out occult metastases, and to determine what type of surgery or therapy is best indicated. Since surgical and even medical therapy may be determined by the overall health of the patient, a complete medical workup is necessary. Since many of these patients have fairly severe underlying liver disease (cirrhosis or hepatitis), they may not tolerate any type of surgery unless a total liver transplant is being considered.

**Staging**

T=Tumor, N=Nodes, and M=Metastasis.

- T0—No evidence of primary tumor. N0–No nodal spread

- T1—Solitary tumor without vascular invasion. N1–Regional node spread

- T2—Solitary tumor with vascular invasion or multiple tumors < 5 cm M0–No distant metastasis

- T3. Multiple tumors or major vascular invasion. M1–Distant metastasis

- T4—Tumor invades adjacent organs

- Stage I—T1–N0–M0

- Stage II—T2–N0–M0

- Stage IIIA—T3–N0–M0

- Stage IIB—T4–N0–M0

- Stage IIIC—Any T–N1–M0

- Stage IV—Any T–Any N–M1

Once the staging has been completed, in many instances the case will be presented to a tumor board or committee and several physicians will discuss the best course of therapy. The course of treatment that has the greatest chance for cure is complete removal of the cancer. There are several options, and in the last few years surgeons have become much more aggressive in theory approach to this disease. With the increasing specialization of surgeons into the liver and biliary-tract fields, and with the excellent success rates in whole or partial liver transplantation, a new age of treatment has commenced.

**Surgery**

The first approach is to determine whether the patient will tolerate any surgery at all. The presence of ascites, impending liver failure with jaundice (and no biliary duct obstruction causing the jaundice), kidney failure, severe coagulation disorders, or extensive spread of the tumor will be contraindications for surgery, and these patients will have to be treated with palliative measures to sustain a comfortable life in their remaining months or years. The role of alternative and complementary medicine will be discussed.

Surgery has many different options and approaches. If the cancer is small, removal of the cancer with surrounding normal liver (lumpectomy) is recommended. If one lobe of the liver is involved with a single or multiple tumors, an entire lobe can be removed (lobectomy), since a normal remaining liver can regrow in several weeks. If there is tumor in both lobes and they can be carefully identified and localized, the surgeon may opt to remove one lobe and then use other means to destroy the tumors in the other lobe. These measures include cryotherapy and radio-frequency ablation of the tumor, and in some cases intratumoral ethanol injection. Another therapy called TACE (trans-arterial chemo-embolization) injects small gel foam or coils and chemotherapy into arteries supplying a tumor to shrink the tumor in anticipation of surgery or transplantation. Surgeons with the appropriate training have been able to do some liver resections laparoscopically through tiny holes, obviating the need for large surgical incisions.

Stereotactic radiosurgery is a newer technique to direct high-powered x-ray beams into a small tumor; another therapy involves proton beam radiation. Sorafenib (Nexavar) is a drug that interferes with VEGF (vascular endothelial growth factor) tumor receptor and may be given prior to and after liver surgery to increase the chance for cure.

The best way to guarantee the highest cure rate is a complete hepatectomy (removal of the entire liver) and a liver transplant. This modality is of course limited by the paucity of available livers for transplant. However, surgeons are now performing partial liver transplants—taking a portion of the liver from a family member or other donor and transplanting this into the patient who has undergone a complete hepatectomy for cancer. The donor's liver and the transplanted liver will both enlarge over several weeks. The major drawback to this treatment is the unfortunate fact that there are some serious complications, and even deaths, in the donor group and some medical centers have even stopped doing partial liver-donor transplantation.

Concerning metastatic cancer to the liver, years ago the spread of a cancer from another primary source, such as the colon, lung, or pancreas, to the liver was a sign of inoperability and incurability. However, in the last few years, with the improvement of liver surgery and the modalities now available to the surgeon, the outlook has changed dramatically. When a patient presents with a metastasis or even several metastases to the liver, the aggressive surgeon will often attempt to remove them with one of the techniques previously mentioned and in many instances can achieve a cure or a significant palliation of symptoms. In many surgical centers, the philosophy consists of continuing to remove cancer metastases (metastasectomy) as long as their removal gives hope for a cure or a marked palliation to extend life. If your surgeon or hospital is not set up to accomplish this kind of surgery, you should seek out a second opinion at a major medical center.

### Radiation and Chemotherapy

For patients who are unable to undergo surgery, those with advanced disease, or postoperative patients with recurrent disease, several therapeutic options are available. Radiation therapy can only be given to a certain limited degree without causing severe liver damage, and the TACE procedure previously mentioned is an option. Intratumor alcohol injection, cryotherapy, and radiofrequency ablation are still available.

Chemotherapy for liver cancer has poor response rates when using cisplatin, doxorubicin, 5-FU, gemcitabine (Gemzar), oxaliplatin (Eloxatin). Hepatic arterial infusion with FUDR (fluorodeoxyuridine) has shown meager results. Bevacizumab (Avastin), erlotinib (Tarceva), and sorafenib (Nexavar) have only been minimally effective. Alpha-interferon (IFN-a) has been of value in preventing liver cancer recurrences, but high doses of this drug are poorly tolerated by patients with cirrhosis. Biochemotherapeutic treatments with combinations of cisplatin, doxorubicin, interferon-a 2a (Roferon-a), and 5-FU have shown a 20 percent response rate and adriamycin, doxorubicin, interferon-a-2b, and (PIAF) Platinol was about the same. Targeted therapies against EGFR (epidermal growth factor inhibitor) using erlotinib (Tarceva) showed a 9 percent response and RAF and VEGF kinase inhibitor sorafenib (Nexavar) showed slight improvement over a placebo. The chemotherapeutic approach to liver cancer shows limited success, but hundreds of clinical trials are in effect and new therapies are being presented every month.

## ■ *Alternative and Complementary Treatment*

Several studies, many of them double-blind clinical trials, were undertaken in China and they affirmed the positive effects of using Chinese herbal medicines and their derivatives for preventing liver cancer. This was accomplished by treating and preventing cirrhosis and fibrosis, improving hepatic blood flow, and also affecting the growth rate of hepatocellular carcinoma. Salvianolic acid B, extracted from a common herbal, *Radix salviae miltiorrhizae,* was found to inhibit several steps in carcinogenesis formation. Oxymatrine, an alkaloid extracted from *Sophora alopecuraides* has antitumor and immunosupression action. Curcumin, a natural antioxidant from *Curcuma longa L* showed antitumor action and apoptosis induction. Glycyrrhizin from licorice root enhances T-cell activity and is active in treating hepatitis and augmenting immune functions. Berberine and trypterigium are two more drugs from herbs that have been effective against hepatic carcinoma.

According to their studies, berberine, celestrol, and curcumin have action to induce tumor apoptosis (death); berberine, glycyrrhizin, and gylcyrrhizic acid are effective against chemical-induced hepatic cancer, and curcumin, glycyrrhizin, oxymatrine, tetrandine, and triptolide have significant immune-augmentation actions. The anticancer effects of arabinogalactans,[30] ginger, selenium, and silymarin (milk thistle extract) have been shown in animal experiments to block or diminish metastases to the liver and other organs. All of these are directly obtained from traditional Chinese herbs and have been put through rigorous double-blind studies as reported in *Liver International,* the official journal of the International Association for the Study of the Liver.[31]

There are several reports describing how Chinese herbal medicines can alleviate pain, ascites, jaundice, and the progression of liver cancer. Many of the American cancer centers are beginning to explore these methods with the view that three thousand years of traditional Chinese medicine (TCM) may well have significant contributions to make to the more recent Western oncologic therapy.

The Ayurvedic literature offers several alternative treatments for liver cancer, which include beta-carotene, catechins, glutathione, lycopene, purple grape seeds, quercetin, resveratrol, selenium, and diets rich in cereals, fish, fruits, legumes, vegetables, and whole grains. They include the use of coenzyme $Q_{10}$, Essaic tea, and raw beet juice, along with acupuncture, massage therapy, meditation, physical therapy, spiritual healing, and visualization. If these seem nonscientific to the Western physician, they have proven effective in ameliorating many of the symptoms associated with liver cancer and its Western therapies and should be examined. This is especially true regarding pain management—acupuncture, acupressure, and massage therapy have been successfully used in combination with standard Western medical therapies.

## LUNG CANCER

If you have to place blame on anyone, you might as well lay the guilt on Sir Walter Raleigh who brought back the first tobacco from the new world to England in the 1580s. In fact, tobacco played a major role in financing the American Revolution and, because of this, it has held a special place in American economics and business. There is no question that tobacco in the form of cigarettes, cigars, and chewing tobacco, as well as secondhand smoke, is responsible for almost 90 percent of all lung cancer. The factual assertions have only been ascertained in the last forty years, and, still, the addictive nature of the product, and the big business industrial organizations behind the product, have kept it popular in the lives of many Americans. My father, a surgeon and an intelligent man, smoked two packs of Camels a day and died of lung cancer at the age of 59. In fact, almost every photograph of him taken as a military surgeon in England and then France during World War II shows him with a cigarette hanging from his lip. He looked cool and casual—like Humphrey Bogart and all the other cool characters in the film world. The adults and the youth of America became addicted by the millions and this led to the overwhelming problem of lung cancer. *Tobacco causes lung cancer.*

Lung cancer, or pulmonary or bronchogenic cancer, can be of two major types according to the physical characteristics of their cells, small-cell carcinoma and non-small-cell carcinoma. The median age for diagnosis is seventy years and the overall survivor rate for all lung cancer is only 15 percent. The disease is rarely caught at an early stage and, surprisingly, chest-x-ray screening for smokers and nonsmokers is not yet a recommendation.

Like most other cancers, lung cancer is initiated by the inactivation of tumor-suppressor genes, or the activation of cancer-causing onco-genes. Substances called proto-oncogenes are transformed into onco-genes when exposed to carcinogens like tobacco. EGFR (epidermal growth factor receptor) regulates cell growth, proliferation, apoptosis (cell death), tumor development, and angiogenesis, the formation of new blood vessels. Changes or mutations in EGFR are found in non-small-cell lung cancer and many treatments are based on finding EGFR inhibitors. Tumor-suppressor gene p53 is inactivated by certain mutations and damage to chromosomes, causing lung cancer. There are many genes that may be altered and thereby lead to lung cancer; among these are BRAF, NKX2-1, PIK3CA—to mention a few and give an idea of the complexity of this process.

The basic types of primary lung cancer and approximate percent-ages are:

◆ Non-small-cell cancer–81 percent

◆ Small-cell lung cancer–18 percent

◆ Carcinoid–0.8 percent

◆ Sarcoma–0.2 percent

Non-small-cell lung cancer is further divided as follows.

◆ Squamous-cell lung cancer (carcinoma)—25 percent of lung can-cers are squamous cell, occurring in the breathing tube called a bronchus

◆ Adenocarcinoma—this accounts for 40 percent of non-small-cell lung cancer and most is due to smoking, though never-smokers also can develop this kind of cancer

◆ Bronchoalveolar carcinoma

◆ Carcinoid

Small-cell lung cancer, originally called oat-cell carcinoma, usually associated with smoking, is less common; it grows rapidly, becoming large and sometimes blocking the breathing tubes (bronchi). These cells often have special granules in them with hormones that can cause paraneoplastic syndrome, phenomena that can affect other areas of the body. One example is Eaton-Lambert myasthenia syndrome, which is a generalized muscle weakness due to auto-antibodies. Another, SIADH (syndrome of inappropriate antidiuretic hormone) can lead to excessive fluid and calcium losses in the urine. Small-cell cancers are usually metastatic when discovered and carry an ominous prognosis, even though they are very sensitive to radiation and chemotherapy treatment if, although rarely, found early.

Often, the signs and symptoms of lung cancer do not appear until the disease has progressed to a more advanced stage—only 15 percent are found in the early stages before a spread to lymph nodes has occurred. The signs include shortness of breath (dyspnea), a persistent cough occasionally with bloody or reddish-brown sputum (hemoptysis), chest pain with deep breathing, wheezing, hoarseness (dysphonia), difficulty swallowing, loss of appetite and weight loss (cachexia), fever of unknown origin, recurring pneumonia, and bronchitis. When the cancer has metastasized to other areas, the symptoms will be related to those areas, namely bone pain (bony involvement), changes in the fingertips (known as hypertrophic osteoarthritis), general weakness, jaundice (liver metastases), masses on the skin, neurological changes in mentation, sensation, weakness, or numbness (brain or spinal cord), and Horner's syndrome from cancer of the lung at the uppermost area of the chest (pancoast tumor), causing drooping eyelid, shoulder pain, a smaller pupil, and absent perspiration on one side. Some men may develop increased breast growth from endocrine-producing tumors. As indicated, common sites for the spread of lung cancer are to the adrenal glands, bone, brain, heart lining (pericardium), kidneys, liver, and opposite lung.

Metastatic cancer is still called lung cancer, not cancer of the organ to which it spreads—lung cancer that spreads to the liver is not liver cancer but metastatic lung cancer to the liver. Other symptoms may include dizziness and drowsiness from hypercalcemia (increased calcium), weakness from hyperkalemia (increased potassium), and arthritis, all part of the paraneoplastic syndromes.

When a lung cancer partially or completely blocks off the vena cava in the chest (vena-caval syndrome), a patient will present with swelling of the upper chest, neck, and arms, along with marked distention of the neck veins. And patients with lung cancer may have anemias, blood clots in their legs and arms (possibly traveling to the lungs and causing pulmonary embolism), and low blood sugar.

Almost 10 percent of lung cancer is asymptomatic and is first diagnosed with routine chest x-rays.

There are also metastatic cancers *to* the lung from other organs, including bones, breast, cervix, colon, liver, rectum, and skin. These cancers usually look different from the primary lung cancer, often appearing as discrete nodules and frequently scattered throughout the lungs.

Although the main cause of lung cancer is tobacco, other causes are radon gas, a breakdown product of naturally occurring uranium in different parts of the world (in the United States, it's highest in Iowa), and viruses, including BK viruses, cytomegalovirus, human papilloma virus, JC virus, and simian virus that apparently all affect the cell cycle and allow uncontrolled cell growth. Also blamed are air pollution, primarily with arsenic, cadmium, chromium, ionizing radiation nickel, and uranium; exposure to asbestos; and diesel fuels—the disease seems more common in urban areas than rural areas. There is also a genetic predisposition in certain individuals, especially those with a rare syndrome called Li-Fraumeni.

Some studies have attributed an increased risk of lung cancer to individuals with low levels of vitamin A, and certain fruits and vegetables seem to have a protective effect.

### ■ Diagnosis and Treatment

Diagnosis is made by chest x-ray, CT scan, needle biopsy, PET scan, MRI followed by bronchoscopy, with possible biopsy (placing a scope through the mouth into the lungs under sedation or general anesthesia), mediastinoscopy or thoracoscopy (examining the lungs and possible biopsy through small scopes placed into the chest under anesthesia), a VATS procedure (video-assisted thoracoscopic surgery), or an open thoracotomy (cutting into the chest) and biopsy, also under general anesthesia.

### Staging

The T=Tumor, N=Node, M=Metastasis system is used. Here is an overview of the fairly complex procedures involved.

### Primary Tumor

- Tx—positive cells, no tumor seen
- Tis—Cancer in situ–local and cannot yet spread

- T1—< 3 m tumor

- T2—> 3 cm–and partially collapsed lung

- T3—Extension to chest wall, diaphragm, heart lining (pericardium), pleura

- T4—Invasion of mediastinum (central chest)

- Malignant pleural effusion (cancer-cell fluid in chest)

**Lymph Node Involvement** (Sorry, but technical terms are necessary)

- N0—no nodal involvement

- N1—Ipsilateral (same side), bronchopulmonary, or hilar nodes

- N2—Ipsilateral, or subcarinal mediastinal nodes, or ipsilateral supra-clavicular nodes

- N3—Contralateral mediastinal hilar, or supraclavicular nodes

**Metastatic**

- M0—No metastasis

- M1—Metastases

| STAGE | T | N | M | 5-YEAR SURVIVAL RATE |
|---|---|---|---|---|
| Occult | Tx | N0 | M0 | |
| Stage 0 | T in situ | N0 | M0 | |
| Stage IA | T1 | N0 | M0 | >70 percent |
| Stage IB | T2 | N0 | M0 | 60 percent |
| Stage IIA | T1 | N1 | M0 | 50 percent |
| Stage IIB | T2 | N1 | M0 | 30 percent |
| | T3 | N0 | M0 | 40 percent |
| Stage IIIA | T3 | N1 | M0 | 00 percent |
| | T1–3 | N2 | M0 | |
| Stage IIIB | Any T | Any N | M0 | <10 percent |
| | T4 | Any N | M0 | |
| Stage IV | Any T | Any N | M1 | <5percent |

The treatment of lung cancer depends on several variables: the type of cancer, whether it is local or has spread; the general condition of the patient, including his or her general health; and the status of the lungs. Frequently patients with lung cancer have been smokers for many years; and their lung function is fair to poor. They might not tolerate having a portion of their lungs removed, so treatment includes surgery, chemotherapy, radiation, palliation, and a number of complementary treatments.

## Surgery

Once the diagnosis has been made, tests must be performed to ascertain the extent of the disease. These will include CT and PET scans. Blood tests, heart studies, and lung studies are performed. The lung studies, called spirometry, evaluate the individual's capacity to take in air and oxygenate the blood. If the person has severe chronic obstructive pulmonary disease from smoking, she/he may not be able to tolerate removal of a lung or even a portion of a lung.

The lungs consist of five lobes, three in the right lung, and two in the left lung. Depending on the condition of the patient and the location and size of the cancer, the options are wedge resection (removal of a triangular portion of the edge of one lobe), segmentectomy (removal of one part of a lobe), lobectomy (removal of the entire lobe or possibly two on the right side), or a one-sided pneumonectomy (removal of either the right or left lung). In many cases, the wider the resection tolerated, the greater the chance of removing the cancer. At the time of surgery, the thoracic surgeon evaluates and often removes lymph nodes, and this helps in the final staging of the disease and often guides the treatment by the radiation therapist.

Another modality as a palliative measure is the use of lasers to open up a blocked bronchus (breathing tube) that has been obstructed by a cancer.

## Complications of Surgery

The complications of lung surgery are air leakage, bleeding, infection, and lung collapse. Some patients may need to have assisted breathing for a while and remain on a ventilator for several days or even several weeks. There are possible incidences of heart problems, strokes, and even kidney problems, with kidney failure in some cases, plus, of course, some pain and discomfort associated with the incision site. The possibility of dying from the surgery is remote, although the risk increases with age and the extent of the procedure; it is at its greatest when a pneumonectomy (removal of one entire lung) is performed. Eventually, though, most patients return to their normal activities within several weeks or months.

With small-cell cancer, patients appear to do better with chemotherapy and radiation than with surgery, except in the rare, very early cases where all three modalities are used.

### Radiation

For non-small-cell cancer, radiotherapy is combined with surgery and chemotherapy with the intent to cure. Sometimes high-intensity radiotherapy (radical radiotherapy, or continuous hyperfractionated accelerated radiotherapy—CHART) is given with chemotherapy in patients who will not tolerate surgery. For noncurable cancers, radiation may be given to control symptoms, and a form of radiation called brachytherapy can be given directly into a bronchus or airway to melt away cancer that is blocking the airway. To prevent mestastases, prophylactic radiation may be given to the brain in some cases.

### Chemotherapy—Small-Cell Lung Cancer

Various combinations of chemotherapy have been used to treat small-cell cancer of the lung. Cisplatin (Platinol) and etoposide, or etoposide and carboplatin are given in combination with radiation therapy. Other regimens include carboplatin, cisplatin (IRINOP), cisplatin (EP), cyclophosphamide, doxorubicin, irinotecan, isosfamide, paclitaxel (CP), VP16 (CDE), VP16 (VIP), and many others, depending on the preference of the oncologist. Even in the best instances, the median survival for patients with this cancer is only three to four months with a five-year survival rate of only 1–2 percent. Therefore, when considering therapy, the age of the patient, the general condition, evaluation of the side effects and must be weighed against the quality of life. For the rare few who have very limited disease, all attempts are made for a cure or at least long-term survival.

### Chemotherapy—Non-Small-Cell Lung Cancer

While still ominous, the overall prognosis for this type of lung cancer is much better than that of small-cell cancer. Many of these cancers are diagnosed early with a better chance for a cure and long-term survival. Stages I and II are amenable to a surgical cure, along with chemotherapy and radiation, whereas Stages III and IV are often relegated to nonsurgical therapies. The newer agents for treatment of non-small-cell lung cancer include docetaxel, gemcitabine, irinotecan, paclitaxel, and vinorelbine. In addition, there are many more regimens with different combinations of carboplatin, cisplatin, ifosfamide, mitomycin, to name a few. Newer agents include bevacizumab, bexarotine, erlotinib, and gefitinib.

Another newer drug for advanced stage non-small-cell disease is Tarceva, but this is used only as a last resort because of its high incidence of complications, such as clotting disorders, eye problems, kidney disease, perforation of the intestine, and skin conditions. The oncologist must weigh the possibility for palliation against the risks involved.

Still one other new drug, Avastin, is used in combination with other chemotherapeutic agents. It is an angiogenesis inhibitor, and starves the tumor by attacking its blood supply. But, as with Tarceva, it has many serious side effects, including bleeding, blood clots, fistulas, heart attacks, high blood pressure, kidney problems, strokes, and others. The oncologist must discuss with the patient the value of using such drugs.

The side effects of this chemotherapy include nausea, pain, and weight loss, which can all be controlled with standard medications, or with a whole host of alternative treatments.

### Gene Therapy

New studies into gene therapy and vaccine therapy for lung cancer are still in the investigational stages. In lung cancer, mutations occur in a gene called the p53 suppressor gene that normally suppresses cancer. Scientists are researching ways to replace the defective gene with a normal one. They are also investigating ways to insert genes into the cell to produce cancer-killing proteins; and in another experiment, they are using a gene for interleukin-2 to stimulate the immune system to destroy cancer cells. These projects are not available for most patients, but those interested can enroll in trials sponsored by the National Cancer Institute (NCI).

**Immune Therapy**

Attempts have been underway to develop ways to stimulate the lung cancer patient's immune system. Certain immune system stimulants, such as Calmette-Guerin Bacillus (BCG), interferon, nocardia rubra cell wall skeleton, thymosin factor V, and others have been tried with little success. Antigens such as p53, ras, erbB2, and surface proteins, such as CEA, MUCI, GD2, and HuD are being explored with limited success.

**Molecular Medicine**

Memorial Sloan-Kettering Cancer Center is one of a few centers involved in the Lung Cancer Mutation Project (LC-MAP) that seeks to identify genetic mutations in non-small-cell lung cancer and to develop new drugs to target these abnormal genes. EGFR mutation responds positively to erlotinib (Tarceva). Other clinical trials are underway for the genes BRAS, EML4-ALK, and KRAS. Patients with these gene mutations may be eligible to enter clinical trials at selected major cancer centers.

**Metastatic Cancer to the Lung**

As mentioned, many cancers in other organs may spread to the lungs. Breast, colon, kidney, melanoma, pancreatic, sarcoma, stomach, and other cancers may metastasize to the lungs. Whereas many years ago this was considered a sign of incurability, today the philosophy has changed significantly. Many surgeons and oncologists advocate surgical removal, and radiation ablation of solitary or a few lesions in the lungs and are seeing some five-year cures as a result. Even in cases of extensive disease, sometimes there is a role for palliative treatment of metastatic disease to prolong life, treat pain, or lower the tumor load upon which other therapy is acting. With less cancer to fight, longer survival and symptom-free survival can be attained.

**■ *Complementary and Alternative Treatment***

With lung cancer, alternative therapy should not be used in preference to standard treatment. A short delay to use a complementary treatment may give lung cancer enough time to upgrade to a higher stage and may result in a previously curable tumor becoming incurable and treatment only palliative. While there are many suggestions for lung-cancer prevention, and therapies to alleviate symptoms or augment the effectiveness of chemo or radiation therapy, alternative and complementary therapy should not be the single first line of treatment for this dangerous cancer. Instead, cancer centers, such as Memorial Sloan-Kettering, Dana Farber, University of California at several sites, M.D. Anderson, and many more, now have programs that are integrating conventional and complementary medicine for lung-cancer therapy.

As one example of integrated Chinese and Western medical treatment for non-small-cell lung cancer, I came upon a very interesting article from the *Hunan Journal of Chinese Medicine*.[32] A very scientific and carefully controlled study described treatment of ninety-two patients with non-small-cell lung cancer (equally staged IIA–IIIB) who were diagnosed via biopsy and after a chest x-ray, a CT scan, and an MRI ruled out other serious disease. Half were treated with Western radiation therapy, the other half with combined Western and Chinese medicine. "While using radiation alone as the Western medical treatment of stage II NSCLC is not considered standard in North America," they felt the study "could serve as a model for the integration of these two medical systems in treating lung cancer." ("Radiation therapy may be used to treat stage II patients who cannot have surgery because of other medical problems; stage III patients may be treated with radiation alone" or with combined modalities.)

The Chinese medicinal formula included a long and complex list of thirty-three-plus herbs. The results of the combined-treatment group showed a significant increase in the two- and three-year survival rates over the radiation-alone group. The study also included thoughts on the Chinese philosophy of lung cancer, discussing *qi* mechanisms that are completely unfamiliar to the Western oncologist. Also, the incidence of radiation esophagitis, bronchitis, and pneumonia were markedly lower in the combined-treatment group.

The important lesson here is that there is a place for the combined use of Chinese medicine and Western medicine to achieve a better outcome. More studies like this are underway in many of the major institutes in the United States, as well as in China and India. Western medical doctors have to join the twenty-first century and stop thinking of this as medicine with no validity.

In another study, Chinese herbal holistic medicine for lung cancer includes scutellaria, taraxacum, ophiopogonis, and oldenlandia. Research facilities, including Heidelberg in Germany, Simon Fraser University in Canada, and the University of Mainz, Germany have tested many regimens.[33,34]

Most major American cancer centers agree that acupuncture and many herbal medications, in the hands of an expert, can alleviate nausea, pain, and other side effects of standard chemotherapy.[35] The American College of Chest Surgeons found that some alternative therapies, including acupuncture, hypnosis, massage, meditation, and yoga, can help people with lung cancer.

The general recommendations that complementary-care practitioners have for prevention and complementary treatment of patients receiving standard cancer care include foods, such as fruits and green vegetables that are rich in beta-carotene (vitamin A), diets with antioxidants, ellagic acid, and vitamin E supplements, and vitamin C to suppress free radicals.

Both sets of practitioners recommend the following.

◇ Quit smoking.

◇ Eat fruits and vegetables.

◇ Have your home tested for radon.

◇ Know what your exposure at work and home is to arsenic, asbestos, coal products, diesel exhaust, ethers, gasoline, vinyl chloride, and other carcinogens.

◇ Keep away from secondhand smoke.

## MELANOMA

Malignant melanoma is a skin tumor that arises from pigmented cells, usually in the skin, called melanocytes, and it is much more dangerous than basal- or squamous-cell cancer. The word melanoma originates from the Greek *melas,* meaning dark, and this tumor usually presents as a rapidly growing, black, asymmetrical skin lesion with irregular borders. There are also some nonblack or amelanotic melanomas, so the diagnosis may not be simple. As a cancer, melanoma has the potential to be one of the most malignant of all cancers in the body, with a nasty propensity to spread and cause death within a year. This cancer can occur in any part of the body where melanocytes are found, and it is more frequent in women and in Caucasians living in sunny climates. Redheads seem to be immune to melanoma because they have the MC1R gene that inhibits melanoma growth. Although it is a relatively rare skin cancer compared to squamous and basal cell, it accounts for more than 75–80 percent of the deaths from skin cancer.

Melanomas are caused by damage to the DNA inside the cells of the melanocytes, and this damage may be from genetic mutation, exposure to UV light from the sun, or tanning booths. The early stage of melanoma forms in the dermis and epidermis of the skin (the upper two layers), is generally 1 mm thick, and is called radial growth. Because the growth is so limited, the cancer cells have not yet reached lymph or blood channels and the potential for cure is high. When the tumor starts to invade other layers, it becomes capable of spreading. Initially called invasive radial, it progresses to frank invasive melanoma with a poorer prognosis. Signs may be bleeding, itching, rapid growth, and conversion of a pale or red lesion to a black one.

■ *Diagnosis and Treatment*

Two named methods are used to describe melanoma of the skin after excision.

**Clark Level:** This measures the depth of invasion when examined under a microscope in five levels. The descriptions are the technical ones used by the pathologist.

◇ I—In the basal layer of the epidermis where it originated

◇ II—Extends to the top layer of the dermis (called the papillary dermis)

◇ III—Extends to the border of the papillary and reticular dermis

◇ IV—Involves the reticular dermis

◇ V—Invades the subcutaneous tissue or fat

**The Breslow Thickness.** This is the other staging system where the thickness of the primary tumor is measured under the microscope with an instrument called a micrometer.

## Staging

An ulceration or a break in the skin surface of a melanoma is a negative predicting sign in terms of long-term survival. The actual classification and staging of melanoma is very complex. This is an abbreviated version.

T=Tumor size, N=Nodes, M=Metastasis

- IA—Localized, melanoma 1mm or less thickness, Clark level II/III (T1a, N0M0)

- IB—Same as 1a with Clark level IV/V with ulceration (T1b, N0M0)

  1–2 mm without ulceration (T2a, N0M0)

- IIA—Localized, 1–2 mm with ulceration (or T2b, N0M0)

  2–4 mm without ulceration (T3a, N0M0)

- IIB—Localized, 2–4 mm with ulceration (T3b, N0M0)

  >4 mm without ulceration (T4a, N0M0)

- IIC—localized, > 4 mm with ulceration (T4b, N0M0)

- IIIA—C-Nodal metastases with or without ulceration (T4, N1–3, M0)

- IV—Distant metastases (Any T, Any N, M1)

When a melanoma develops, the human body elicits an immuno-logical response against the cancer that can be evaluated by the presence of tumor-infiltrating lymphocytes (TILs). Sometimes these cells can even destroy the tumor. The actual mutations that cause melanoma are complex and may involve gene CDKN2A, destabilization of transcription factor p53 and CDK4, and mutations to MC1R—all complex science more germane to a medical textbook than this overview.

Melanomas may be superficial spreading, and less dangerous, or nodular and more dangerous, the latter usually being elevated, firm, and growing rapidly. Diagnosis requires a skin biopsy done under local anesthesia, with enough tissue removed to make the diagnosis and staging.

There are nine types of melanomas.

1. Acral lentiginous melanoma
2. Amelanotic melanoma
3. Desmoplastic melanoma
4. Lentigo maligna
5. Mucosal melanoma
6. Nodular melanoma
7. Polypoid melanoma
8. Soft tissue melanoma
9. Superficial spreading melanoma

The treatment of melanomas depends on the staging. Stage I can be cured, in most cases, by wide excision. Higher stages may be treated with wide excision and sentinel-node biopsy. The sentinel node is the first lymph node draining a particular area of the body. This is found by injecting the cancer or the area where it was excised with a radioactive material and observing where it travels, using lymphosyntography or a blue-dye method. Once the sentinel node has been localized by nuclear medicine or the blue-dye technique, it is removed and examined for cancer cells. If there are none, the disease is call N0; if tumor cells are found, it is N1. When N1 is present, a radical dissection of the lymph nodes in that area is sometimes performed, depending on the surgeon or oncologist.

Recent reports at the American College of Surgeons stressed the importance of continual and vigorous removal of metastatic melanoma tumors in the lung, liver, and other areas, with resultant longer survival and even a few cures.

When lymph nodes are positive for a tumor, a full radiological evaluation of the entire body is needed to determine the presence or absence of metastasis.

Depending on the stage, chemotherapy (BiCNU taxol, dacarbazine, DTIC, taxotere, temodar, ternozolomide, velban) or immunotherapy (with interleukin-2, IL-2-proleukin), or high-dose interferon may be indicated. Radiation therapy is often used for the site of the original tumor after it has been removed, or for shrinkage of metastatic disease.

Combination therapy, using DTIC and ipilimumab (a monoclonal antibody that targets CTLA-4 antibodies) appears to offer increased survival for metastatic melanoma. Unfortunately, the drug ipilimumab (Yervoy) costs a staggering $120,000 for a course of therapy. In advanced cases of melanoma involving one limb, isolated limb perfusion has been done using high-dose chemotherapy (melphalan-Alkeran). Newer agents for therapy include dendritic cell therapy, sorafenib (BAY 43–9006, Nexavar), and thalidomide that blocks angiogenesis.

## ■ Complementary and Alternative Treatment

In addition to the previously mentioned standard treatments, patients with melanoma are offered acupuncture, dietary counseling, massage therapy, medications for pain, palliative care, physical therapy, and yoga. Complementary methods, such as acupuncture to relieve pain, meditation to reduce stress, and peppermint tea to relieve nausea, are also effective. Non-standard methods should never delay rapid evaluation and surgical removal of the primary tumor and any lymph nodes that may possibly be involved.

Alternative modes of therapy have been used in China with excellent results. Harmine, a beta-carboline alkaloid from *Peganum harmala* inhibits the metastasis of yttB16f-10 melanoma cells by activating intrinsic and extrinsic pathways for cell apoptosis (cell death). Another traditional Chinese herbal medicine, keishi-ka-kei-to (containing *Cinamomi cortex, Glycyrrhizae radix, Paeoniae radix, Zingiberis rhizome,* and *Zizyphi fructus*) inhibited metastasis in mice with B16 F10 melanoma cells.

A retrospective study showed marked improvement in cure and long-term survival of patients with melanoma who used Gerson's diet therapy, which is lacto-vegetarian, with low sodium, fat, and somewhat low protein, high potassium, phytochemicals, $CoQ_{10}$, flaxseed oil, vitamins A, $B_3$, C, pepsin, fluid, nutrients, raw liver, and carrot juice. (Derived from studies at U.C. San Diego for advanced melanoma in 157 patients on the Gerson regimen.[36])

Recommended herbal treatments include astragalus, which increases the effectiveness of IL-2 and natural killer cells, cat's claw tincture, which stimulates natural-killer cells, kudzu-containing diadzein to halt melanoma growth, lentinan to slow metastasis, polysaccharide kureha (PSK) to slow the metastasis to the lungs, and reishi, to increase the body's production of IL-2.

Other practitioners recommend acupuncture to stimulate the immune system, and naturopaths say that ultrasound and diathermy, massage, heat and cold treatments, gentle electrical therapies, and exercise can help relieve pain and musculoskeletal disorders related to melanoma.

Maintaining weight and nutritional health is important in later stages of the disease and may increase the length of survival. People are encouraged to eat fish, poultry, fruits, legumes, vegetables, whole grains, and cereals. The recommendations also include supplements of beta carotene, selenium, vitamins C and E, and EPA (eicosapentaenoic acid). Other therapies include cartilage therapy, herbal teas (with Essiac), and $CoQ_{10}$.

Mind-body advocates offer programs in stress management, spiritual meditation, humor therapy, and relaxation and imagery training. If the patient feels better with these, and does better, all the better.

## MESOTHELIOMA

Mesothelioma is a malignant disease affecting the membrane that covers and protects many of the internal organs of the body. In the chest, this would involve the pleura (lining of the chest cavity), the pericardium (lining of the sac around the heart), or the peritoneum, (the lining around the peritoneal cavity). The disease is five times more common in men than women, and its etiology has been directly related to asbestos exposure, with an incubation period between thirty to forty years. Asbestos is divided into two major groups, serpentine and amphibole, and the latter contains crocidolite, the most carcinogenic form of the substance.

### ◼ Diagnosis

When the chest is involved, patients present with chest pain, fever, hoarseness, loss of appetite, shortness of breath, and weight loss, and when the peritoneum is involved, symptoms include nausea, swelling of the legs, urinary or intestinal obstruction, and vomiting. The laboratory workup usually reveals nonspecific findings, including anemia, eosinophilia, hypergammaglobulinemia, and frequently thrombocytosis, a condition where there is a marked increase in platelets (a blood-clotting substance).

Since none of these are diagnostic, further workup will include x-rays, CT scans (computer axial tomography), MRIs (magnetic resonance imaging), PET scans (positron emission tomography), and a special radionucleotide study called FDG (fluorodeoxyglucose). A definitive diagnosis is made with a thoracentesis (removal of fluid from the chest with a needle) and examination of the cells obtained; a pleural biopsy with a needle, or through a small incision; or by using thoracoscopy (inserting a fiberoptic scope into the chest).

Once the diagnosis has been confirmed, staging is done to clarify the type of treatment. Staging has been designed by several different groups and no one system is generally accepted. Overall, the disease is rarely cured, and the staging only assists in directing the type of therapy for palliation.

## Staging

The simplest system I have found is according to Butchart:

- Stage I—Tumor confined to one side of the pleura, lungs, diaphragm

- Stage II—Tumor invades chest wall and involves mediastinum (esophagus, heart, opposite pleura, lymph nodes)

- Stage III—Tumor penetrates through diaphragm to involve peritoneum, opposite pleura, and lymph nodes

- Stage IV—Distant blood-born metastases

## *Treatment*

With a median survival rate between four and eighteen months, the objective is to make the patient as comfortable and productive as possible. While attempts may be made in the rare, early-stage mesothelioma to completely eradicate the disease through surgery and chemotherapy, a realistic approach warrants focusing on the least destructive and compromising procedure so as not to decrease the amount of quality-of-life time remaining. A chest tube is often inserted to remove accumulated fluid and resolve breathing difficulty.

Aggressive surgical approaches may dictate the removal of large portions of the chest contents, including a lung, pleura, and even diaphragm. Unless there is a definite advantage to this approach, a more reasonable palliative procedure may be the best choice. Discussion at a tumor conference will include the use of radiation therapy, as well as various combinations of chemotherapy, including cisplatin, cyclophosphamide, doxorubicin, and pemetrexed (Alimta). There are several clinical trials in progress, including hyperthermic pleural perfusion with chemotherapy, photodynamic therapy (light-activated sensitization of tumor cells), and complex gene and cytokine therapies that appear to prolong life, up to two years in several cases. Newer agents include raltitrexid (Tomudex) and ranpurnase (Onconase).

### ■ Complementary and Alternative Treatment

Because of the dismal results with standard treatment for this cancer, many individuals have sought alternative and complementary, as well as Chinese, Ayurvedic and other, treatment options. Several modalities have helped to relax and reduce the stress of the disease, and others have relieved the side effects of the protracted chemo- and radiation therapy involved.

The Ayurvedic medicine and herbs have anti-inflammatory, immunomodulatory, and some anticancer capabilities and should be examined in conjunction with the standard Western therapies. Use of these medicines with names strange to Westerners, such as kantakari, manjishtha, amalaki, and mahamanjisthadi qadha, may add something beneficial to the armamentarium of drugs in this very lethal disease.

Other alternative treatment options include acupuncture, aromatherapy, art therapy, biofeedback, feng shui, hypnotherapy, homeopathy, massage, naturopathy, reflexology, yoga, and vitamin and herbal supplements. In a Japanese study, antioxidants, such as boysenberries, chocolate, olive oil, red wine, and walnuts with polyphenols, have been shown to inhibit mesothelioma growth.

Additional complementary recommendations include astragalus, celandine, mistletoe, cat's claw, and vitamin C. The patient with this serious cancer should look into all available therapies in consultation with his oncologist in a search for increased palliation for the disease.

## PANCREATIC CANCER

The pancreas is an elongated, flounder-shaped organ that lies across the back and upper portion of the midabdomen, below and behind the stomach, in front of the aorta, and behind the colon and omentum (the fatty apron of the abdomen). It is divided into four parts, a head, neck, body, and tail.

This organ has two functional types of cells. One is called endocrine, or ductless, which means it secretes hormones directly into the bloodstream. The endocrine portion consists of clumps of cells called islets of Langerhans with alpha and beta cells. The alpha cells produce glucagon, which raises blood sugar (glucose), and the beta cells produce insulin, which lowers blood sugar and prevents diabetes mellitus. The other division is the exocrine pancreas that produces enzymes, such as amylase and lipase, that flow through pancreatic ducts directly into the intestine and help digest carbohydrates, fats, and proteins.

Cancer of the pancreas is the fifth leading cause of cancer death in the United States, and it usually occurs in the seventh decade of life. It is more common in blacks than whites and is slightly more common in men than women. Because it remains asymptomatic in its early stages, most pancreatic cancer is diagnosed late and the five-year survival rate with any type of therapy is poor.

The factors associated with development of pancreatic cancer are:

◇ Advancing age

◇ Alcohol

◇ Ashkenazi Jewish heritage

◇ Cirrhosis

◇ Diabetes mellitus

◇ Diets low in vegetables and fruits

◇ Environmental toxins, such as ammonia, carbon monoxide, hydro-carbons, nicotine, nitrosamines, secondary smoke, and smog

◇ Exposure to aliphatic solvents, chromium silica dust, insecticides, nickel

◇ Exposure to tobacco smoke

◇ Genetic predisposition and genetic syndromes with genetic alter-ations

◇ Infection with the Helicobacter pylori bacterium

◇ Low socioeconomic status

◇ Obesity

◇ Pancreatitis

◇ Soft drinks with sugar

Pancreatic cancer appears to be associated with inherited or acquired genetic abnormalities, such as inactivation of the tumor-suppressor genes p53, BRCA2, DPC4, and p16, as well as the presence of the oncogene K-ras. However, pancreatic-cancer cells may have several of the over twenty-five different genetic aberrations.

Pancreatic cancer can be categorized as originating from the exocrine or endocrine cells. The exocrine have two basic malignant types —solid and cystic. Of these, the most common is the solid adenocarcinoma, accounting for almost 95 percent of all pancreatic cancers. Cystic cancers (mucinous cystic carcinoma and mucinous cystic neoplasm) have a tendency to be less invasive and thereby have a much better long-term prognosis after surgical removal.

Endocrine pancreatic cancers are often called neuroendocrine (islet cell) tumors. They account for only 1 percent of pancreas cancers, have a less ominous progression, and are often curable with surgery. Gastrinoma is a rare tumor that may cause severe ulcers to develop in the stomach and other areas of the intestinal tract (Z-E–Zollinger-Ellison tumor). This tumor is often localized and removed without extensive pancreatic surgery, and the cure is complete. Another rare endocrine tumor, the insulinoma, which causes lowered blood sugar, can be removed and cured.

In general, discussion of pancreatic cancer in this chapter is focused on exocrine cancer.

Pancreatic cancer usually presents with abdominal pain going into the back, anemia, diabetes mellitus, diarrhea, fever, lethargy, loss of appetite, thrombophlebitis (Trousseau's sign), and weight loss. If the head of the pancreas is involved, there may be distention of the gallbladder (called Courvoisier gallbladder), and obstruction of the ducts from the gallbladder and liver, causing yellow skin (jaundice), dark urine, and pale-colored stools.

### ■ Diagnosis and Treatment

Pancreatic cancer is strongly suspected when many of the above symptoms are present and is confirmed with several studies. A tumor marker, Ca19–9, is often elevated, another enzyme, CEA, may be elevated, and in cases of bile-duct obstruction, the serum bilirubin is markedly elevated. The definitive diagnostic test is the CT (computerized tomography) scan. Other studies include an MRI (magnetic resonance imaging), the ERCP (endoscopic retrograde cholangiopancreatography—looking into the bile and pancreatic ducts with a fiberoptic scope passed through the mouth into the stomach and duodenum), and an direct biopsy through the skin into the tumor with a fine needle. The tissue removed is examined by the pathologist to make the final diagnosis.

## Staging

The staging of pancreatic cancer uses the TNM method. T=Tumor, N=Lymph Nodes, M=Metastasis.

- Tis—Carcinoma in situ—N0–No nodes

- T1—Limited to pancreas and < 2 cm—N1–Nodes involved

- T2—Limited to pancreas and > 2 cm

- T3—Extends beyond pancreas, but not to celiac—M0–No distant metastases—superior mesenteric arteries

- M1–Distant metastases

- T4—Extends beyond pancreas to celiac and superior mesenteric arteries

- Stage 0—T1a—N0 M0

- Stage IA—T1—N0 M0

- Stage IB—T2—N0 M0

- Stage IIB—T1—N1 M0

- T2—N1 M0

- T3—N1 M0

- Stage III—T4 Any N M0

- Stage IV—Any T Any N M1

Due to its intimate relationship with several anatomical structures, surgery on the pancreas is fairly complex. After determining that the cancer is resectable (removable for cure), the location dictates the type of surgery. Cancer in the body and tail can be treated with a distal pancreatectomy (removal of pancreas); this usually requires removal of the spleen, which is intimately attached to this area. Cancer of the head and neck of the pancreas involves a complex surgery called the Whipple procedure where most of the pancreas, the surrounding lymph nodes, possibly the spleen, the duodenum (first part of the small intestine that wraps around the pancreas head), the omentum (fatty apron in the abdomen), the gallbladder, a portion of the bile duct, and sometimes part of the stomach are removed. The surgeon must then use portions of the intestine in complicated connections to put everything back in working order, and this requires expertise in the hands of the surgeon doing many of these procedures. Whereas most surgeons are trained to do Whipple procedures, those who do many of them will have better results, and the trend is shifting toward having special pancreatico-biliary surgeons do most of this work. In some centers, extended Whipple procedures are done, actually removing and replacing involved major arteries in an attempt to completely remove all the cancer. The five-year survival rate for all pancreatic cancer is only 5 percent, but when the tumor is resectable in the hands of a skilled surgeon, the five-year survival rate may be as high as 21–25 percent.

In situations where a curative operation cannot be performed, palliative procedures are done, including bypassing an obstructed intestine or stomach, stenting the blocked bile duct (bypassing with an internal tube) to alleviate jaundice. Several studies have also shown that, in the hands of skilled surgeons, a Whipple procedure followed by chemotherapy can afford the patients a longer survival time, even in cases of advanced disease.

The complications of Whipple and other pancreatic surgery are bleeding, leakage at the many connections, heart problems, infection, the need for ventilator assist (being on a respirator for a period of time), and difficult-to-control diabetes mellitus.

Chemotherapy and radiation may be given prior to surgery (neoadjuvant) in an attempt to shrink the cancer and make it more easily removable. Most often, chemo-radiation is given postoperatively. This may destroy any residual cancer cells not removed at the time of surgery and offer a greater chance for cure. In patients who cannot tolerate surgery (for medical reasons—heart or lung problems, generalized weakness, etc.) chemo-radiation can provide increased length of survival and diminish pain.

The agents used for chemotherapy include capecytabine (Xeloda), cisplatin (Platinol), erlotinib (Tarceva), 5-FU (fluorouracil), gemcitabine (Gemzar), interferon, mitomycin, and oxyplatin (Eloxatin). Newer treatments, including bevacizumab, an angiogenesis inhibitor that destroys tumor blood vessels, cetuximab, monoclonal antibodies, and trastuzumab. Other new therapies directed against cancer oncogenes include ras and the epidermal growth factor (EGFR). Immunotherapy using vaccines is at the forefront of cancer research. Some of those who have advanced disease may be candidates for clinical trials with new drugs or combinations of drugs, and patients with this kind of extensive disease should ask their physician about the possibility of being enrolled in one of these trials.

## ■ Complementary and Alternative Treatment

The serious and frequently rampant nature of pancreatic cancer often precludes any recommendation to attempt alternative therapy prior to seeing an oncologist who practices Western medicine. The window of opportunity for therapy and cure is so narrow that delay can only mean tragedy. One of the most intelligent businessmen of the present century opted for alternative treatment of a potentially curable pancreatic cancer, delaying definitive surgery and chemotherapy until the tumor had grown beyond the bounds of curative resection.

This does not imply there is no place for alternative and complementary medicine in the treatment of this disease. The role of naturopathic recommendations regarding diet and behavior can certainly have a significant impact on preventing this disease. There are many regimens of herbs and vitamins that may well lower the possibility of developing the disease, and these should be examined by those in high-risk categories (to lower their odds of developing this disease).

The main focus should be on the complementary use of alternative and complementary medicine to augment the standard Western medical and oncological therapies, and to lessen the side effects of the tumor, of surgery, and of the chemotherapy and radiation therapy.

Chemo-preventive neutraceuticals and phytochemicals recommended for pancreatic cancer include isoflavones (soy, red clover), vitamin D (salmon, sardines, tuna), curcuminoids (turmeric), and green tea. *The American Cancer Society Complete Guide to Complementary and Alternative Cancer Therapies* has hundreds of listings for therapies under the headings of "Mind-Body-Spirit Therapies, Manual Healing and Physical Touch Therapies, Herb-Vitamin-and-Mineral Therapies, Diet and Nutrition Therapies, and Pharmacological and Biologic Therapies."

After many of the chapters, come watchwords that state, "Relying on this type of treatment alone and avoiding or delaying conventional medical care for cancer may have serious health consequences." This advice, in an otherwise open-minded book on complementary and alternative care, stresses that the patient who already has pancreatic cancer should seek out second opinions, including complementary approaches *in conjunction with* standard Western cancer therapy.

As an example, the semisynthetic drug Ukrain, derived from the herb celandine, is used in Russia. Clinical studies have shown that when used alone, it slows the progression of pancreatic cancer, and when used in combination with the standard chemotherapeutic agent gemcitabine (Gemzar), it doubled the survival time, although other studies showed there were harmful side effects. The combined use of some of the alternative herbs and drugs pose a delicate balancing act between what is effective, at what dose, and how frequently it is to be given. Standard chemotherapeutic drugs often have severe toxicities when used at recommended doses and may be lethal at higher dosages or with more frequent regimens.

Traditional Chinese medicine (TCM), with its medicinal herbs, acupuncture, massage, exercise programs, and dietary recommendations, has much to offer the patient with pancreatic cancer. While the modalities of *qi* energy, acupuncture, and various herbal preparations may seem bizarre to the Western patient and physician, evidence is steadily mounting as to the effectiveness of these therapies.

The general principles they uphold are repeated in almost every cancer here discussed, namely detoxifying carcinogenic substances, supporting the immune system, promoting apoptosis (death of cancer cells), and blocking invasion and angiogenesis.

Prevention, then, is focused on eliminating carcinogenic substances, such as avoiding the N-nitroso compounds found in processed meats, drinking alcohol in moderation, minimizing exposure to environmental toxins, losing weight if obese, and smoking, or exposure to secondary smoke. And if there is a genetic propensity toward pancreatic cancer, prevention includes making sure to have the appropriate tests and screening.

# PERITONEAL CARCINOMATOSIS

Peritoneal carcinomatosis is the spread of cancer throughout the abdominal cavity. The tumor cells may come from cancers in the abdomen or from distant sites. These patients present with abdominal distention, ascites (fluid in the abdomen), malaise, obstruction, pain, weakness, and weight loss. The most common cancer sources are ovarian, gastrointestinal, pancreatic, mesothelioma, liver, gallbladder, appendix, and even melanoma and breast cancer. Whereas this phenomenon was previously felt to be incurable and untreatable, newer therapies have been developed to palliate, and, in rare cases, cure this disease. The treatment is often a combination of therapies: treating the primary tumor, and treating the problem that has arisen (i.e., ascites, infection, and obstruction).

## ■ Diagnosis and Treatment

The diagnosis is usually made with a CT scan, an MRI, paricentesis (withdrawing ascites fluid and examining the cells), a laparoscopy, or a laparotomy if emergency surgery is needed.

Treatment may be systemic chemotherapy using the following drugs: carboplatin, cisplatin, doxorubicin, methotrexate, mitomycin-C, and paclitaxel.

Occasionally, surgical debulking of the tumor is performed to present a smaller tumor load for treatment. In some cases, intraperitoneal chemotherapy is recommended, sometimes as hyperthermic continuous intraperitoneal perfusion, or, most recently, with the placement of time-release chemotherapy-impregnated microspheres.

This disease may progress with nausea, obstruction, and pain and may require a gastrostomy (placing a drainage tube in the stomach) to drain the stomach for relief. The ascites can sometimes be relieved by diuresis (increased urine excretion), and by shunting the intra-abdominal fluid back into the bloodstream using special shunts (LeVeen and Denver shunts).

## ■ Complementary and Alternative Treatment

Complementary medicine is helpful in allaying the symptoms of nausea, pain, and inanition (lack of vigor, exhaustion). The positive effects of good nutrition, abstaining from alcohol and tobacco, and supplemental nutrients and vitamins will be of benefit.

## PROSTATE CANCER

The prostate gland is a chestnut-shaped reproductive organ that wraps around the first part of the male urethra. It is richly supplied with arteries, nerves, and veins, and produces a secretion that when added to the sperm from the testicles, is called semen. As men get older (fifty-plus years), the prostate enlarges, either from a benign disease, benign prostatic hypertrophy (BPH), or cancer, the gland tightens its grip around the urethra, making urination more difficult to start, and causing the stream to be less forceful (older men never win pissing contests). But a decrease in the urinary stream is certainly not diagnostic of prostate cancer. Cancer of the prostate is the most common cancer after skin cancer, and the second leading cause of cancer death among men (after lung cancer).

It has been said that if men live long enough, they will all develop prostate cancer, and, while this may be a bit of an exaggeration, it is true that many men are found to have foci of cancer in the prostate when examined for other reasons after an autopsy. The disease usually occurs after age sixty-five, is more common in African Americans (close to a 10 percent lifetime risk; 8 percent for American whites); it is high among Scandinavians and lowest in Japanese and other Asians. The risks are higher for those with relatives who have prostate cancer. Most prostate cancers are slow growing; however there are occasional cases that are very aggressive. More advanced prostate cancer can metastasize to bones and lymph nodes and may cause pain along with difficulty urinating.

Genetic changes are apparent in prostate cancer and the presence of BRCA1 and BRCA2 (also important in breast and ovarian cancer in woman) have been implicated in prostate cancer. Other genetic abnormalities include the loss of the tumor-suppressor genes PTEN and KAI1, P53 mutations, and the presence of cancer gene HPC1 (hereditary prostate cancer gene1), androgens, and vitamin-D receptors, and the loss of E-cadherin and CD44—all in all, a very complicated genetic system that most oncologists don't even fully understand.

The risks are higher after a vasectomy (1.85 greater risk) and lower among men with high ejaculatory frequency, and may be more common with high-fat intake and low physical activity. A number of other studies have shown increased risk with smoking, low consumption of tomato sauce, high consumption of calcium and alpha-linoleic acid; others suggested a relationship between prostatic infections (prostatitis), STDs (sexually transmitted diseases), and cancer.[8]

Research on prostate-cancer prevention has indicated that men have less incidence of cancer after receiving finasteride (Proscar), a drug to decrease the size of the prostate when urinary symptoms are severe. Other agents under study are vitamin E, selenium, and omega-3 fatty acids, found in some coldwater fish, most beneficially in wild salmon.

The disease is usually asymptomatic in the early stages, and not until later stages do symptoms of urine retention, increased frequency, decreased potency, nocturia, dribbling, anemia, and general weakness occur. At later stages, there may be enlarged lymph nodes in the groin, causing swelling of the legs and, in some cases, the spine, resulting in paralysis from spinal-cord compression.

### ▉ Diagnosis and Treatment

Cancer screening is done by digital rectal examination (DRE) and, every two years, with the PSA blood test (prostate-specific antigen)—in recent years, many cases are diagnosed at an early stage before symptoms develop. While there is no normal level for PSA that ranges from 0.1 ng/ml to 4.0 ng/ml, more attention is paid to the rate of rise of the level. There is still much controversy about when a patient should undergo a prostate biopsy, and it needs to be discussed with a urologist. The UPM-3, a newer test performed on urine directly after a rectal exam, is being used to evaluate the need for a repeat biopsy in men with elevated PSAs who have previously had negative biopsies.

Further studies include TRE (transrectal ultrasound), a CAT scan (computerized axial tomography), an MRI (magnetic resonance imaging), PAP (prostatic acid phosphatase), ultrasound, and IVP (intravenous pyelogram).

Most prostate cancer is adenocarcinoma and is staged according to two programs, the usual TNM system, the Gleason grading system, and one called the D'Amico system.

## Staging

The TNM method is used. T=Tumor, N=Node, M=Metastasis.

- T1—Tumors not palpable on rectal or transrectal ultrasound. Further subclassified a, b, c by incidental findings at TURP (transurethral resection of the prostate gland) for benign disease, and biopsy for elevated PSA

- T2—Tumors confined to the prostate. Further subclassified a–confined to one half of one lobe, b–confined to one lobe, c–confined to both lobes

- T3—Tumor extends through prostate capsule

- T4—Tumor fixed or invading adjacent structures (bladder, rectum, levator muscles)

- N1—Presence or absence of cancer in nodes

- M1—Presence of distant metastases

## Gleason Grading System

The Gleason score is a numerical method of evaluating the seriousness and extent of prostate cancer based on a pathologist's evaluation of the needle biopsy and may be variable because it is based on the pathologist's subjective interpretation of what he sees. The range is between two and ten and results from adding a primary and secondary grading (adding the results from two areas).

◇ Grade 1—Cancer resembles normal prostate tissue glands

◇ Grade 2—Many normal glands, larger cells, and a few definite changes of cancer

◇ Grade 3—Some recognizable normal glands, but many cancer cells

◇ Grade 4—Very few normal glands, mostly cancer tissue

◇ Grade 5—No normal glands, all cancerous

Adding the grades of the Gleason score together gives clinicians an idea of the seriousness of the disease and assists in determining the therapy. Very low scores may dictate no therapy, whereas high scores indicate a need for treatment. (This is a broad example and varies with age.)

Since the Gleason score is a composite of the two most common cell types described by the pathologist after several biopsies, the general rule is that any combined number below 6 is probably not treatable as cancer. Discussions with urologists support the premise that most, if not all, prostate cancers they treat are at least Gleason 6 or above. The treatment varies tremendously with age. A man of seventy-five with a Gleason score of 6 will probably not need therapy and has a low risk for dying of prostate cancer. A man in his early fifties with the same Gleason score of 6 has a much higher probability of dying from prostate cancer and thereby needs some type of treatment, or careful observation if he declines treatment. Needless to say, the treatment of prostate cancer is complex and should be discussed with a urologist, and followed up with second and third opinions.

### D'Amico System for Localized Cancer

This system assists the patient as well as the urologist. It consists of categorizing the relative risk of the disease and is stratified as low, intermediate, and high.

**Low risk:**

> PSA > 10
>
> Gleason less or equal to 10
>
> Clinical Stage T1c–T2a

**Medium Risk:**

> PSA > 10 but < 20
>
> Highest Gleason–7
>
> Clinical Stage T2b

**High Risk:**

> PSA > 20
>
> Highest Gleason equal or less than 8
>
> Clinical Stage T2c/T3

The decision about what therapy to undertake is still a hot topic of discussion between urologists, radiation therapists, oncologists, and patients. Given all the information listed above, including the patient's age and sexual activity, and the expertise and experience of the treating physicians, several options are available.

First would be just active surveillance, continuing to monitor the disease, watching for the extent and rate of progression to avoid over-treatment and its side effects. If the cancer is very slow growing, and the scores very promising, no therapy may be the choice.

More aggressive treatment includes surgery (prostatectomy), one of several types of radiation therapy, chemotherapy, cryosurgery, hormonal therapy, or a combination of the above. Most men are concerned about the loss of sexual activity, and each of these therapies has inherent risks and complications.

## Surgery

Radical prostatectomy removes the prostate gland and the seminal vesicles. There are several methods, depending on the training and expertise of the surgeon. Most modern surgeons are becoming well-versed in nerve-sparing procedures, to preserve to a certain degree the ability to have an erection and somewhat normal sexual function. The surgical procedures include:

◆ Radical perineal prostatectomy—a surgical incision is made between the base of the scrotum and the anus

◆ Radical retropubic prostatectomy—an incision in the low mid-abdomen

◆ Laparoscopic prostatectomy—with 5–6 small incisions

◆ Robotic prostatectomy—5–6 small incisions

These surgeries, which can take from two to seven hours, may also include extensive lymph-node excisions. There are also the potential complications of bleeding that may require transfusions, impotence, injury to adjacent organs, such as the bladder, rectum, and ureters, varying degrees of incontinence (loss of urine with coughing or strain-ing), and erectile dysfunction.

Unfortunately, in my personal discussion with urologists and radia-tion therapists, I do not often get a straightforward answer about sexual dysfunction, and patients are frequently reticent to discuss their inabil-ity to have intercourse after a surgical therapy. Lack of an erection, or a weak erection, can be significantly improved by the use of such drugs as sildenafil (Viagra), tadalfil (Cialis), and vardenifil (Levitra), as well as penile injection therapies, suction devices, and implanted prostheses. These serious emotional and psychosocial side effects need to be more openly addressed, but, when the decision for treatment pits one specialist against another, and when turning down multiple prostatectomy surgeries may significantly impact a urologist's ability to make a living, the patient's best interest may not be served.

### Radiation

Radiation therapy works by giving a high enough dose of radiation energy to kill cancer cells without destroying too much normal tissue.

*External beam radiation*—This delivers the radiation from outside the body and may be done in several ways. External landmarks, along with CT guidance, allows the radiation therapist to deliver the beam to a limited area. However there is always exposure to surrounding tissue.

New therapies have given the advanced capability of limiting the peripheral damage to normal tissue while focusing more selectively on the cancer.

*Conformal radiation therapy (CRT-3D)* and *Intensity modulated radiation (IMRT)* involve the complex mechanics of physics to allow more discrete focusing of the radiation.

*Proton beam irradiation*, emitting high energy radiation to a small field, is another application.

In conjunction with these therapies, the patient may receive hormonal deprivation therapy before, during, and/or after treatment to enhance the effect of the radiation.

Radiation, like surgery, does have side effects, usually related to urinary bowel and sexual function, but these are less significant than those found after surgery. The downside is that the sexual side effects may develop as long as two years after the treatment.

### Brachytherapy

This is the placement of radioactive material into or near the prostate gland. In a procedure that takes about an hour, iodine-125 or palladium-103 seeds are injected by needles through the skin of the perineum directly into the prostate gland. Patients go home the same day and have few side effects, namely a temporary burning sensation during urination, with very little effect on continence or sexual function. The seeds are left in place, and because the half-life of the radioactive material is so short (iodine–60 days, palladium–17 days), there is minimal concern about exposure. (Don't let kids sit on your lap for those few weeks.)

*High-dose-rate brachytherapy* is another modality where small temporary rods are placed through the perineum into the prostate and high doses of radiation are delivered (iridium 192), using careful CT guidance. Two or three sessions are needed and then the patient is sent home. This technique delivers the higher dose of radiation needed for larger tumors.

It is important to add that patients with metastatic disease to bone may be candidates for palliative external beam radiation therapy to the bony metastases, or, in extreme cases, intravenous administration of strontium-89 chloride (Metastron), or samarium 153 (Quadramet), both bone-seeking radioactive substances.

## High-Intensity Focused Ultrasound

This technique uses a rectal probe to heat the prostate to 185°F, destroying normal as well as cancerous prostate cells. Patients usually require a TURP (transurethral resection of the prostate) in conjunction with this procedure because of the frequent development of urethral obstruction from the heat therapy. This procedure is not permitted in the United States, except in certain clinical trials.

## Cryosurgery

This technique involves placement of small tubes into the prostate under transrectal ultrasound (TRUS), then infusing liquid nitrogen, and freezing the cancer. Although several physicians advocate this technique, there are apparently several side effects, including prolonged urinary symptoms and erectile dysfunction. Most of the time this therapy is reserved for cases of local recurrence. There is also much work being done on more focal cryosurgical techniques.

## Hormonal Therapy

Hormonal therapy attempts to obliterate the delivery of androgens (testosterone) to the prostate and over time cause prostate cancer cells to lie dormant or die. The drugs used for this are luteinizing hormone-releasing hormones—abarelix (Plenaxis), goseralin, and leu-prolide (Lupron), which has the side effect of causing cardiac prob-lems—surgical castration (removal of testicles), and the antiandrogens (bicalutamide, flutamide, nilutamide), diethylstilbestrol (DES), and ketoconazole (Nizoral). These agents are best prescribed under the aegis of an oncologist or urologist who is familiar with prostate cancer, not an internist or general practitioner.

### Chemotherapy

For prostate cancer that is resistant to the previous therapies, several chemotherapeutic regimens have been used, including mitoxantrone (Novantrone) in conjunction with the steroid prednisolone, and doc-etaxel and prednisolone. Newer therapies include the endothelial receptor antagonist atrasentan plus vitamin D (calcitrol), epidermal growth-factor-inhibitor bevacizumab (Avastin), sunitinib (Sutent), and immunotherapy (Provenge). Numerous clinical trials are underway for advanced disease and some patients may be recommended for these trials. I always recommend that patients with cancer obtain second opinions, and this should be a major priority because of the tremen-dous variation in approaches to this particular disease.

### ■ *Complementary and Alternative Treatment*

There are many alternative treatments advocated for prostate cancer and because of the desire to maintain sexual function, men may choose treatments that might not be in their best interest. These therapies should be used only after consultation with certified specialists along with Western-trained oncologists or urologists.

One of the most strongly recommended alternative therapies for the prostate is the addition of a lycopene-rich diet. Lycopene is the antioxidant that gives tomatoes, fruits, and vegetables their color; these are the carotenoids. Although diets rich in tomatoes have a definite effect in preventing cancer, their effectiveness in treating cancer of the prostate has not been well-established. And, since tomatoes also con-tain vitamins, potassium, other carotenoids, and antioxidants, the lycopene alone may not be the only active ingredient, but lycopene-rich foods are believed to help repair damaged DNA through the gene XRCC1.

Pomegranates are also helpful in preventing prostate cancer. Saw palmetto inhibits 5-alpha reductase, which converts testosterone to dihydrotestosterone, a substance that stimulates the growth of prostate cancer.

Other examples of the alternative approach to prostate cancer therapy include the following recommendations.

◇ Modified citrus pectin (MCP) interferes with the ability of the prostate-cancer cell to aggregate and inhibits cancer growth.

◇ Curcumin, a strong anti-inflammatory, will reduce swelling during therapy.

◇ Genistein, an isoflavone, acts as an antioxidant.

◇ Green tea inhibits cancer-cell growth and induces apoptosis (death of cells).

◇ Zinc, vitamins E and D, and selenium inhibit cancer-cell growth.

◇ Melatonin inhibits cancer-cell growth and potentiates the effects of chemotherapy and radiation.

In addition to direct anti-prostate-cancer effects, the following are recommended to avoid or facilitate standard care problems.

◇ Avoid products that increase bleeding, such as aspirin, ginkgo, St. John's wort, and vitamin E.

◇ Avoid alcohol.

◇ Take increased doses of vitamins A, B, C, zinc, and citrus pectin.

◇ The NIH is investigating the use of shark cartilage, plant extracts such as palmetto, and a complex combination of eight herbs, including chrysanthemum, *ganoderma lucidum, isatis, scutellania*, and saw palmetto, all said to cause prostate cancer to regress.

Most alternative practitioners recommend acupuncture, meditation, movement therapy, music and art therapy, and relaxation therapy, all modalities of great benefit while undergoing treatment for prostate cancer. And every natural cancer treatment recommends a good diet, which includes cruciferous vegetables, such as broccoli and cauliflower, fresh fruits, a reduction in saturated fats, and lycopene-containing vegetables, as discussed.

# SKIN CANCER—BASAL CELL, SQUAMOUS CELL, AND OTHERS

Twenty percent of Americans will develop skin cancer at some time in their lives and 97 percent are nonmelanoma skin cancers. These are called basal-cell and squamous-cell cancers, depending on their origin and appearance microscopically. As the adult population ages, the incidence of skin cancer increases.

## BASAL-CELL CANCER (CARCINOMA)

Basal-cell cancers are slow-growing tumors that arise from the basal cells of the skin and are the most common cancers seen in humans. They have the capacity to grow locally and after long periods may spread deeply or widely into other tissue and very rarely metastasize. Ultraviolet radiation (UVR) is felt to be the major inciting cause and light-skinned individuals are more prone to the disease. People who were exposed to atomic radiation have a high incidence of these skin cancers, as well as those with familial genetic tendency. UVR damages the DNA, and cumulative damage causes mutations and cancer. People with immune suppression from diseases (such as advanced age, AIDS, any other form of cancer, chronic disease, living at high altitude with increased sun exposure, organ transplantation, or x-ray treatment for acne) are more prone to develop skin cancers, and men are more prone than women. Avoidance of direct sunlight, protective clothing, and topical sunscreen with high SPF levels are the greatest deterrents to this cancer that can develop many decades after continued exposure occurs. Beachgoers and those who opt for tanning-salon tans in their teens and twenties may start to see skin cancer in a few years, or many years later. It is usually found on the areas of the body most exposed to sun—the face, arms, and neck.

These cancers present in many guises, usually as a small lump, frequently thought of as a pimple, with a raised center and skin-colored, dark or red pigmentation. A superficial form may appear pink and scaly and mimic psoriasis or eczema, but it is rarely itchy, and a nodular form may ulcerate as it grows.

## ■ *Diagnosis and Treatment*

Because this cancer mimics other diseases, a diagnosis can only truly be made by a biopsy. At this juncture it is important to understand there are several acceptable surgical methods for removal of this lesion. Since the skin is involved, local anesthetics are used—as a surgeon, I prefer excising the entire tumor with a very small margin of clear skin, then suturing it in a plastic fashion. This results in complete cure in 98 percent of the cases. Other methods include shaving the surface and/or an incisional biopsy (cutting out only part of the lesion to make a diagnosis), and the Mohs method of micrographic surgery, which is more time-consuming, more expensive, and rarely indicated unless the lesion is on the nose or eyelid.

Further modes of treatment include laser therapy (another form of cutting) for lesions that may be bloodier, and cryosurgery, using liquid nitrogen that eliminates the lesion without getting a pathological diagnosis. Some dermatologists make it a practice of freezing or lasering lesions, stating they are treating cancer, without having a definitive diagnosis, or telling the patient, "You have skin cancer and it must be treated."

There is curettage with and without electrodessication, a treatment method for nonaggressive small basal-cell cancers. Since skin cancer cells are not as strong and cohesive as normal nonmalignant skin cells, this method may be a viable treatment method that removes only the skin cancer while the normal skin stays intact. The treated area appears like a circular scab that can resemble a cigar burn. The cure rate for appropriately selected small nonaggressive basal-cell cancers is between 90–95 percent, depending on the technique of the surgeon.

There is chemotherapy (5-FU-5 fluorouracil cream) that causes an inflammatory reaction, which destroys the tumor. The skin eventually heals, but frequently with a scar or without complete obliteration of the tumor, requiring further treatment. This method is often used to avoid scars on the face of individuals with many tumors. Along with the 5-FU, imiquimod and aldara are effective chemotherapeutic topical creams.

Radiation is occasionally used for patients over fifty (younger patients exposed may be prone to develop other cancers), or those with large tumors.

Immunotherapy using *Euphorbia peplus* (garden weed) may be

effective, and photodynamic therapy, with methyl aminolevulinate as a photosensitizer, is used in Europe.

### ■ Complementary and Alternative Treatment

Prevention and avoidance are the best methods to use and it's advisable to avoid the primary contributing factors to this type of cancer. These include ultraviolet radiation (UVR) that damages the DNA, x-ray treatments for acne, and overexposure to harmful rays of the sun.

There are a few alternative modes of treating skin cancer, predominately diet and nutritional supplements, although nutritional therapy is not generally recommended as a cure for skin cancer. A suggested healthy diet for preventing skin cancer is one rich in fresh fruits and vegetables, antioxidant foods, such as carrots, cruciferous vegetables, potatoes, green tea, and citrus fruits. Supplements mentioned are vitamins B, C, and E, selenium, and beta carotene, grapeseed extract, and evening primrose.

The use of 5-FU crème as a chemotherapeutic agent may be considered complementary medicine by some. Chinese practitioners use acupuncture to relieve cancer symptoms and reduce pain levels, or to ease chemotherapy-related nausea and vomiting.

Herbs should not be used to treat skin cancer once it has developed. A number of herbs, such as ginkgo biloba, hawthorn, milk thistle, and the polyphenols found in green tea, may have skin-protective and antioxidant properties, but some of these interfere with conventional cancer treatments and should not be used without consulting a physician.

## SQUAMOUS-CELL CANCER (CARCINOMA)

Less common than basal-cell cancers, squamous-cell cancers are, however, more malignant, with increased risk for spreading locally, and certain types have the potential for distant metastases. The name squamous comes from the Latin word *squama* meaning fish scale because the cells, which originate in the middle and upper layers of the skin, often have a flat scaly appearance. The squamous-cell cancer that is only superficial may be called Bowen's disease and these cells are noninvasive. The seriousness of the cancer depends on the pathologist's evaluation as to the depth of invasion and the nature of the cells, i.e., how differentiated (different) the cancer cells appear from normal skin cells. Those that look very little like normal cells are called poorly differentiated and have a higher incidence of local and distant spread.

Squamous-cell cancers have the same causes as basal-cell cancers. Individuals exposed to UV radiation may first develop a reddish, angry-looking skin lesion called actinic keratosis that is often difficult to distinguish from cancer and that may progress to squamous-cell cancer. Patients with cancer, HIV, or those who have immuno-suppression from chemotherapy or radiation, are more prone to developing this cancer. This slow-growing skin cancer, though more common in exposed areas, such as the face, nose, lip, scalp, and back of hand, can also be found anywhere on the body.

The cancer usually appears as a scaly, slightly raised, reddish lesion with recurring irritation from rubbing or scratching. As the lesions grow, the edges become raised and turned inside out, and the central portions ulcerate and present with a rugged base. They often have bleeding and can develop secondary infections.

## ■ Diagnosis and Treatment

When this cancer spreads, it may invade locally or spread to regional lymph nodes, so a complete exam of surrounding tissue and a drain of lymph node areas must be done. Sometimes very small cancers can spread locally and distally.

The treatment, similar to that of basal-cell cancers, is preferably a complete removal with a small margin of normal tissue to insure that it is completely removed. Recurrent squamous-cell cancers may need more surgery, or, in certain cases, radiation therapy.

In individuals with extensive cancers of the scalp, or people who cannot tolerate surgery, focal and local radiation may be the best choice. In cases where the cancer has spread locally, wide excisions of the skin, surrounding tissue, and underlying muscle are indicated, unless severe deformity (as on the face) precludes this treatment. In those cases, radiation may be an option.

When the cancer has spread to the lymph nodes, excisional biopsy of the nodes followed by radiation is usually indicated. Depending on the extent, location, and age of the patient, this is, in turn, followed by some type of systemic chemotherapy.

While rare, metastasis of squamous-cell cancers to other parts of the body do occur and present difficult treatment options. Solitary or multiple metastatic lesions may be removed surgically if they are in feasible, accessible locations, such as the brain, liver, or lungs.

When seeing a surgeon or dermatologist, it is important to stress that both basal-cell and squamous-cell carcinomas, while they have many distinctive characteristics, are definitively diagnosed by pathological examination. While it may be the custom of some physicians to remove lesions by freezing, lasers, or cauterization without a pathological diagnosis, this is not always a standard of practice that should be accepted. When you have a skin lesion, be sure to ask whether the specimen, when removed, has been examined by a pathologist or someone with pathology training, ask for the report, and make sure that what you had was truly a cancer. Skin lesions should not become an annuity for physicians. Many lesions need not have extensive surgery and might best be treated conservatively, especially if similar lesions have been excised and shown to be nonmalignant.

### ■ *Complementary and Alternative Treatment*

Prevention is important and is the same as with basal-cell cancers: avoidance of UV radiation, covering exposed areas, and staying out of bright sun. Many individuals who work outside at manual labor and have recurring sores or skin injuries may be at increased risk for squamous-cell cancers. Chronic scarring, irritation, and prolonged skin irritation by chemicals are also increased risks.

The alternative treatments are the same as those listed above for basal-cell carcinomas.

## MERKEL CELL CARCINOMA

This rather rare tumor is a very aggressive, fast-growing cancer of the skin that derives from what is called neural crest origin. Though not specifically related to UV radiation, there is an increased incidence with immunosuppressive diseases, such as HIV, chemotherapy, and in patients with other malignancies. These cancers usually occur in the sixty to eighty-year-old group and have a nasty habit of spreading locally to lymph nodes and metastasizing, so they need to be excised widely. Sentinel lymph-node biopsies must be done and radical node dissection may be indicated. Radiation therapy and systemic therapy with chemotherapeutic agents has been of limited success using such drugs as carboplatin, cisplatin, cytoxan, doxorubicin, and etoposide. The prognosis is poor for metastatic disease and most do not respond well to treatment. There are no recommended alternative treatments except, as with all cancers, to help keep the immune system strong.

## OTHER, RARER MALIGNANCIES OF THE SKIN

There are several relatively obscure cancers with long complex names that are included for the sake of completeness. They include atypical fibroxanthoma, malignant fibrous histiocytoma, microcystic adnexal carcinoma, sebaceous carcinoma, and dermatofibrosarcoma protuberans (a mouthful, to be sure). These all need to be widely excised and further therapy may be indicated.

Angiosarcoma, a cancer of the blood vessels in the skin, is an aggressive and often fatal disease that does not usually respond to treatment, even after complete local excision.

Kaposi's sarcoma is an indolent skin cancer usually associated with HIV/AIDS, and sometimes with the herpes virus. It may also be categorized as iatrogenic (inadvertantly induced by a physician or surgeon, by medical treatment, or by diagnostic procedures). Endemic African Kaposi's sarcoma is common in parts of Africa and is one of the most widespread types of cancer in that region. It may occur in Ashkenazi men or persons of Mediterranean descent and appears as a purplish lesion that may become raised and nodular. The treatment usually depends on the stage: I—locally indolent, II—locally invasive, III—disseminated, and IV—systemic. Early stages may respond to complete excision, while later stages need treatment with interferon and chemotherapy.

Some cancers in other organs may spread to the skin. They are called carcinomas metastatic to skin and may be the first indication there is cancer elsewhere in the body, so identification and tissue diagnosis may lead to treatment of the primary cancer. Cancers that may spread to the skin include kidney, lung, and ovary, and leukemias and lymphomas can spread from other skin cancers. The best known skin manifestation of an internal cancer is called the Sister Mary Joseph nodule where cancer is found at the umbilicus (bellybutton) in some patients with stomach cancer. (Sister Mary Joseph was a surgical assistant to the famous physician Dr. Henry Mayo.)

## SMALL INTESTINE CANCER

The small intestine is that part of the gastrointestinal tract between the stomach and the colon, beginning with the duodenum, then the jejunum and the ileum. Primary cancer of the small intestine is very rare, but many malignancies in other areas can involve the small intestine and often need to be addressed because of the symptoms of pain, obstruction, or bleeding they present. The small intestine is fifteen to twenty feet long, accounting for more than 75 percent of the gastrointestinal system and 90 percent of the surface area of the intestines. The function of this intestine is the further breakdown and digestion of food, and absorbing minerals, vitamins, and other nutrients. Yet, oddly enough, cancer of the small intestine is very rare (2 percent of gastrointestinal tumors) when you consider the small size of the colon and the much higher incidence of cancer there—cancer of the colon is fifty times more common.

The reason for the low incidence of malignancy in the small intestine is felt to be related to the following facts.

◇ The pH of the liquid in the small intestine is neutral to very alkaline; an acid milieu is more conducive for carcinogens to act.

◇ The contents are liquid, flowing through very quickly; the mucosa have less exposure to carcinogens.

◇ Bacterial content is less anaerobic, causing less degradation of bowel salts that may have a effect on cancer development.

◇ The small bowel has a high level of lymph nodes, lymph system, and immunoglobulin A that may prevent cancer formation.

◇ There is a high level of benzopyrene hydroxylase, an enzyme that breaks down the cancer-causing substance benzopyrene (a common food additive).

◇ There are fewer stem cells that would lend themselves to attack by carcinogens.

There are four major types of primary small bowel cancer

1 Adenocarcinoma, which arises from the inner lining or mucosa of the bowel. This usually occurs in men fifty to seventy and most tumors are advanced stage when diagnosed.

**2** Sarcoma (leiomyosarcoma) and GIST (gastrointestinal stromal tumors), which arise from the muscle wall layer of the intestine.

**3** Carcinoid, which starts in the hormone-producing cells.

**4** Lymphoma, which starts in the lymph tissue of the bowel and can be subclassified into diffuse large B-cell lymphoma, MALT lymphoma, Burkitt's lymphoma, and peripheral T-cell lymphoma.

The other small intestinal cancers, much more common than those previously mentioned, are the metastatic cancers from other areas of the body. Common areas are the breast, colon, liver, ovaries, pancreas, and stomach.

The causes of small-intestine cancer remain unknown, although certain conditions increase the risk. These include immunodeficiency diseases like AIDS, celiac disease, Crohn's disease (an inflammation of the small intestine), Gardner's syndrome, neurofibromatosis, and Peutz-Jegher syndrome, plus alcohol abuse, hereditary multiple polyposis, smoking, and certain foods with heterocyclic amines (fried bacon, ham, smoked, and barbecued meat and fish).

## ■ *Diagnosis and Treatment*

Symptoms do not develop until late in the disease, unfortunately, and diagnosis is often delayed for several months because of the vagueness of the symptoms. These may include bleeding, bowel obstruction and even perforation, nausea, pain, and weight loss. Although there are several classical findings on a barium study called enteroclysis, as well as on CT scans, more than half the cancers are missed on these tests. Endoscopy is often not effective because the scopes cannot go that far down the intestine, and a capsule endoscopy (having the patient swallow a tiny camera that photographs the inner wall of the intestine as it passes) has been of limited success. Rarely, a colonoscopy can extend into the last portion of the small bowel (ileum) to make the diagnosis, and, likewise, an upper endoscopy can advance to the first portion of the intestine (the duodenum), but diagnosis is often left to a high index of suspicion and after ruling out cancer in other areas of the GI tract.

Most times the diagnosis is made at surgery when the pathologist gets the specimen and examines it under the microscope.

**Staging**

The staging of small-intestinal cancer is: T=Tumor, N=Nodes, M=Metastasis.

- T1a—Invades lamina propria—N0–No spread to lymph nodes—M0–No metastases
- T1b-Invades submucosa—N1–1–3 nodes with cancer—M1–Metastasis
- T2—Invades muscularis propria—N2–4 or more nodes with cancer
- T3—Invades through wall into mesentery and retroperitoneum
- T4—Perforates the wall and invades nearby structures
- I—T1–T2, N0, M0
- IIA—T3, N0, M0
- IIB—T4, N0, M0
- IIIA—N1, N0, M0
- IIIB—N2, N0, M0
- IV—Any T or N, M1

Surgery is the main treatment for these cancers, removing the involved segment of intestine and connecting the rest back together (using surgical stapling devices). Sometimes, when the disease is extensive, bypass procedures may be done to alleviate obstruction as a palliation to prevent pain and allow the patient to eat. Sometimes there is so much cancer that extensive lengths of bowel must be removed, and, if intestinal continuity cannot be reestablished, then the proximal intestine has to be brought out to the skin as a permanent ileostomy.

Chemotherapy is of limited use, predominately with lymphomas that respond well to this treatment. There are too few studies on this rare cancer to adequately judge the effectiveness of the usual gastrointestinal regimens with 5-FU, irinotecan, and oxaliplatin. Similarly, radiation therapy has very little role in treatment of this cancer. Interferon has been used in a few cases with limited success.

## ■ Complementary and Alternative Treatment

Alternative and complementary medicines are of limited value with this rare cancer, except to offer palliation for the side effects of other therapy, or to enhance the general health and nutrition of the patient.

## SOFT-TISSUE SARCOMAS

Soft-tissue sarcomas are a diverse group of cancers that occur in the soft tissues throughout the body and represent less than 1 percent of all newly diagnosed cancers. More common in the extremities, these rare tumors are also found in the abdomen and chest. Small, early diagnosed tumors are often highly curable, whereas the larger cancers are often difficult to manage, with frequent recurrences, repeat surgeries, and innovative therapies. The two forms involving bony tissue are covered under bone tumors.

Regrettably, many of these tumors remain asymptomatic in their early stages, often appearing as soft, painless masses that are initially ignored. They can grow very rapidly and often become difficult to manage because of their size or the involvement of adjacent tissue, or even distant metastases. They can develop from fat, muscle, fibrous, nerve, or deep skin tissues, as well as from blood vessels, and they take the name of their tissue of origin as delineated in the following.

◇ Dermatofibrosarcoma—From tissue under skin in trunk and limbs

◇ Gastrointestinal stromal tumor (GIST)—From stomach and intestines

◇ Hemangiosarcoma—From blood vessels

◇ Kaposi's sarcoma (*see* chapter on AIDS and cancer)

◇ Leiomyosarcoma—From smooth muscle (uterus, stomach, intestinal tract or the lining of blood vessels)

◇ Liposarcoma—From fatty tissue in the legs or abdomen

◇ Lymphangiosarcoma—From lymph vessels

◇ Malignant fibrous histiocytoma—From fibrous tissue usually in the legs

◇ Malignant mesenchymoma—From connective tissue

◇ Neurofibrosarcoma—Around peripheral nerves

◇ Rhabdomyosarcoma—From skeletal muscles in the arms and legs

While the general etiology is unknown, except for Kaposi's related to AIDS, there is a higher incidence related to previous radiation for malignancy, and it is postulated that there is a hereditary basis for some sarcomas with the following unusual syndromes: Li-Fraumeni, Gardner's, neurofibromatosis, retinoblastoma, tuberous sclerosis, and Werner's syndrome. Chemical exposure to dioxin, certain herbicides (phenoxys), vinyl chloride (substance in PVCs), wood preservatives (chlorophenols), and agent orange (during the Viet Nam conflict), have been implicated in increasing the risk for sarcomas. Soft-tissue sarcomas have been reported after exposure to certain chemotherapeutic drugs, including chlorambucil, cyclophosphamide, melphalan, nitrosureas, and procarbazine. Chronic swelling of the legs (lymphedema) has been implicated, and even trauma and foreign bodies have been suggested, although no direct causal relationship has been proved.

## ■ *Diagnosis and Treatment*

As the tumor grows, it generally pushes adjacent tissue aside, eventually causing discomfort. In the abdomen, symptoms may mimic indigestion, constipation, or menstrual cramps. In the arms and legs, eventual pressure on the nerves and muscles will cause soreness, and the tumor will be brought to the attention of a physician. At this juncture, tests will be taken to determine the characteristic, extent, and diagnosis. These include an MRI (magnetic resonance imaging), a CT scan (computer axial tomography), x-rays, and needle or open biopsies.

### Staging

The staging of these cancers is complex but has been simplified in the Mayo clinic discussion below.

* Stage I—Tumors < 5 cm where the cells appear normal (like tissue of origin), and without a spread to lymph nodes or distant sites.

* Stage II—Tumors larger (often over 5 cm) with cells that begin to look abnormal but still have no spread to nodes or distally

* Stage III—Cells look more abnormal and also have spread to lymph nodes.

* Stage IV—Cells are severely abnormal and cancer is found in lymph nodes and other parts of the body

Surgery is the most common treatment for sarcomas, with an attempt to remove the entire cancer, along with a small amount of normal surrounding tissue. Sampling or removal of adjacent lymph nodes may be indicated in staging and treatment of the disease. In some cases this may involve radical surgery, including amputation. If the tumor has spread, attempts may be made to remove the metastases in a procedure called metastasectomy. In some cases, neoadjuvant (treatment before surgery) chemotherapy and radiation therapy may be used.

Additionally, after surgical removal, these cases are often discussed at tumor conferences and decisions are made about whether postoperative chemotherapy and radiation therapy are indicated, but the truth is, these cancers are not very responsive to chemotherapy and only poorly responsive to radiation. Newer drugs, such as bevacizumab as an anti-angiogenesis drug and imatinib (Gleevac) for GIST, have been studied and used, but with limited success. Chemotherapy for unresectable advanced or metastatic disease may also include dacarbazine, doxorubicin, ecteinascidin, gemcitabine, ifosfamide, mesna, and combined therapies with these drugs.

A number of clinical trials are in progress and patients with advanced disease should inquire about joining these studies. They include high-dose chemotherapy, stem-cell transplant, targeted therapy against epidermal growth factor (EGFR), and many other complex new therapies that can be reviewed through the NCI (National Cancer Institute) of the NIH (National Institutes of Health).

### ■ Complementary and Alternative Treatment

The side effects of therapy may include hair loss, increased risk for infection, mouth sores, nausea, vomiting, and weakness. Many of these can be treated with standard, as well as complementary, medicine therapies. Many traditional Chinese and Ayurvedic treatments are offered in conjunction with standard Western medical management.

## STOMACH CANCER

Stomach, or gastric, cancer is a classic example of the dietary and environmental impact on cancer. The disease, relatively uncommon in the United States, is the number one cancer in China and is very common in Japan and Korea. This is associated with the Eastern dietary habit of a low consumption of vegetables and fruit, and a high intake of nitrites, salts, smoked and pickled fish, and other similar foods. When an Asian-born individual moves to the United States, if the diet changes, her/his risk decreases sharply over five to ten years, eventually reaching that of the Westerner.

Exposure to coal mining and the processing of rubber, nickel, timber, and tobacco smoke also increase the risk for this disease. And those with a family history of stomach cancer have a higher incidence of developing the disease.

Stomach cancer is attributable to changes or abnormalities in the tumor-suppressor gene TP53, and overexpression, or mutation, in the oncogenes Her-2/neu and c-Ki-ras, or a mutation in the E-cahedrin gene. A substance called cyclo-oxygenase 2 (COX-2) has been implicated in gastric cancers by causing immune suppression, stimulating blood-vessel growth for tumors (angiogenesis), inhibition of natural cell-death occurrence (apoptosis), and increasing invasion and metastatic potential. This is the basis for the use of COX-2 inhibitors in the prevention and treatment of stomach cancers (and other gastrointestinal malignancies). The bacteria helicobacter pylori (H pylori) is believed responsible for many cases of stomach cancer.

Most gastric cancers occur in people between ages sixty-five to seventy-five; twice as many are men and there is a higher mortality rate among the men; among African Americans, it is twice as common. Only 20 percent of the patients present with localized disease and therefore the five-year survival rate for all stages combined is only 25 percent. Oddly enough, the disease is more common in individuals with blood type A and in patients who have a family member with stomach cancer.

Most gastric cancers are discovered at an advanced stage with vague symptoms—decreased appetite (especially for meat), indigestion, nausea, occasional abdominal pain, occasional vomiting, and weight loss. A few patients vomit up blood. There may be a bloating sensation, and blood in the stool appearing black (a tarry stool), fatigue, and weakness.

### ■ Diagnosis and Treatment

Since the disease is so common in Asia, the Japanese and Koreans have instituted screening for the disease, and this has accounted for a significant improvement in the survival rates compared to the United States. Because of the low incidence of the disease in Western countries, routine screening is not practiced.

The definitive diagnosis is made by endoscopy or barium swallow x-ray. Further evaluation of the extent of the disease is accomplished with CT scans, endoscopic ultrasound, a bone scan, and a PET scan, the latter to show distant metastatic disease. Prior to definitive surgery, many surgeons prefer to do a laparoscopy, looking through a small incision into the abdomen with a scope to evaluate the extent of the disease. Often, even with negative or limited findings on an x-ray, endoscopy, laparoscopy, or scans, the patient may turn out to have extensive disease and that would preclude any major surgical intervention.

Adenocarcinoma tumors arise from the gastric glands that contain mucous and they account for more than 95 percent of stomach cancer. Other cancers include carcinoids, lymphoma, small-cell cancer, and squamous-cell cancer. An interesting tumor called GIST (gastrointestinal stromal tumors), arising from the interstitial cells of Cajal in the stomach, have mutations in the C-KIT or PDGFR genes. Blood studies on patients with stomach cancer who have high levels of VEGF (vascular endothelial growth factor) and CEA (carcinoembryonic antigen) usually predict a poor prognosis after surgery.

## Staging

The staging of gastric cancer uses the TNM system. T=Tumor, N=Node, M=Metastasis.

### Tumor

- T0—No evidence of primary tumor

- Tis—Carcinoma in situ–No invasion of the lamina propria (superficial layer)

- T1—Tumor invades the lamina propria or mucosa

- T2a—Tumor invades the muscularis propria

- T2b—Tumor invades the subserosa

- T3—Tumor invades through the serosa

- T4—Tumor invades adjacent structures

### Lymph Nodes

- N0—No nodes with tumor
- N1—Cancer in 1–6 nodes
- N2—Cancer in 7–15 nodes
- N3—Cancer in > 15 nodes

### Metastasis

- M0—No metastasis
- M1—Metastasis

### Stage—Five-Year Survival Treatment

- 0 Tis, N0, M0, 90 percent

### Surgery

- IA T1, N0, M0, 00 percent

### Surgery

- IB T1, N1, M0, 00 percent

### Surgery and Chemo-Radiation

- T2a/b, N0, M0
- II T1, N2, M0, 00 percent

### Surgery and Chemo-Radiation

- T2a/b, N1, M0
- T3, N0, M0
- IIIA T2a/b, N2, M0, 20 percent

### Surgery and Chemo-Radiation

- T3, N1, M0
- T4, N0, M0
- IIIB T3, N2, M0, 10 percent

### Preoperative Radiation Then Surgery and Chemo-Radiation

- IV T4, N1–2, M0, 5 percent

### Palliative Chemotherapy

- Any T, N3, M0

### Possible Surgery, Radiation

- Any T, Any N, M1

As seen above, the treatment is based on the stage of the disease. Sometimes there is no evidence of distant spread, but the cancer is locally invading several important structures, making curative surgery impossible. Other cases may employ surgery to bypass an obstruction, even though there is no possibility for cure, in order to palliate the symptoms and allow the patient to eat and avoid obstruction.

#### Surgery

The various conventional types of surgical approaches are: Total gastrectomy (removing the entire stomach), subtotal gastrectomy (removing the proximal or distal stomach), liver resection (removing an adjacent portion of the liver to which a cancer is attached, or removing a single, or several, metastatic tumors), HIPEC (hyperthermic intra-peritoneal chemo-perfusion), and radiofrequency ablation (destroying cancer with a radiofrequency probe).

Standard surgery involves removing varying amounts of the stomach and then reconnecting the gastrointestinal tract by one of several methods. This may involve making a partial pouch from the intestines and connecting this with the esophagus, or reconnecting one segment of the remaining stomach with another, or with the duodenum, the first part of the small intestine just after the stomach. For some very early cancers, the Japanese have been using endoscopic mucosal resection, removing just the inner lining of the stomach in a much simpler and better tolerated procedure. This is more feasible in Japan where early diagnosis and lower-stage disease is more common than in the West.

After stomach surgery, patients often have iron-deficiency anemia and need vitamin $B_{12}$ and iron supplements. They may have upset stomach (gastritis after partial removal) because of bile or intestinal secretions backing up into the esophagus and may need antacids, such as Mylanta, Maalox, or Riopan; they may need Carafate to coat the stomach. If the distal stomach is left in and the patient still produces acid, an acid blocker (H-2 blocker) will be needed, such as Prilosec or Zantac.

The dumping syndrome can occur after stomach surgery, when food passes too quickly into the intestine after part or most of the stomach has been removed. It is characterized by dizziness, fast pulse, nausea, vomiting, and weakness and usually goes away on its own, but it can be treated by taking in fewer carbohydrates, eating smaller meals, and avoiding chocolate.

Cancer support groups are helpful for the patient as well as the family, and most major hospitals and medical centers have trained therapists to assist patients and family through every stage of the cancer diagnosis and treatment.

## Chemotherapy

With gastric cancer, oncologists use combination therapy involving several drugs. There are several newer regimens—DCF (docetaxel, cisplatin, and 5-FU), ECF (epirubicin, cisplatin, and 5-FU)—the older regimens include FAMTX (5-FU, doxorubicin, and methotrexate) and MCF (mitomycin, cisplatin, and 5-FU).

Newer agents and protocols are always coming out. Most recent regimens use adriamycin, BCNU (carmustine), fluoropyrimidine, methyl-CCNU (semustine), and taxotere. In patients who test positive for overexpression of the gene HER2, trastuzumab (Herceptin) has been used along with chemotherapy. Molecular profiling of the tumor helps the oncologist decide upon the therapy. Other procedures involve intra-arterial chemotherapy (injection of drugs directly into the artery supplying the cancer) and chemo-embolization.

## ■ *Complementary and Alternative Treatment*

Several approaches are used to offset the side effects of standard chemotherapy, surgery, and radiation therapy. Chemotherapy kills cells that have the high rate of cell division seen in cancer. Unfortunately, other *normal* cells with a high rate of turnover, such as blood-cell producers in the bone marrow, hair, and gastrointestinal tract, and mucosa (lining of mouth and vagina) may also be affected. The side effects here are anemia from decreased blood production, bleeding, dysphagia (difficulty swallowing), gastrointestinal symptoms, such as nausea and vomiting, hand-foot syndrome (tingling pain and numbness in hands and feet), hair loss, loss of appetite, and ulcerations in the mouth and vagina, all of which lead to depression, emotional problems, and fatigue.

The dysphagia can be helped by taking supplements in protein shakes, puddings, and applesauce, along with a number of homeopathic remedies, vitamins, and minerals. Acupuncture and acupressure has been effective in decreasing nausea, along with ginger products. The pain is alleviated with intravenous and oral medications as well as hot packs and hydrotherapy. Naturopathic regimens are often helpful: mouth sores can be treated with L-glutamine powder in water or mixed with baking soda, diarrhea responds to charcoal capsules, and L-glutamine, the B-vitamins, and topical lotions are recommended for hand-foot syndrome.

Traditional Chinese medicine (TCM) strongly recommends soybeans and soy products (one of the five sacred foods in China), along with garlic, ginger, and sesame. Green tea contains catechins that are considered strong anticancer substances. Other traditional Chinese foods recommended for cancer patients are carrots, cauliflower, kelp, and shiitake mushrooms.

In view of the high incidence of gastric cancer in Asia, several dietary regimens are recommended (along with conventional treatment) to inhibit progression of the cancer and relieve the symptoms. A popular herbal medicine, Zooncan, contains *sarcandrae;* most Chinese formulae contain six to twelve herbs. A number of studies have found success using fu-zhen therapy for immune-compromised conditions. Nearly all the traditional Chinese medicines used today are tonic herbs stimulating the immune system, toxin-clearing herbs clearing waste and toxins, and blood-activating herbs that reduce inflammatory reactions. Kampo, the Japanese version of Chinese herbal medicine has many herbal recommendations, including tai chi and other behavioral techniques.

Ayurvedic herbs include isatis leaf for reducing inflammation, triphala that contains antioxidants, and turmeric for irritable bowel syndrome—all three are used at Memorial Sloan-Kettering.

General recommendations for patients with stomach cancer include black cohosh, chamomile, dong quai, echinacea, garlic, ginkgo biloba, ginseng, St. John's wort, and yohimbe.

Before, during, and after standard Western treatment, and in consultation with his oncologist, the patient with gastric cancer may want to consult with a complementary care doctor to enhance his treatment and recovery.

## TESTICULAR CANCER

Cancer of the testicle is the most commonly occurring malignancy in young men ranging from fifteen to thirty-five years old. The disease has caught the public eye because of such notables as cyclist Lance Armstrong and many other internationally recognized sportsmen, businessmen, and politicians who have made their experience with the cancer public knowledge. This open approach to a once *closet* disease has led to early diagnosis and successful treatment of a once-devastating cancer, with cure rates, depending on the stage, between 90 and 100 percent. Even in cases where the cancer has spread to distant organs, such as the liver or brain, cure rates of well over 80–90 percent have been achieved. Testicular cancer is more common in Caucasian than African Americans, but the disease is usually more severe in blacks and Asians, with Scandinavians having the lowest incidence.

These cancers are placed under the heading of germ-cell tumors (seminomas), meaning they originate from cells that have the ability to form other reproductive cells. Most testicular cancers are seminomas, the focus of this section, and the very rare few that remain are non-seminomas, which include embryonal carcinomas, teratomas, trophoblastic tumors, yolk sac tumors, and about a dozen more obscure cancers.

This disease is more often found in individuals with an incomplete or undescended testicle (cryptorchidism), a family history of this cancer, exposure to DES (diethylstilbesterol) in utero, individuals who have Klinefelter syndrome (47,XXY genetic abnormality), and Down syndrome. Technically, many patients have an isochromosome 12p on chromosome 12, and testicular-cancer cells are often triploid and have too many chromosomes.

The first signs of this disease are swelling of the testis, or a lump identified by the patient on self-examination. The lump may not be painful, but there may occasionally be sharp shooting pain or achiness and heaviness in the scrotum. There may also be blood in the scrotum in a sac (hematocele), distended vein (varicocele), or inflammation of the testicle (epididymitis). With more advanced disease, gynecomastia (enlargement of the male breast) may occur. Aside from the scrotal mass, some patients present with a scrotal hydrocele (fluid-filled mass), which in and of itself is a benign finding. When this disease is more advanced, there may be enlarged lymph nodes or symptoms relative to the area where the cancer has spread—for bones, bone pain; for the brain, neurological disorders; for lungs, a shortness of breath.

### ■ *Diagnosis and Treatment*

Diagnosis is made by digital exam—an ultrasound can determine the size, location, and characteristics of the cancer. Once a diagnosis has been made, a CAT scan of the abdomen and pelvis (computerized axial tomography) will also be necessary to determine whether cancer has spread beyond the scrotum, as well as a routine chest x-ray and CT scan of the chest, plus a possible PET scan (positron emission tomography).

Several serum-tumor markers, including AFP (alpha-fetoprotein), BHCG (beta-human chorionic gonadotrophin), and LDH (lactic dehydrogenase), are helpful in making the diagnosis. Needle biopsy of a testicular mass is not recommended, and, if a cancer is suspected, the surgeon must remove the entire testicle through a groin incision. It may seem a radical way to make a definitive diagnosis, but using a needle biopsy has a high incidence of spreading the cancer to the scrotum or systemically. Cutting into the scrotum itself is contraindicated.

### Staging

The staging system for testicular cancer uses the TNM system. T=Tumor, N=Nodes, M=Distant Metastases.

Depending on the text and source, it can be very complicated, so to make it as simple as possible, I have limited it to four stages adapted from the Royal Marsden System.

- Stage I—Cancer is localized to the testicle

- Stage II—Cancer involves the testicle and has spread to lymph nodes in the abdomen below the diaphragm

- Stage III—Cancer involves testicle and lymph nodes above and below the diaphragm

- Stage IV—Cancer has metastasized to other organs—liver, lungs, brain, bone

The three basic types of treatment for testicular cancer are surgery, with or without radical lymph node dissection, chemotherapy, and radiation therapy.

## Surgery

A radical orchiectomy consists of removal of the testicle as well as the spermatic cord, extending the dissection into the retroperitoneum (back of the lower abdomen). In certain cases, especially nonseminomatous cancers, an extensive lymph-node dissection may be undertaken. Surgeons regularly attempt to perform nerve-sparing surgery that requires special technical ability so the patient can continue to have good ejaculatory function. In the hands of well-trained surgeons, these sympathetic nerve plexuses can be preserved during complex surgeries.

Only one testis is needed for adequate hormone production, to maintain sexual function and fertility. The radical orchiectomy may be all that is needed for the cure of stage I disease, and, in many centers, further treatment is deferred pending evidence of a recurrence of the disease.

## Radiation

Radiation therapy is used to treat some Stage I and most Stage II seminomas. Seminomas are very sensitive to radiation, and, because the spread up the abdominal para-aortic retroperitoneal lymphatic chain is so predictable, the direction and total dosages used are low and the success rates very high.

The side effects of radiation are nausea and vomiting, occasionally diarrhea. Because of the effects of scatter radiation on the remaining testicle, the recommendation is made for the individual who wants to have children to store his sperm before the treatment, since there might be an absence of sperm production from the remaining testicle for up to a year. The testicle usually recovers and can eventually produce normal sperm.

## Chemotherapy

Chemotherapy is becoming more popular as an alternative to radiation therapy for seminomas, and one or two doses of carboplatin appear to have the same success rates as the radiation. Recurrences are treated with all three modalities, surgery to remove to recurrence, radiation to the area, and another regimen of chemotherapy, with excellent results.

The handling of the nonseminomatous testicular cancers are more difficult and often require combination radiotherapy and chemotherapeutic regimens that include bleomycin, cisplatin, etoposide, ifosfamide, mesna, paclitaxil, and other compounds.

The unpleasant side effects of chemotherapy can include myelosuppression (effect on bone marrow) from ifosfamide causing anemia, nephrotoxicity (kidney damage) from cisplatin, neutropenia (decreased white blood cells) and a related fever, thrombocytopenia (decreased platelets and bleeding problems), all of which require special drugs and are a good place for complementary medical therapies. There may be severe effects on the lungs from bleomycin, peripheral neuropathy, vinblastine, and hearing problems from cisplatin. Delayed toxicities include other cancers, heart disease, Raynaud's phenomenon (cold extremities), sarcoidosis, and of course infertility.

### ■ Complementary and Alternative Treatment

The efficacy of herbs and supplements in warding off some of the toxic side effects of the therapies for testicular cancer is well known. Glutathione reduces the renal and neurological effects of cisplatin, and quercetin increases the number of cancer cells killed by cisplatin.

Traditional Chinese herbal supplements are offered in conjunction with orthodox Western medical therapy. Among these are *Bulbus iphigeniae, Herba hedyotis diffusae, Herba scutellariae barbatae, Radix gentianae, Rhizoma liguistici chuanxiuong, Spica prunellae, Thallus laminariae,* and while these might sound obscure and bizarre to the Western patient, trained herbalists in China have used them with excellent results for over a thousand years.

There is a long list of complementary therapies available, and patients with this and other cancers should avail themselves of their benefits. Find a qualified holistic, herbal, Chinese, or Ayurvedic specialist, listen to what is offered and make an intelligent decision about further adjunctive treatments.

Overall, seminoma is a highly malignant, but also very curable, disease and the main focus should be on standard Western medicine, with the assistance of complementary medicine to offset the side effects of the usually very successful therapy.

## THYROID CANCER

The thyroid gland is a butterfly-shaped organ that straddles the front of the trachea in the neck. It consists of a right and left lobe and a connecting, or isthmus, lobe. Thyroid cancer is the most common of the endocrine cancers, more common in women than men, and often seen in younger individuals in their twenties and thirties. There are four main types: papillary, follicular, medullary, and anaplastic. The papillary and follicular types make up 90 percent of thyroid cancer, medullary about 5 percent, and anaplastic < 3 percent.

Papillary cancers have an excellent prognosis and even if they spread to local lymph nodes, they have an almost 100-percent cure rate with combination surgery and radioactive iodine therapy. The follicular tumors tend to be slightly more serious, with a lower survival rate and a tendency to be spread by blood vessels rather than lymph nodes. Hurthle-cell follicular tumors are a variant with a slightly more malignant potential. Medullary carcinoma is rare and more prone to regional and distal metastases, requiring more vigorous therapy. The anaplastic carcinomas, occurring in older people (from seventy years on), is always diagnosed when in stage IV and is unresponsive to surgery, radiation, or other measures.

The signs and symptoms of thyroid cancer are a nodule in the thyroid, or node enlargement in the neck; a voice change (due to invasion of the tumor into the larynx or injury to the recurrent laryngeal nerve that courses near the thyroid gland and can be irritated by tumor growth); or a neck mass felt by the patient or a physician.

### ■ Diagnosis and Treatment

A diagnostic workup includes a history and physical examination, followed by an ultrasound, then a fine-needle aspiration biopsy to determine the nature of the lump. The pathologist can make a diagnosis 80 percent of the time, but sometimes an exploration of the thyroid and an open biopsy must be done to confirm the diagnosis. Radioactive iodine scans may be helpful.

## Staging

The staging of papillary and follicular thyroid cancer follows the TNM method. T=Tumor, N=Lymph nodes, M=Metastasis.

- T0—No evidence of primary tumor, N0—No regional lymph-node spread, M0—No metastasis

- T1—Tumor < 2 cm in thyroid, N1—Regional lymph-node spread, M1—distant metastasis

- T2—2–4 cm in thyroid (1a and 1b depending on location)

- T3—> 4 cm in thyroid

- T4—Any size–outside thyroid gland (a and b depending on location)

| STAGING OF PAPILLARY AND FOLLICULAR THYROID CANCER (ABBREVIATED) | |
|---|---|
| **UNDER AGE 45** | **OVER AGE 45** |
| Stage I—Any T, Any N, M0 | Stage I—T1, N0, M0 |
| Stage II—Any T, Any N, MI | Stage II—T2, N0, M0 |
| Stage III—T3, N0, M0 | T1,2,3, N1a, M0 |
| Stage IVa—T4a, | T1–3, N0-N1a, M0 |
| Stage IVb—T4b | Any N, M0 |
| Stage IVc—Any T | Any N, MI |

There is much debate about the proper handling of papillary and follicular thyroid cancer. The general consensus is that in a patient under forty-five years of age, with a tumor less than 1 cm, the side of the gland containing the mass should be removed. Over 1 cm and older than forty-five, the recommendation is for a total thyroidectomy.

Medullary carcinomas of any size require a total thyroidectomy. In many cases, lymph-node sampling and, rarely, a complete neck-node dissection is indicated. To perform the surgery, an arcuate collar incision is made in the front of the neck that usually leaves a very fine line scar easily covered with makeup or a necklace.

After surgery, a determination is made whether any further therapy with radioactive iodine is needed to kill any remaining or circulating cancer cells.

Thyroid surgery presents several potential complications because of its location in the neck. Four tiny parathyroid glands (two on each side of the thyroid) must be identified, and at least one or two preserved. These glands control the calcium and phosphorus levels in the body, and complete removal of these glands means the patient will need life-long calcium replacement. In some rare instances of extensive cancer, this may be unavoidable, but it is not the usual occurrence. Running on either side, and slightly behind the thyroid are the recurrent laryngeal nerves that stimulate the vocal cords. Injury to one will cause hoarseness, and if both are injured a tracheostomy will be required in order for the patient to breathe (a rare and severe complication). In general, patients undergoing partial or complete thyroidectomy remain in the hospital for twelve to twenty-four hours to be sure no postoperative bleeding occurs. Pain is moderate to minimal and easily controlled with pain pills. Some transient mild hoarseness may occur, but it clears in a few days to a few weeks.

## ■ Complementary and Alternative Treatment

The role of complementary medicine for thyroid cancer is debated between the adherents of conventional and natural medicine. Complementary practitioners feel that natural thyroid medication can strengthen the immune system and ward off malignant change when used in appropriate dosages. Natural therapeutic disciplines, such as breathing exercises, meditation, and yoga, enhance the body's well-being and thereby inhibit the development of cancer. Other therapies include Ayurveda, traditional Chinese medicine (TCM), herbal dietary supplements, and massage. It is generally recognized that most individuals have cancerous cells in their bodies at all times and these are eliminated by naturally occurring killer (NK) cells. Weakening of the autoimmune system prevents this process from functioning adequately and leads to cancer formation.

Dr. Dharmananda, director of the Institute for Traditional Medicine in Portland, Oregon, has an excellent article on the *Treatments for*

*Thyroid Disease with Chinese Herbal Medicine.*[37] He describes eighteen clinical trials on the efficacy of materials from the sea including oyster shell, seaweeds (laminaria and sargassum), as well as clam shells, arca shells, and pumice for use in maintaining thyroid gland health. He quotes articles from the book *Practical Traditional Chinese Medicine and Pharmacology Clinical Experiences* in outlining several methods of maintaining thyroid health and preventing, and even curing, thyroid cancer. He emphasizes the differences between the Eastern and Western medical approaches to thyroid disease and cancer. In one instance he focuses on hyperthyroidism noting the focus on 1) Disturbance of *qi*, 2) Heart fire disorder marked by emotional disturbance, 3) Extreme anger, and 4) External factors—food and water deficiencies.

The Eastern approach may seem bizarre and unprofessional to the Western-trained physician, nevertheless it must be examined since it has centuries of knowledgeable adherents and positive outcomes. Many herbal remedies and complex formulas have been evaluated and found effective by Chinese practitioners.

Chinese doctors treat thyroid tumors with a wide range of herb formulas, as cited in *An Illustrated Guide to Anti-Neoplastic Chinese Herbal Medicine.*[38] Among these are preparations named luffa decoction, xiao ying tang, huangyaozi, and thyroid tumor formula. In the text, *Treating Cancer with Herbs,*[39] bao jin san, wu ying fang, and ying jie san are listed, and most of them contain gentian, laminaria, and sargassum. The text *Anticancer Medicinal Herbs*[40] lists other formulas containing kalimera, scutellaria, and solidago. This last formula was tried for fifty-three cases of thyroid cancer and twenty-eight of the patients were cured without surgery. In cases not cured with Chinese herbal medicine, the patients were subjected to standard Western surgical and medical management. The article emphasizes that the action of Chinese herb therapy is unknown when expressed in Western pharmacological terms. When the Chinese philosophy of medicine uses terms like yin/yang, and *qi*, most Western physicians are unable or unwilling to even look into the matter because it is so far from their view of what is standard, accepted medical care. But the fact remains that most of these remedies have been used for over a thousand years and have been reported as clinically successful in Chinese journals and anecdotal reports.

Complementary medical care has been used to treat the side effects of surgery for thyroid cancer, and, in terminal cases, such as those seen with anaplastic carcinoma, the various modalities of acupuncture, herbal supplements, massage, meditation, and yoga have been used to offset the pain and emotional suffering.

The Indian Ayurvedic approaches to thyroid cancer have been oriented toward understanding and correcting certain internal imbalances in our lives. While difficult for the Western medicine advocate to understand, this philosophy stresses the importance of restoring homeostasis by correcting the doshas or humors. They recommend drinking hot ginger tea, eating raw fruits and vegetables, and avoiding dairy, salty foods, and wheat products. The recommendation for yoga as an effective therapy is very difficult for a Western physician to understand or accept if he/she has not been exposed to its benefits. Several herbal and dietary regimens are recommended for treatment, and even cure, of thyroid cancer at the Divyajyot Ayurvedic Research Foundation in India. Their programs can be examined online and decisions about complementary care evaluated. They always recommend using Ayurvedic regimens with the knowledge and approval of standard medical doctors.

# PART 3

# ALL OTHER CANCER-RELATED MATTERS

# ALL OTHER CANCER-RELATED MATTERS

Events that create emergencies and need to be acutely managed before the underlying causes are addressed here.

## Hemorrhages

Rapid and excessive bleeding is obviously an emergency and must be attended to on an urgent basis to prevent exsanguination and death. Of course, there are many surgical situations that can result in an intraoperative hemorrhage and even result in postoperative hemorrhagic situations that must be managed by the surgeon. The most common are procedures connected to the colon, esophagus, lung, prostate, as well as some gynecological procedures.

There are, however, several occurrences related to cancer growth or therapy that can result in the acute, or even chronic, onset of bleeding, leading to a drop in blood pressure and an eventual, or rapid, progression to death. The relatively slow, but progressive, fall in the blood count due to chronic blood loss, or to diminished blood production due to cancer, or to chemo- or radiation therapy can be treated by a blood transfusion and timely management of the underlying cause. This is not what is meant by hemorrhage, the rapid and life-threatening loss of blood that, if not attended to immediately, will have a fatal outcome.

Visible arterial bleeding where there is pulsatile (pulsating with each heart beat) high-pressure flow must be instantly controlled in the best way possible by firm manual (with the hand or palm) pressure at the bleeding site, regardless of the pain, to prevent immediate exsanguination. Venous bleeding, while not pulsatile, may still be massive and should be compressed with a palm or folded washcloth against the area until help arrives. On extremities, a tourniquet may be used for short periods of time only.

Patients with a hemorrhage must be taken to a hospital emergency room rapidly, preferably by calling 911 and having immediate, urgent resuscitation and fluid replacement in transit by emergency medical technicians (EMTs), or by able family members if other resources are not available.

The following situations may arise in the individual with cancer and must be addressed immediately upon their occurrence and recognition.

◇ Direct external hemorrhage from a tumor: head and neck tumors (direct involvement of the carotid artery or jugular vein), melanomas, skin cancers

◇ Internal hemorrhage from the gastrointestinal tract (esophagus, small and large intestinal cancers, stomach), intraperitoneal hemorrhage (liver, ovarian, splenic cancers)

◇ Complications of bronchoscopy

◇ Complications of endoscopy

◇ Due to herbs and supplements (ginkgo biloba, garlic, saw palmetto) especially when used with anticoagulants

◇ Acute leukemia

◇ Brain cancers

◇ From use of angiogenesis inhibitors (bevacizumab)

◇ From bladder cancer

The only concern is the propensity of many of the alternative and complementary herbs and medications, in addition to the ones mentioned above, to cause changes in blood coagulation. Relatively simple procedures can be made complex and dangerous if the patient has used certain herbs that have caused increased bleeding, and the use of all complementary medicine should be shared with the patient's oncologist and surgeon prior to any procedure.

## Increased Intracranial Pressure

This condition is a common occurrence in patients with brain cancer. Because the brain is in the skull, a nonexpandable cavity, any increase in contents there will cause pressure on the normal brain tissue. The cause may be an enlarging malignant tumor or may be causes secondary to the presence of cancer. These include a coagulation problem that can result in intracerebral bleeding and increased pressure, an infection due to a tumor, an immuno-compromised state, an edema (swelling) of the brain due to a tumor, or a hypercoagulable state causing vein thrombosis and swelling.

The most common causes are brain metastases, a tumor from other sources spreading to the brain (and secondarily from primary brain tumors), growing, compressing, and pushing on normal brain tissue. The most frequent complaint is a severe, unrelenting headache. Increasing pressure on the brain can cause lethargy, slow responses, confusion, and, eventually, coma and death. Other neurological deficits include vomiting, vision and eyeball-position changes, weakness and even paralysis, diminished intellect, and urinary and rectal incontinence.

The cranium, or skull, contains brain tissue, CSF (cerebrospinal fluid that surrounds the brain and spinal cord), and blood. The Munroe-Kellie hypothesis states that in the cranium there is a balance of these contents that creates a volume equilibrium, and an increase in any one of the constituents will be compensated for by a decrease in volume of the other. This explains why a growing cancer or secondary infection in the brain will have a compressing and devastating effect on the brain's functioning.

Diagnosis is made by physical exam and by a CAT scan (computer axial tomography).

When a tumor or swelling blocks the normal flow of CSF, urgent surgical intervention with a ventricular-peritoneal shunt may be indicated. In this procedure, a neurosurgeon places one end of a tube into the obstructed fluid channel in the brain and the other end into the abdominal peritoneal cavity so the flow of brain fluid (CSF) can continue.

Generally, intracranial pressure can be alleviated by simply elevating the head of a bed, by intravenous injection of corticosteroids and diuretics, and by using medications to control the symptoms of headache and vomiting. More definitive therapy focuses on diminishing or eliminating the cause, either with radiation, chemotherapy, or in selected cases, neurosurgery.

## Metabolic Emergencies

This is a group of medical emergencies caused by the presence of cancer or by the therapy that has been initiated. Their management is complex and difficult and often poses diagnostic and therapeutic problems for the oncologist. Among the more common are:

◇ Adrenal gland failure

◇ Hyperammonemia. Increased ammonia in the blood when the liver fails to detoxify it

◇ Hypercalcemia or hypocalcemia. An increase or decrease of calcium in the blood

◇ Hyperuricemia. An increase of uric acid in the blood

◇ Hypoglycemia. Low blood sugar

◇ Hyponatremia. Lowered sodium level in the blood

◇ Lactic acidosis. This occurs in patients with extensive disease, in advanced leukemia and lymphoma

◇ Tumor lysis syndrome. This is caused by the death of cells either from a growing, degenerating cancer, or from chemotherapy-killing cancer cells—it puts dead cells and their tissue into the blood and taxes the kidney's ability to excrete the waste, resulting in kidney failure with all its side effects

## Obstructions

As a cancer grows, the mass may cause external compression with resulting obstructing blockage of blood vessels, or a portion of the intestinal tract, the bronchial tract (breathing tubes), or the urological tract.

### Blood-Vessel Blockages

Blockage of a blood vessel by cancer, or a cancer-induced blood clot may lead to a brain infarct (loss of limb, fingers, toes, or stroke), infarction (death) of an organ or tissue (i.e., a spleen infarct), an intestinal infarction leading to perforation and peritonitis, or ischemia (decreased blood supply).

Vascular occlusive emergencies (blockage of a blood vessel, usually with a clot) often require surgical intervention to remove dead tissue and occasionally to revascularize (improve the circulation) in an area. Endovascular stenting is becoming more popular with the growing specialty of interventional radiology and the expertise of endovascular surgeons and interventional cardiologists. Unfortunately vascular occlusive occurrences in the brain are often catastrophic, resulting in permanent neurological deficits, and are usually not manageable except to prevent further problems by using radiation and chemotherapy.

### Bronchial Obstructions

Blockage of the bronchi causes respiratory distress. Bronchial obstruction is a dire situation and, if it is not corrected, you die.

### Intestinal Blockages

Tumor blockage of the intestine will cause abdominal distention, obstruction, and pain, along with nausea and vomiting. Intestinal obstruction may respond to chemotherapy or radiation therapy while the patient is being treated with a temporizing decompression of the distended abdomen via a nasogastric tube, to gain time. But often a surgical intervention is required, necessitating removal or bypass of the obstructed area of intestine.

### Urological Blockages

Blockage of ureters due to cancer can cause kidney failure; a blockage of the urethra in men and women can cause an inability to urinate, pain, and eventual kidney damage. Blockage of the ureters requires a placement of catheters through the obstruction, and urethral obstruction necessitates a placement of a catheter into the bladder through the abdomen (cystostomy). Radiation and chemotherapy may relieve these obstructions, but surgical intervention by a urologist is frequently required.

Other urological emergencies include infection, which can cause sepsis (blood infection with dire systemic effects, lower blood pressure, or shock), and requires vigorous antibiotic therapy. It can also cause a bladder hemorrhage that may require a cystoscopy (examining the bladder with a fiber optic scope), evacuation of blood clots, and cauterization of the bleeding sources.

## Spinal-Cord Compression

When a primary or metastatic cancer compresses the spinal cord, the initial symptom may be pain followed soon after by neurologic deficit (an umbrella term for a problem with nerve, spinal cord, or brain function). If it's not attended to rapidly, permanent damage and paralysis may ensue. Because back pain is a common complaint in the general population, early signs of the cancer that is causing the spinal-cord compression may be ignored or entirely missed, leading to catastrophic outcomes. Frequently, undiagnosed patients are advised to take analgesics or have bed rest, which may even temporarily alleviate the symptoms, giving a false sense of security to both the health-care provider and the patient. In most cases, however, almost a month passes between the initial onset of pain and a rapid progression of the symptoms, at which time the window of opportunity for treatment and reversal of the neurological deficit may have significantly narrowed. Individuals with known cancers, and those with rapidly progressing back symptoms must seek out medical help on an urgent basis. Immediate workup includes an MRI (magnetic resonance imaging) and an urgent biopsy of the suspected primary cancer or metastasis and is followed by the initiation of a definitive therapy. The spinal cord will not tolerate compression for very long without permanent damage.

Other symptoms associated with spinal-cord compression are constipation, loss of sensation or sense of position, numbness, tingling or coldness of the extremities, urinary retention, and weakness.

Initial treatment may consist of a rapid intravenous infusion of corticosteroids to decrease the edema (swelling), alleviate pain, and prevent further cord damage while other therapies are being instituted. A few cancers that are extremely sensitive to chemotherapy, such as non-Hodgkin's lymphoma, may respond so rapidly to intravenous chemotherapy that surgery or radiation will not be needed.

However, many patients will be subjected to immediate radiation therapy to *melt* the tumor and diminish the cord compression. Patients with metastatic breast cancer and lymphoma, both of which are frequently very sensitive to radiation, often have an excellent response to external-beam radiation therapy with a reversal of the neurological symptoms.

About 10 to 20 percent of those with spinal-cord compression will require immediate surgical decompression in an attempt to alleviate symptoms and prevent permanent nerve damage. Depending on the location, extent of the disease, and general condition of the patient, there are several surgical approaches. Some surgeons will opt for posterior approaches, through the back, while others may decide on an anterior approach, through the abdomen, chest, or neck.

One of the most important determinants of functional outcome is the extent and severity of the neurologic damage at the time of diagnosis and initiation of treatment. Those who are not treated and relieved of the compression usually deteriorate within a month of diagnosis, and those treated by one of the modalities discussed may survive for extended lengths of time, depending on the type of tumor and the response to therapy.

There are patients who fall into the category of terminally ill, and, after discussion with the patient and the family, vigorous treatment of their spinal-cord compression may be relegated to palliative care and pain management because of debility and widespread metastatic disease.

## Superior Vena Cava Syndrome

The superior vena cava is the large vein in the chest formed at the confluence of the veins coming from the arms and the head (subclavian veins/innominate veins, jugular veins), to bring venous blood back to the heart. (The inferior vena cava brings blood from the lower limbs and abdomen to the heart and combines with the superior vena cava at the right atrium of the heart.)

Certain tumors and lymph-node enlargement with cancer can cause partial, and then complete, blockage of the superior vena cava (SVCS—superior vena cava syndrome), resulting in a backup of blood in the head and neck, as well as the arms. The blockage to the vessel may come from external compression on the thin-walled vena cava from a tumor or lymph nodes, or from blood clots forming in an already compromised cava. If the process occurs slowly, over many weeks or months, collateral veins (extra small veins) may enlarge and partially take over the function of the superior vena cava. However, when the process is fairly rapid and there is no time for the body to adjust to the process, an acute emergency occurs, with massive swelling of the head, neck, face, and upper extremities.

The symptoms of SVCS are chest pain, coughing, cyanosis (bluish skin discoloration), difficulty swallowing (dysphagia), facial swelling, distention of neck veins, shortness of breath (dyspnea), and swelling of arms.

Diagnosis is made on a clinical exam and history and augmented with a chest x-ray, a CT (computerized axial tomography) scan, and occasionally venography (x-ray of veins with intravenous contrast). The most common malignant causes of this syndrome are lymphoma and lung cancer, and the latter may be curable.

On some occasions, the obstruction in patients with cancer may be caused by vein thrombosis due to the placement of an intravenous catheter, although this is usually in conjunction with an already narrowed vessel or a hypercoagulable state (where the patient's blood clots more easily, as with certain cancers).

The treatments of this emergency are designed to alleviate the signs and symptoms and then eradicate the underlying cause. Radiation therapy to the area, along with chemotherapy; steroids to decrease swelling; anticoagulation; and diuretics to increase urination and decrease fluid in the veins are all often successful at relieving the acute situation. Success is excellent with non-Hodgkin's lymphoma, but the success and prognosis with non-small-cell lung cancer only temporarily relieves the signs of obstruction.

In urgent situations, endovascular stenting is becoming an additional therapy. This involves placing a wire through the area of obstruction (either from the thigh vein or the jugular vein in the neck), dilating the area of blockage with a special balloon catheter, and then placing a rigid stent in the vena cava to allow the blood flow to return to normal.

Surgery with a direct-bypass graft has essentially been eliminated as a feasible manner of handling this acute condition and is used only in noncancerous conditions after the failure of other modalities. There is no role for complementary medicine in the handling of this acute situation.

## THE REST OF THE STORY

### Venous-Access Ports and Lines

During treatment for cancer, patients may have a continuing need for intravenous medications and blood products. If the patient has very small veins, if the veins have been used so often that access is difficult, or if the substance infused requires a large vein, then a venous-access port or a special access line is indicated.

This can be done by a hospital specialist who places a PIC (peripherally inserted central line) in the arm under local anesthesia and ultrasound guidance, or by a physician placing an access port or catheter, also usually in the arm. The line consists of an intravenous catheter placed in a large vein (via the jugular vein or subclavian vein) under local anesthesia and may either have a capsule (Port A Cath) under the skin that can be accessed using a special needle, or the catheter itself (Permcath) may exit the skin and be accessible for injections.

Care must be taken to prevent infection or thrombosis of the lines, which would require special treatment or removal and replacement of the access line. When treatment is completed or concluded, these lines can be easily removed.

### Tumor Ascites

Ascites is an accumulation of excess fluid in the peritoneal cavity, the fluid-filled gap between the abdomen and the organs contained in the adomen. In noncancerous situations, this occurs when there is severe liver disease, as in cirrhosis from alcoholism. In cancer, the cause of ascites may be twofold. The liver may be so involved with the primary or metastatic cancer that it behaves like the cirrhotic liver, producing ascites. The other cause is direct tumor involvement of the intraperitoneal structures (surface of the intestines, peritoneum, and omentum). In women this often occurs with ovarian or other gynecological cancers, whereas in men the source is gastrointestinal or pancreatic cancer spread into the abdomen. The accumulation of ascites fluid may be massive, causing debility and discomfort.

Before instituting therapy, a diagnosis of the etiology is necessary and is usually accomplished by removing and examining some of the fluid using a needle (paracentesis), or by means of a laparoscopy where, additionally, the extent of tumor involvement can be ascertained. The fluid will usually contain cancer cells and a pathologist can often determine the site of origin. This will lead to the use of the appropriate chemotherapeutic agents (in some cases injected directly into the abdomen), along with diuretics. Recurring paracenteses (removal of fluid) may be undertaken to relieve symptoms. On rare occasions, at special cancer centers, radical surgical procedures to remove cancers have been done with some success, but the morbidity and mortality of such procedures usually precludes their use in community hospitals.

Aside from repeated paracentesis, another procedure, the peritoneal-venous ascites shunt, is available. Under anesthesia in an operating room, one end of a special catheter is placed in the abdomen while the other is tunneled up under the skin into the jugular vein in the neck (there is a one-way valve preventing backflow of blood). The abdominal fluid passes through the catheter into the venous system, then to the kidneys to be excreted. With this technique, there is an increased risk for bleeding because of the diluting of the coagulation factors in the blood, but there is a saving of the protein in this fluid that would be lost during repeated paracenteses. The peritoneal-venous ascites shunt is, in most surgeons' experience, only 50 percent successful and should be reserved for cases where other treatment modalities have failed.

## Stem-Cell Transplantation

Stem-cell transplantation is a procedure that involves the repopulating, or infusion, of healthy stem cells into a recipient's body. Stem-cell transplantation, also known as bone-marrow transplantation or umbilical-cord transplantation, depending on the source of the cells used, is a method of infusing healthy blood-producing cells into a damaged or nonfunctional bone marrow through a vein or special intravenous port. In the progression of a cancer, or as the result of chemotherapy and radiation therapy for the cancer, bone marrow may stop working and thereby become unable to produce red blood cells (that carry oxygen to tissue), white blood cells (that help fight off infection), and platelets (that are important in blood clotting).

When a patient with cancer is not cured or has not responded well to regular oncologic treatment with radiation and chemotherapy, an extreme method of therapy that involves high doses of chemotherapy and/or radiation therapy to kill all the remaining cancer cells can be used. In the course of this therapy, normal bone-marrow cells are destroyed and must be replaced by healthy stem cells that repopulate the marrow and eventually start producing blood products. Stem-cell transplantation is a high-risk procedure that is only done as a last measure when all other therapies have failed.

The process of destroying cancer cells and suppressing the immune system involving chemotherapy and/or radiation therapy is often called conditioning and can itself cause several acute side effects. These include anemia, bleeding, cataracts, diarrhea, fatigue, hair loss, infections, infertility, mouth sores and ulcers, nausea and vomiting, pneumonia, and even secondary cancers. Many of these can be treated and alleviated using standard and complementary therapies already described. So patients need to understand that the interim between the time the cancer cells have been destroyed by the high-dose therapy, and the repopulation and regrowth of new bone-marrow cells, is a dangerous one because patients are at risk for severe anemia, bleeding, and infections. This procedure is therefore done in a highly specialized cancer center equipped to anticipate and handle all the complications and side effects.

Stem cells can come from a patient's own body (an autologous stem-cell transplant), or they may come from a donor (an allogeneic stem-cell transplant). They may either come from blood drawn from a vein or taken from bone marrow using a large bore needle with local or general anesthesia. Of note is that the new infused cells themselves may act to help destroy any remaining cancer cells.

There are many risks and long-term complications associated with stem-cell transplantation, and their extent and severity may vary from patient to patient. Among the problems encountered are the following.

◊ Graft-versus-host reaction. This is a condition where the infused new stem cells see the recipient's body as foreign and react against it; anticipated to some degree, it is treated with steroids, such as prednisone, and special immuno-suppressive medications—the condition can occur soon after the transplant, or even years later, and may consist of abdominal pain, diarrhea, nausea, skin rashes, and vomiting—in rare cases it may be life-threatening

◊ Stem-cell failure. A failure of the transplanted cells to survive and/or repopulate the bone marrow is an ominous occurrence and repeat attempts may be tried

◇ Organ damage. This extreme therapy may in some instances cause damage to certain organs, such as the heart, the kidneys, the liver, and the lungs

◇ Cataracts. Blurring of the cornea may be a side effect of the treatment and require surgical treatment

◇ Development of other cancers, including leukemias, lymphomas, and oral (mouth) cancers

◇ Growth retardation, especially in young children

◇ Joint problems

◇ Kidney and lung problems

Suffice it to say that stem-cell transplantation is a complex and involved procedure and a patient will need to have comprehensive discussions with the oncology team at the time of this procedure to help clarify the procedure, the risks, and the long-term side effects.

## Organ Transplantation

The placement of a normal organ to replace one with cancer is not done except in the case of hepatic malignancy. Patients who have been treated and cured of cancer, however, may be eligible for various types of organ transplants, such as corneal, heart, kidney, liver, and lung. Since there is a long waiting list for these donors, a patient who still has a possibility of residual cancer may not be at the top of the recipient list, for obvious reasons. However, this does not preclude any living (often related or familial) donors who wish to donate a kidney or even a portion of a liver for transplantation.

The patient with a solitary, or even multiple, primary liver cancer may be a candidate for liver removal and transplantation if the evaluation team believes there is a strong possibility of cure. However, if the liver cancer is metastatic, even if only one or a few lesions are present, the decision may be to ablate (remove) the metastasis as previously described because of the possibility and probability of recurrence in the transplanted liver or elsewhere.

On the downside, there are noted instances where financial influence or the notoriety of wealthy or famous individuals have resulted in inappropriate salvage transplants that eventually failed, where the donated organ might have benefited an individual not dying of cancer. In the United States, compensated donations (organs for sale from living donors, as with kidney or partial liver) is illegal. It is well known that throughout the world, organs are offered for sale through the Internet and private organizations, resulting in illegal and often unethical procedures.

Organ transplantation is fraught with many potential and real problems, as well as the complications of stem-cell transplantation, discussed in the section above.

## Infections In Cancer Patients

The objective of this section is to emphasize that patients with cancer may have decreased resistance to infection because of their cancer, or due to the therapy they are receiving. Once the cancer is gone, however, the increased risk for infection usually disappears with it. For this reason, the individual with cancer needs to be proactive in recognizing and preventing infections. This means avoiding exposure to dangerous germs, taking appropriate drugs after exposure to germs, and seeking out professional help as soon as an infection is apparent. Obviously, radiation, chemotherapy, and the cancer itself may all increase the risks for infection.

The body's defense against infection consists of natural barriers, including the immune and blood systems, intact intestinal tract, mucous membranes, skin, and overall general nutrition. Any breakdown or diminution of these that occurs in patients with cancer can lead to severe infections.

Skin is the largest organ in the body (it's not usually thought of as an organ, but it is), and it is also the main barrier keeping germs from getting into the body. So careful inspection of cuts or bruises, and keeping it from drying out or developing any other skin irritation is important. Maintenance of good nutrition and supplementation with complementary modalities is important as well, as is having an oncologist who follows the status of the immune system and augments it with immunotherapy when deficits are found.

These parts of the body are the most prone to infection.

◇ The bones—osteomyelitis

◇ The brain—meningitis

◇ The eyes—conjunctivitis

◇ The heart—myocarditis and pericarditis

◇ The intestines—colitis, gastroenteritis

◇ The liver—hepatitis

◇ The lungs—bronchitis, pneumonia

◇ The mucous membranes—mucositis, stomatitis

◇ The skin—cellulitis

◇ The urinary tract—cystitis, pyelonephritis, urinary tract infection–UTI

◇ Any skin and tissue around a vascular-access device, such as a PIC line or another IV-access device

When infection is suspected, cultures are taken from the area and laboratory studies are done to determine the kind of organism present and what appropriate therapy should be instituted. The cultures may be from blood, spinal fluid, sputum, urine, or wound drainage (pus).

Some of the organisms may be bacterial, including E. coli, klebsiella, MERSA—methicillin-resistant staphylococcus aureus, pseudomonas, staphylococcus, or streptococcus. There may be fungus (including Aspergillis, candida, pneumocystis) protozoa (cryptosporidium, toxoplasma), or viruses (cytomegalovirus, herpes, varicella). It's clear there are a number of different organisms, and often the treatment is highly specialized; in otherwise compromised patients, a specialist in infectious diseases may be needed to treat the disease appropriately.

Augmenting nutrition with the help of a nutritional specialist is always helpful, and many highly regarded complementary regimens are recommended and effective.

## Nutrition and Cancer

Patients lose weight and fail to thrive under the influence of a growing cancer. And in the course of treatment for their cancer, they tend to lose more weight, either due directly to the cancer, or to the consequences of the therapy, whether it be surgical, oncologic, or radiotherapeutic. Nutrition is a major focus of oncologists in the standard Western tradition, in many of the alternative or complementary fields, including Chinese, Indian Ayurvedic, and a whole host of other modalities, and they all advocate many approaches to improving the nutrition of individuals with cancer who are undergoing therapy.

Although the approach may be quite different, the objectives are basically the same. In this particular area the Eastern and Western, naturopathic and holistic, and other complementary modalities can agree to agree. And it is in just this area that the major cancer centers in the United States and abroad are developing active programs in complementary medicine because they have grown to understand and appreciate how an integrative approach toward cancer and nutrition, examining all modalities, can only help in the management of patients with cancer.

The National Cancer Institute notes that patients with cancer often have decreased absorption of carbohydrates, fats, and proteins, and, although they eat their usual diet, they tend to lose weight. Tumors make chemicals that change the way the body accepts and uses ingested food. The Institute emphasizes that chemotherapy, immunotherapy, radiation therapy, stem-cell transplantation, and surgery, all affect nutrition. Cancers of the esophagus, head, neck, and stomach directly affect how many nutrients can be ingested. A number of therapies cause loss of appetite (anorexia), constipation, depression, diarrhea, dry mouth, nausea and vomiting, and trouble swallowing, all of which result in diminished caloric intake and weight loss. Cancers and their treatment also can cause changes in the sensations of taste and smell and decrease the appetite.

The broad field of nutrition deals with all these problems by increasing the appetite, treating mouth sores, preventing and treating pain, treating nausea and vomiting, and other problems. When adequate nutrition cannot be taken by mouth, other methods are instituted.

◇ **Feeding tube.** A tube through the mouth into the stomach

◇ **Gastrostomy.** A tube through the abdominal wall into the stomach placed under anesthesia by a surgeon or under heavy sedation by a gastroenterologist

◊ **Enterostomy.** A surgical procedure to initiate feeding by a tube placed into the intestine

◊ **Hyperalimentation (parenteral nutrition).** An intravenous infusion of high-calorie feedings via IV access sites (a Port A Cath or a PIC line—see section above on Venous-Access Ports and Lines)

There are several very effective standard and complementary approaches to the problems of nutrition, and there are several websites in back that present Ayurvedic, Chinese, holistic, and other complementary modalities.

## Steroids—Their Uses and Problems

Steroids are hormonal substances naturally produced in the adrenal cortex of the body. Basically, there are two medically important steroids, corticosteroids and androgenic, or anabolic, steroids, the latter often heard about in connection with their illegal role in increasing athletic performance. Both these substances are now produced synthetically.

Corticosteroids, such as cortisol, have powerful anti-inflammatory effects and depress the immune system. They are used medically for treatment of asthma, arthritis, and painful joints, certain allergic reactions and skin rashes, and to make the immune system less active when fighting off the possibility of the transplants being rejected. They can decrease the inflammatory response around cancers and are acutely useful in the treatment of brain tumors, reducing the swelling and alleviating the symptoms of intracranial pressure. They are used to treat Addison's disease (adrenal insufficiency), autoimmune diseases, inflammatory bowel disease, and spinal cord trauma. They are effective in decreasing the itching, pain, redness, and swelling of inflammation. Another effect of steroids is the creation of delusions, euphoria, and frank psychoses.

Prolonged usage can lead to bone thinning and muscle wasting, development of diabetes, and even glaucoma and cataracts, and continuing use can exacerbate severe infections and cause nonhealing of wounds, with a severe diminishing of the immune system's ability to fight off cancer and infections. Extended use of steroids can result in increased fat accumulation in the upper back (buffalo hump) and a swelling of the face (moon face).

Anabolic steroids, androgenic steroids, or testosterone steroids have some beneficial uses for cancer patients. They can induce an increased appetite and subsequent weight gain, help breathing in those with chronic obstructive pulmonary disease (COPD), and possibly produce euphoria in terminal cancer patients.

Because of their ability to improve performance, these anabolic steroids are universally, and illegally, used by bicycle racers, body-builders, professional wrestlers, and other professional sportsmen. An industry has grown up around the development of anabolic steroid analogs that are easy to expel from the body, or easy to conceal in drug testing. There are many harmful side effects of these drugs, including acne, enlarged breasts, infertility, loss of hair, smaller genitalia, rage, and an increased incidence of hypertension, kidney disease, and prostate cancer. Women who use these steroids start looking like men, with baldness, beard growth, enlarged clitoris, lowered voice, and sterility.

## Hemopoietic (Blood) Growth Factors

One of the major side effects and complications of chemotherapy and radiation therapy is the effect on the blood-producing system of the body. Often the bone marrow doesn't produce enough blood products to maintain a healthy body. With recent advances in drug development, it is now possible to stimulate production of several elements found in the blood, namely erythrocytes (red cells that deliver oxygen to cells and remove $CO_2$), neutrophils that help fight infection, and platelets that help clotting. These substances have a long name: recombinant human hematopoietic growth factors or hemopoietic cytokines.

The following is a list of drugs and indications for use.

| TABLE 6.1. DRUGS AND INDICATIONS FOR THEIR USE | | |
|---|---|---|
| DRUG NAME | CELLS STIMULATED | INDICATION |
| Epogen/ Procrit/Aranesp | Erythrocytes (red cells) | Anemia from cancer or cancer treatment |
| Neumega | Platelets | Low platelets from cancer or cancer treatment |
| Neupogen/Neulasta | Neutrophils | Cancer patients receiving myelosuppressive therapy |

## Treatment Complications

I include this to emphasize that people are not machines. Removing and treating cancer is a far cry from changing a muffler or a faulty carburetor. Even similar cancers have remarkably different behaviors in different individuals. Similarly, surgery, medicine, and radiation therapy are all fraught with risks and complications. All the cancer doctors I work with try their best to use the information and experience at hand to give the best care to their patients. True, some physicians are better than others, have more experience, better hands in surgery, different personalities. That is the problem with humanity—humanness.

Many of the side effects and complications with cancer growth and treatment have been discussed here. But be aware that patients with cancers are often in poorer than normal health and are prone to bleeding, complications from wound healing, constipation, depression, diarrhea, fatigue, infections, nausea, pain, unusual immune system reactions, as well as the catastrophic occurrence of a tumor spreading (metastasizing) or returning after a period of expected cure.

Those who denigrate the drug companies and the medical profession as insensitive, bilking the patients, and looking only to themselves and their profits are usually barking up the wrong tree. Sure, there are charlatans and greedy practitioners in every area of the world, and medicine is no haven for saints. But an informed, open-minded approach benefits the patient as well as the treating physician. Often anger at the disease projects onto the treating physician, and a patient or family member may want to blame someone, especially if complications and adverse events occur. Although batting 500 percent may be great in baseball, anything less than 100 percent in medicine is often deemed a failure.

## Heart Complications

Some chemotherapy drugs, as well as radiation therapy, can cause damage to the heart, and as a result the heart may be unable to pump as much blood efficiently. This complication may occur during, or directly after, completion of therapy and may persist and become chronic. Sometimes the damage may only be apparent months, or even years, after the cessation of treatment.

The problems may be mild or severe and are detectable by measuring the left ventricular ejection fraction (LVEF), a percentage measurement of the amount of blood pumped out of the heart with each contraction. The damage may be so minimal that it is only detected by an LVEF measurement, or so severe that a patient develops heart failure, treatable with medications. In extreme cases a heart transplant may be needed.

The tests used to measure LVEF are the echocardiogram (sound wave study of the heart) and a nuclear medicine scan called a multiple gated acquisition scan (MUGA). When heart failure occurs, it is treated the same as in other situations, with strong medications, bed rest, and careful observation. Other cardiac complications include arrhythmias and EKG changes.

A specific class of chemotherapy drugs called anthracyclines cause most cardiac toxicity, among them daunomycin, doxorubicin, epirubicin (Ellence), idarubicin (Idamycin) and mitoxantrone (Novatrone). These drugs may be combined with others (alkylating agents and vinca alkaloids) that also contribute to heart damage. Radiation to the chest wall around the heart in conjunction with anthracyclines, as is sometimes done with breast cancer and lymphoma, can cause heart damage and in some cases a heart attack.

The toxicity of the chemotherapeutic agents is related to the cumulative dose and the speed and timing of delivery. The risk has been reduced by using anthracyclines prepared in a different fashion, where the drug is encapsulated in a globule of fat called a liposome. For biochemical reasons, this form of the drugs is not as toxic to the heart and is now being used more frequently as liposomal daunorubicin (Daunoxome) and liposomal doxorubicin (Doxil). In addition to this, the drug dexrazoxane (Zinecard) has been shown to prevent or reduce the severity of the heart damage caused by these drugs.

## Lung Complications

Pulmonary toxicity or lung damage is a side effect of some chemotherapy and radiation therapy for cancer. Any chemotherapy drug can damage the lungs. And radiation to the chest wall or the lungs, as used for breast cancer, Hodgkin's lymphoma, and lung cancer, can cause damage as well.

The damage may be due to inflammation that causes swelling of the large and microscopic breathing apparatus (bronchi and alveoli) and affects the absorption of oxygen into the bloodstream. The inflammation, also known as pneumonitis, pneumonia, or bronchitis, results in the lungs diminished ability to exchange oxygen in the air with carbon dioxide in the blood, thus reducing the amount of oxygen reaching the body tissues. This is often a reversible process.

Another cause of lung damage is scarring that also reduces the amount of air breathed. Pulmonary fibrosis, or scarring, damages the elasticity of the lungs and reduces a person's ability to breathe in and out. This complication can occur soon, or several months after cancer treatment, and can get progressively worse with time. This damage may be temporary or long-term and treatment is focused on relieving the symptoms and helping to alleviate the underlying pathology.

The diagnosis and the severity is determined through chest x-rays, pulmonary (lung) function tests, and, occasionally, bronchoscopy (a fiberoptic tube to examine the airways and lungs).

Chemotherapy drugs associated with lung damage are arsenic trioxide (Trisenox), bleomycin (Blenoxane), idarubicin (Idamycin), mitomycin, and some alkylating agents (busulfan), antimetabolites (methotrexate), and nitrosoureas (BCNU or carmustine).

The uncomfortable symptoms of lung damage include breathlessness during exercise, chest pain, dizziness, dry cough, fatigue, shortness of breath, and a worsening of symptoms when lying on your back.

Treatment of lung damage is with, first, oxygen therapy, then antibiotics, calcium channel blockers (medications that treat high blood pressure in the lungs—Verapamil–Calan, Diltiazem–Dilacor), corticosteroids (to decrease inflammation and swelling), cough medications and decongestants, diuretics (water pills to prevent lung congestion by urinating off fluid), immune-suppressing agents (azothioprine–Imurancy, clophosphamide–Cytoxan), pain medication, and pulmonary rehabilitation. Obviously, cessation of smoking and avoiding smoke-filled environments is important, as is participating in daily exercises and the use of an incentive spirometer, an apparatus that helps a person breathe slowly and deeply to expand the lungs and help oxygenation.

## Hair Loss

Not surprisingly, one of the most emotionally unsettling side effects of cancer, radiation, and chemotherapy is the temporary, and sometimes permanent, loss of hair (alopecia). No single occurrence is more apparent than the unwanted loss of hair, almost screaming out that an individual has cancer. It directly impacts a person's self-image and is also traumatic because it psychologically ties in with loss of self and is a blatant daily reminder of the presence of the disease and the risk of dying.

Some cancers (acute myeloid leukemia, breast, lung, squamous cancer of the tongue, stomach, T-cell lymphoma, and trophoblastic) can cause hair loss even without chemotherapy or radiation therapy.

Hair growth can be divided into three phases, anagen, telogen, and catagen. The early phase, anagen, is when the hair is being produced in rapid cell growth and is most susceptible to genetic change, therefore most affected by radiation and chemotherapy. This hair loss occurs within two to three weeks of therapy and usually regrows within two to three months after cessation of therapy. However, when the hair regrows there is sometimes a thinning and incomplete regrowth.

There are several old therapies for decreasing alopecia, including head tourniquets and scalp hypothermia during chemotherapy sessions to decrease the blood flow of chemotherapeutic agents to the scalp, but these have unwanted side effects and are generally not recommended by physicians. Five agents used to decrease alopecia are AS101, a-tocopherol, cyclin-dependent kinase, thiol, and topical minoxidil. However, these are often unsatisfactory, leaving patchy hair growth that is often more unpleasant than a total loss of hair.

Several medications to prevent or diminish hair loss are under study, among them are a Japanese drug called alopestatin, and a German product, Thymuskin. Several complementary treatments are recommended but are not generally considered as effective.

The best approach is to understand what is occurring and prepare for it with a visit to the American Cancer Society Look Good Feel Better Program, which provides information about wigs, head scarves, and hats. Cancer support groups are also very helpful in emotionally and physically dealing with this occurrence.

## Sexual Dysfunction

Cancer, and the treatment of cancer with surgery, radiation therapy, and chemotherapy may cause sexual side effects in both men and women. These effects may be limited to an inability to have children or may also include sexual dysfunction and the inability to have normal physical sexual relationships. While the eradication of a cancer may be foremost in the mind of the patient and the physician, changes in self-image, as with hair loss and loss or decrease of sexual function, may strongly impact an individual emotionally and needs to be addressed by both the patient and the treating physician.

### Treatment for Women

Women undergoing any type of pelvic surgery, followed by pelvic radiation and chemotherapy, will usually have changes in, or a temporary absence of, their menstrual cycle. Women treated for breast cancer, Hodgkin's disease, certain leukemias and lymphomas, and other cancers often have temporary or permanent failure of their ovarian functions. In younger, premenopausal women, there may be impacts on the ability to have children because of the effects on the ovaries, and in some instances harvesting (removing and storing) eggs for later use is indicated.

Although many women with cancer are in the postmenopausal age group, loss of their remaining ovarian function may affect their ability to have normal sexual relations physically, psychologically, and emotionally. Loss of libido and desire, pain with intercourse (dyspareunia), or vaginal dryness may be due to decreased estrogen hormone production or secondary to anxiety, changes in pelvic blood flow, depression, and stress. While these may also be directly related to age, successful management of the patient with cancer by a physician or sex counselor is important for maintaining psychological and emotional wellness. Embarrassment or a hesitancy to bring up these issues must be overcome and wise physicians or complementary medical practitioners should be alerted to the important side effects when cancer therapy uses testosterone.

The drugs and therapies often associated with temporary or permanent ovarian failure are procarbazine-containing substances, busulfan, chlorambucil, cyclophosphamide, melphalan, mitomycin-c, and radiation. All the combined treatment regimens—MOPP, MVPP, COPP, ChIVPP (*see* glossary)—induce ovarian failure.

Sexual dysfunction due to anxiety, decreased circulation, depression, and hormonal imbalance may be reduced with standard and complementary medicines. Psychotherapy and antidepressants may be indicated. Vaginal estrogen creams may help with dryness and dyspareunia. Nutritional supplements include DHEA (dehydroepiandrosterone—

must be used under physician supervision)—essential fatty acids (borage oil, evening primrose, fish oil), magnesium (supports hormone production), and vitamins B-complex (to reduce stress), C (to increase libido), and E (to support hormone production). Herbal supplements are arginine, damiana, ginkgo biloba, and ginseng; yohimbe with argenine may increase libido. Also effective are acupuncture, contrast sitz baths (alternate hot and cold water), massage, meditation, traditional Chinese medicine (TCM), and yoga. Participation in women's cancer support groups, and/or sexual therapy is recommended.

### Treatment for Men

Sexual dysfunction in men includes ED (erectile dysfunction), premature, delayed or retrograde ejaculation, loss of libido and sexual desire, and infertility. This may be due to a direct effect from the tumor (involving the gonads, pituitary or other brain involvement, and reproductive tract), from chemotherapy (loss of hormones), radiation therapy (loss of hormone production, nerve damage), or surgery (bladder surgery, colon and rectal surgery, impotence, injury to nerves, loss of orgasm, lymph node dissection, penis surgery, prostate surgery, and removal of testicles). Even so-called nerve-sparing procedures have a high incidence of nerve injuries. Other causes may be anxiety, depression, and other psychological issues, other medical problems (diabetes, heart disease), alcohol and drug abuse, use of some antidepressants, and progressing older age.

Standard treatment options include sildenafil (Viagra), tiadalafil (Cialis), and vardenafil (Levitra). More vigorous options are placement of a penile prosthesis, vacuum devices and surgery to improve blood flow, or vasodilators that can be injected into the penis. As with women, alternative therapies can help with anxiety, decreased circulation, depression, or hormonal imbalance. Nutritional and supplemental options include essential fatty acids, magnesium, and vitamins B-complex, C, and E. Herb therapy includes chaste tree, ginkgo biloba, panax ginseng, saw palmetto, and yohimbe. Since these may interact with chemotherapeutic drugs, they should be used with the consultation of a physician. Additionally, acupuncture, contrast sitz baths, massage, meditation, traditional Chinese medicine (TCM), and yoga have been shown to be helpful. Men should seek out psychological counseling from their physician or a sex therapist. Testosterone hormone therapy for men may be contraindicated in patients with prostate cancer, but this should be discussed with the oncologist.

## Secondary Malignancies

Secondary malignancies are cancers caused by treatment with chemotherapy or radiation therapy. They differ from the original treated cancer and can occur within months or years of the former therapy. The unfortunate quandary is that the same therapies that kill cancer cells can also injure normal cells and induce malignant transformation.

A classic example is Hodgkin's disease for which there is a very high cure rate. However the combination therapies using alkylating agents (cyclophosphamide, nitrogen mustard, procarbazine), anthracyclines (doxorubicin), bleomycin, corticosteroids (prednisolone, prednisone), and vinca alkaloids (vinblastine and vincristine) can result in the formation of a second cancer. Among the cancers seen *after* this treatment for Hodgkin's disease are, in order of frequency, breast, thyroid, bone, colorectal, lung, stomach, non-Hodgkin's lymphoma, and acute leukemia. The risk was as high as 10 percent over twenty years.

Secondary cancers after treatment for non-Hodgkin's lymphoma occur in 2.75 percent of patients and are felt to be due to CHOP therapy. CHOP is an abbreviation for a combination of drugs—cyclophosphamide (Cytoxan), doxorubicin (or adriamycin), vincristine (Oncovin), and prednisolone. The incidence of secondary cancers after breast cancer treatment with alkylating agents (cyclophosphamide), anthracyclines (doxorubicin, epirubicin, mitoxantrone), antimetabolites (5-FU, methotrexate), and taxanes (Taxol, Taxotere) is 3.8 percent at 10 years. Children with acute lymphoblastic leukemia treated with radiation therapy have a twentyfold increase in developing a second cancer. Patients treated for testicular cancer with the combination therapy of cisplatin, etoposide, and bleomycin (PEB) have an increased risk for leukemia.

The most common secondary cancers are usually low-malignancy skin cancers of the basal- and squamous-cell types. When diagnosed early, they are easily detected and cured. The important principle to understand is that treatment of primary tumors can, in a small percentage of cases, result in the development of a secondary cancer, and part of a routine follow-up should be a thorough exam to determine if any such occurrences have developed.

## Neurotoxicity

Chemotherapeutic agents may cause a variety of acute and chronic neurological toxicities. The effects may be on the brain where they can cause long-term developmental problems in children, or on the peripheral nerves.

Impaired brain function, central neurotoxicity, or chemo brain refers to alterations in memory, thinking, and concentration; motor, sensory, and reflex function in adults; and learning and developmental difficulties in children. Peripheral neuropathy refers to numbness, pain, or tingling in the arms or legs. All these toxicities are usually related to the dosage and time interval between treatments.

Aside from problems with the arms and legs, symptoms can include agitation, difficulty learning new things, difficulty handling money and financial matters, drowsiness, memory lapse, sleep problems, or severe confusion. It should be emphasized that many of the neurological changes and abnormalities may not be directly related to the chemotherapy, or even the cancer, but to other concurrent conditions, such as anemia, electrolyte imbalance, endocrine and metabolic problems, heart problems, or infections.

The workup for neurotoxicity consists of a comprehensive physical examination by a physician or neurologist that includes an evaluation of cranial nerves 1–12 (see glossary), motor function (movement), reflexes, and sensory function (pain, position, temperature, and touch). Further studies may include a CT (computerized tomography) scan, an EEG (electroencephalogram-records brain waves), an EMG (electromyelogram–electrical conduction in nerves and muscles), and an MRI (magnetic resonance imaging).

Treatment of neurotoxicity is often related to decreasing, altering, or stopping the chemotherapy, or treatment with biphosphonates, corticosteroids, narcotics for pain, and NSAIDS (nonsteroidal anti-inflammatory drugs—ibuprofen, naproxen, Tylenol). In addition, practical therapies for confusion or transient memory loss, such as getting enough sleep, getting physical therapy, keeping a quiet environment, making notes and a calendar of a schedule and events, not being alone, and wearing hearing aids or glasses to decrease confusion are important and helpful. In these circumstances, it is best to avoid alcohol and too much pain medication. Most of all, stay in close contact with your physician.

## TABLE 6.2. COMMON CHEMOTHERAPEUTIC AGENTS ASSOCIATED WITH NEUROTOXICITY

| AGENT | NEUROTOXICITY |
|---|---|
| Vinca alkaloids, Vincristine, Vinblastine, Vinorelbine | Diminished reflexes, paresthesias of hands and feet, weakness, facial weakness, cranial nerve problems, sexual dysfunction, GI problems |
| Cisplatin and Oxyplatin | Sensory deficits, vision problems, seizures, encephalitis (inflammation of brain) |
| Thalidomide | Paresthesias arms and legs |
| Cytarabine | Seizures, encephalopathy, ataxia, peripheral neuropathy |
| Ifosfamide | Hallucinations, dizziness, peripheral neuropathy, cranial nerve dysfunction |
| 5-fluorouracil | Ataxia, Nystagmus, confusion, coma, peripheral neuropathy |
| Methotrexate lethargy, | Meningeal irritation, headache, nausea, vomiting, transient paralysis |
| Paclitaxel/ Docetaxel | Peripheral neuropathy, weakness, visual defects, confusion, burning mouth |
| Procarbazine | Lethargy, depression, confusion, hallucination, paresthesias |
| Interleukin | Hallucinations, disorientation, agitation, seizures |
| Interferon | Decreased short-term memory and attention span, depression, sleep problems, lack of coordination |
| Taxanes | Distal neuropathy |

There are many alternative/complementary therapies for these symptoms, and they should be discussed with your oncologist or internist prior to use.

## Nephrotoxicity—Kidney Problems

The kidneys function by filtering blood and excreting waste in the form of urine. Chemotherapeutic agents in the blood may result in minor changes in kidney function detectable only in blood and urine tests, or severe kidney damage and complete kidney failure requiring renal dialysis. The drugs most responsible for this are carboplatin, carmustine, cemcitabine, cisplatin, ifosfamide, methotrexate, mitomycin, and streptozosin, and the toxicity is related to dosage, frequency, and length of therapy. Unless there is underlying or preexisting kidney disease prior to therapy, such conditions as diabetes mellitus, hypertension, heart disease, kidney toxicity, and even kidney failure resolve slowly after the chemotherapy has been stopped.

## Hepatotoxicity—Liver Problems

The liver functions as a filter to separate out harmful substances from the blood. The liver produces a substance called bile that aids in the removal of these substances. Chemotherapy uses toxic agents to destroy cancer cells and these toxic substances are eventually filtered through the liver. If there is preexisting liver disease or any liver damage, the organ will not filter out enough of the chemotherapy drugs and the liver can get overloaded and have its own cells destroyed by the chemotherapy. This is called hepatotoxicity.

For this reason, the oncologist needs to evaluate the function of the liver prior to starting any chemotherapy and then adjust the dosages appropriately if there is evidence of any preexisting liver disease, such as hepatitis or cirrhosis due to alcohol, bacteria, or a virus. Even so, patients may develop signs and symptoms of hepatotoxicity under the best of circumstances.

These are the signs and symptoms of liver dysfunction.

◇ Abdominal pain, nausea, vomiting

◇ Itching

◇ Jaundice (yellowish appearance of skin and whites of eyes due to increased accumulation of bilirubin in bile)

◇ Light-colored stools

◇ Swelling hands and feet

◇ Tendency to bleed more easily

◇ Weakness, fatigue

◇ Weight gain due to fluid in abdomen (ascites)

Tests for liver toxicity are: Bilirubin blood levels (> 3.0), liver function tests that include alanine aminotransferase, alkaline phosphatase, LDH (lactic dehydrogenase), SGOT, and SGPT.

The following is a list of some chemotherapeutic drugs likely to cause hepatotoxicity.

◇ **Alkylating agents.** Busulfan, cisplatin, nitrogen mustards (chlorambucil, cyclophosphamide, ifosphamide, mechlorethamine, melphalan), nitrosoureas (BCNU, CCNU, streptozosin), oxaliplatin (Eloxatin)

◇ **Antimetabolites.** Azathioprine, cytosine arabinoside (Ara-C), 5-fluorouracil (5-FU), gemcitabine, 6 mercaptopurine, methotrexate

◇ **Antitumor antibiotics.** Bleomycin, dactinomycin, daunorubicin, doxorubicin, mithramycin, mitomycin

◇ **Platinums.** Carboplatin, cisplatin

◇ **Spindle inhibitors.** Docetaxel (Taxotere), paclitaxel (Taxol), vincristine

◇ **Topoisomerase inhibitors.** Etoposide, irinotecan (Camptosar), topotecan (Hycamptin)

◇ **Tyrosine kinase inhibitors.** Imatinib (Gleevec), lapatinib (Tykerb), nilotonib (Tasigna)

◇ **Others.** A-interferon, interleukin II, tamoxifen

The treatment for hepatotoxicity is to discontinue or alter the dosage of any chemotherapy drugs that are responsible for the condition. Patients should avoid acetaminophen, alcohol, and drugs that control high blood-cholesterol levels. The liver has a high capacity for repair and regeneration if the hepatotoxicity is recognized and the responsible agent or agents are adjusted or eliminated.

## Hypersensitivity Reaction

Hypersensitivity reaction is another name for allergic reaction—an overactive response of the immune system to foreign substances that cause a local or full-body reaction. Although there are four types of allergic reactions, the discussion here is limited to the TYPE I reaction, the one most commonly associated with allergic reactions to drugs, such as chemotherapy medications. The usual symptoms are hives, flushing, itching (pruritis), a mild or severe rash, and swelling. An extreme reaction is called anaphylaxis, which can cause low blood pressure, shock, and even death.

The chemotherapy drugs most often associated with hypersensitivity reactions are carboplatin, cytarabine, docetaxel, L-asparaginase, procarbazine, monoclonal antibodies (bevacizumab, cetuximab, rituximab, and trastuzumab), oxaliplatin, paclitaxel, and teniposide.

Treatment for chemotherapy-based allergic reactions includes antihistamines (Benadryl), bronchodilators to open up the breathing passages (Proventil or Brethine), and corticosteroids (Beclovent).

## Vascular Toxicity

There are several forms of blood-vessel abnormalities that can occur as a result of cancer or chemotherapy for cancer. These include bleeding, blood clots blocking arteries and veins (thrombosis), clotting of tiny kidney blood vessels causing kidney failure, or ischemia (diminished or lack of arterial blood flow to an organ).

Irinotecan can increase the risk for venous thrombosis (clotting) in the presence of metastatic cancer, and the chemotherapy drugs cisplatin, in association with tamoxifen, have been found to increase blood clots in the brain, heart, and legs. Thalidomide along with chemotherapy increases the risk of blood clots.

Patients receiving continuous 5-FU can develop heart attacks and heart failure, and bleomycin and cisplatin regimens have been known to cause Raynaud's (cold extremities) syndrome, although this is more severe in smokers.

The new angiogenesis inhibitors may cause bleeding, such as intestinal bleeding and nosebleeds, and, conversely, bevacizumab can cause venous thrombosis (blood clots in legs).

The toxicities must be identified and treated early to prevent major problems. Their diagnosis is based on routine examinations and questioning by the patient's oncologist or family physician.

## Paraneoplastic Syndrome

A paraneoplastic syndrome is a disease or symptom triggered in response to the presence of a cancer in the body. The syndrome may be due to humoral substances secreted by the tumor or due to the body's cancer fighting antibodies, or white blood cells (T-cells) responding to the presence of the cancer. This occurs in middle-aged and older patients and is most common in individuals with breast, lung, lymphatic, or ovarian cancer.

There are four main categories of neoplastic syndrome: endocrine, neurological, mucocutaneous, and hematological.

**1** **Endocrine Symptoms.** These are mediated by hormones and, depending on the organ and the hormones, they produce symptoms found in such conditions as hypo-/hyperthyroidism or diabetes mellitus.

- Causal mechanism. Symptoms produced by hormones from a gland

- ACTH (Adrenal cortico-trophic hormone). Cushing's syndrome, lung, pancreas, thymoma

- Antidiuretic hormone. SIADH lung (Syndrome of inappropriate anti-diuretic hormone), CNS (central nervous system) cancer

- PTHrP (Parathyroid type hormone). Hypercalcemia, lung, breast, kidney, myeloma (increased calcium) leukemia, lymphoma, ovary

- Insulin/insulin-like substances. Hypoglycemia, liver, sarcoma, insulinoma (low blood sugar)

- Serotonin Carcinoid syndrome, bronchial adenoma, pancreas, stomach

**2** **Neurological Symptoms.** Autoimmune reactions causing brain dysfunctions. These are found with breast, lung, and ovarian cancers and have a host of complex neurological symptoms including weakness and encephalitis (brain inflammation) with motor and sensory symptoms, and intellectual, cognitive deficits.

**3** **Mucocutaneous Symptoms.** Autoimmune reaction causing skin reactions. These are most common with cancers of the breast, kidney, lung, stomach, and uterus.

**4** **Hematological Symptoms.** These syndromes cause anemia and increased coagulation that can lead to heart and kidney disease

There are no cures for (para)neoplastic syndromes. Treatment is first directed toward treating the cancer and then to decreasing the immune response with intravenous immunoglobulins, plasmaphoresis (a process that cleanses antibodies from the blood), radiation, or steroids.

## Pain and Pain Management

Most patients with cancer have a certain degree of pain related to the growth and spread of their cancer and/or to the therapy they receive for their cancer. The pain may be acute or chronic, mild to severe, or varying in intensity. This area of cancer evaluation and therapy is one that often results in inadequate treatment because of patient and physician ignorance or fear, and it often results in inappropriate and unsatisfactory pain control. This is an area of treatment that welcomes the complementary approaches to therapy, with many contributing recommendations from holistic, Ayurvedic, traditional Chinese, and other disciplines. The use of alternative approaches to pain management has opened a whole new world of therapeutic modalities, with acupuncture, herbal and nutritional treatments, massage, meditation, yoga, and other therapies added to the standard surgical and drug regimens.

But consider the barriers to pain management in cancer. The patient may not understand the nature of the pain, may fear addiction from opiates, may feel that pain is inevitable, may fear the side effects of the pain medicine, may be unable to pay for medication, or may not have access to pain management specialists, to name a few potential barriers. On the physician side, he or she may not have an adequate understanding of the pain mechanisms or their assessment and management, may have undue fears about addiction, overdose, and side effects, or may not have the time or desire to treat this complex and often difficult area of cancer care. And finally, the patient may live in an area where pain management is low on the list of priorities—there may not be any organized pain management teams, the cost of adequate pain treatment may be prohibitive, or there is just a lack of appreciation concerning the importance and crucial nature of pain management.

Pain makes work and thought more difficult, it impairs intellectual pursuits and day-to-day normal functioning, and it leads to anger, depression, anxiety, fear, and hopelessness.

Given all the above, it is important for the patient to find a physician and a cancer center or network that has an excellent pain-management program. Unmanaged intractable pain from cancer or its treatment makes life unbearable, and at this juncture patients often contemplate suicide.

There are several aspects of pain to consider, including etiology, nature of the pain, and the panoply of available treatments available.

Eighty-five percent of pain is illness-related. In the case of cancer, it may be directly related to the growth of the cancer and secondarily to infection and inflammation, and it may involve the nervous system, bone, pelvis, intestines, skin, or soft tissue. Treatments such as surgery and radiation can cause acute pain that usually resolves after the treatment. And radiation can cause nerve damage in the brain or spinal cord resulting in pain.

Similarly, chemotherapeutic agents, including bortezomib, cisplatin/oxyplatin, docetaxel/aclitaxel, and thalidomide, can cause chemotherapy-induced peripheral neuropathy (CIPN) that, in turn, causes intense pain, numbness, tingling, and hypersensitivity to cold that, in some cases, may last for a long time after the treatment has ceased. Some drugs can cause severe irritation to the nose, mouth, and throat, making eating and drinking unpleasant and difficult.

Pain management must be preceded by a complete physical and psychological evaluation, as well as a pain assessment. This latter may be done by having a patient rate the pain from one to ten, or grade it on a sheet of paper from minimal to most severe. The physician needs to understand the source of the pain. Does it originate from the bones, the central nervous system, the intestines, or the skin? Is it acute, chronic, or transient? With this guideline and an understanding of the patient's needs, the physician can design a treatment program to alleviate the pain without completely incapacitating the patient.

Pain management is often difficult because pain is a subjective issue and because, in chronic and even acute situations, different patients require different drugs and dosages for similar disease presentations. Also, prolonged use of strong medications, such as opioids, often leads to dependence and a need for increasing dosages of medications.

After relieving the acute pain, the first line of therapy is to treat the inciting cause of pain. This can be done with radiation therapy (for bone pain, soft-tissue tumor growth, or to reduce the size of the tumor that may be pressing on nerves), chemotherapy to diminish the tumor size, and nerve blocks, usually done by a pain management specialist (often an anesthesiologist) who can inject medications directly into a nerve or nerve plexus and block the nerve, relieving the pain (celiac axis block, continuous epidural injections, nerve blocks that are back injections, and trigger point injections). Long-term pain control can be delivered by a patch worn on the skin or through placing special pain-infusion catheters connected to small machines that can pump in pain-killing medicines. Neurosurgeons can place wires deep in the brain to deliver electrical currents that completely block pain centers and eliminate pain sensation.

The appropriate use of drugs often presents a problem and should be delegated to physicians who are familiar with the need and the side effects. Elimination of pain supersedes any concern about addiction. However, the wise physician starts with a lower dose and a less addictive drug, increasing strength as needed, and making sure to eliminate most, if not all, the discomfort experienced by the patient. Treatment often begins with non-opioid medications and advances to the more powerful opioids as the pain progresses. Medications may be taken by mouth, rectal suppositories, transdermal patches, or injections—subcutaneous (in skin), subdermal, intramuscular (deep tissue or muscle), intravenous, epidural, or intrathecal (medicine placed directly into the spine area).

Below is a list of progressively more powerful drugs used for pain management.

## TABLE 6.3. DRUGS USED FOR PAIN MANAGEMENT

| NON-OPIOID ANALGESICS FOR MILD TO MODERATE PAIN | OPIOID DRUGS FOR CANCER PAIN |
|---|---|
| Aspirin | Codeine |
| Acetaminophen | Dihydrocodone |
| Ibuprofen, fenoprofen | Hydromorphine |
| Naproxen | Methodone |
| Ketorolac (Toradol) | Meperidine, mefenamic, Gavapentin |
| | oxymorphone |
| | Levorphanol |
| | Fentanyl-patch/ |
| | inhaled/transderm cream |
| | Nucynta |

Aside from the pain medications, patients will often benefit from other medications that help with the management of their pain-related symptoms. These include the following.

◇ Anti-anxiety-Clinazopam

◇ Anticonvulsants, such as Gavapentin

◇ Antidepressants, such as Cymbalta and Prozac

◇ Antiemetics (antinausea). Compazine, ondansetron (Zofran), metoclopramide (Reglan), Emend

◇ Bone pain medications. Biphosphonates, calcitonin, strontium 89, gallium nitrate, denusomad-xgeva

◇ Corticosteroids

◇ Laxatives

◇ Local anesthetics

◇ Neuropathic pain (brain- and nerve-centered pain). Caffeine, dextroamphetamine, methylphenidate, Provigil, Lyrica (pregabalin)

◇ Stimulants

The informed physician and patient will be well aware of the side effects and complications of any of these drugs and will modify or stop the usage if problems arise.

The Ayurvedic pain-management regimen includes proper nutrition, removing the buildup of toxins, balancing nervous-system activity, stress management, exercise and flexibility education, and certain herbs and additives. There are many programs available.

The Chinese management of cancer pain includes acupuncture, food therapies, herbal remedies, and massage. Other modalities include guided imagery, heat and cold treatments, individual and group therapy, physical therapy, and self-hypnosis.

## Nausea and Vomiting

The side effects of chemotherapy depend on the type of drug used and the amount given. New medications have made these side effects far less common and, when they do occur, much less severe. This is an area where a close collaboration between standard and complementary medicine can give the patient a tremendous advantage.

Individuals are prone to develop nausea and vomiting from different aspects of the disease: the cancer itself; anxiety about the disease or therapy; the chemotherapy and radiation treatments.

In addition to the unpleasantness of the condition, nausea and vomiting can cause a number of physical and mental problems.

◇ Chemical changes in the body

◇ Dehydration

◇ Esophageal tearing

◇ Fractured bones

◇ Loss of appetite

◇ Malnutrition

◇ Mental changes

◇ Surgical wound opening (dehiscence)

There are four described types of nausea and vomiting.

1. **Anticipatory**, where the patient has had previous therapy and a reminder of this through smells, sight, sound, or even the treatment room triggers nausea and vomiting even before the therapy has begun

2. **Acute**, occurring within twenty-four hours of chemotherapy

3. **Delayed**, after twenty-four hours of therapy

4. **Chronic**, usually with advanced cancer and connected to the following situations:

- Brain tumors
- Colon tumors
- Constipation
- Dehydration
- Infections in the mouth or airway
- Medications (narcotics and antidepressants)
- Radiation therapy
- Stomach ulcers

Certain chemotherapeutic drugs are more likely to cause nausea and vomiting. Among these are the following.

◇ Altretamine (Hexalen), estramustine (Emcyt)

◇ Busulfan (Busulfex, Myleran), etoposide

◇ Carmustine (BCNU), ifosfamide (Ifex)

◇ Cisplatin (Platinol), lomustine (CeeNu)

◇ Cyclophosphamide (Cytoxan), mechlorethamine (Mustargen)

◇ Dacarbazine, procarbazine (Matulane)

◇ Doxorubicin (Adriamycin), streptozosin (Zanosar)

◇ Epirubicin (Ellence), temozolomide (Temodar)

The standard drug treatments for nausea and vomiting include the following.

◇ Aprepetant (Emend)

◇ Cannabinoids (marijuana, nabilone)

◇ Dexamethasone (Decadron), methylprednisolone (Medrol)

◇ Dronabinol (Marinol)

◇ Haloperidol (Haldol)

◇ Lorazepam (Ativan), alprazolam (Xanax)

◇ Metoclopramide (Octamide, Reglan)

◇ Olanzapine (Zyprexa)

◇ Ondansetron (Zofran), granisetron (Kytril), dolasetron (Anzemet)

◇ Palonasetron (Marinol)

◇ Prochlorperazine (Compazine)

In addition to these drugs, there are complementary therapies for nausea.

◇ Acupressure                    ◇ Guided imagery

◇ Acupuncture                    ◇ Hypnosis

◇ Behavioral modification        ◇ Relaxation therapy

◇ Biofeedback

Plus, here are some recommendations to deter nausea and vomiting.

◇ Avoid caffeinated drinks.

◇ Avoid strong smells, and especially cooking odors.

◇ Avoid sweet, fatty, and fried foods.

◇ Breathe deeply and slowly.

◇ Chew food well.

◇ Drink most liquids an hour before or after meals.

◇ Eat and drink slowly.

◇ Eat mints and tart candies.

◇ Have small meals multiple times throughout the day.

◇ Prepare and freeze foods in advance of therapy.

◇ Rest, but don't lie down for a few hours after eating.

◇ Watch TV or movies, listen to music, and chat with friends.

◇ Wear loose-fitting clothes.

Other alternative and complementary treatments include aloe vera juice, chamomile tea, ginger (tea), goldenseal (pill or tea), and peppermint tea or oil.

Ayurvedic recommendations also include noncarbonated syrups, cardamom, cinnamon, cloves, lemon with rock salt, and several other substances, such as apple cider vinegar with honey, cumin in various preparations, red raspberry, slippery elm, and wheat germ.

A study by Joseph A. Roscoe, PhD, Peter Bushunow, M.D., et al describes the effectiveness of acupressure bands in reducing nausea related to radiation therapy.[1]

There arc many resources in alternative and complementary medicine to research for other methods of alleviating nausea and vomiting. As with other situations, any modality should be discussed with the patient's primary treating physician to ascertain there are no contraindications to the therapy.

## Depression and Anxiety

An article by the National Cancer Institute[2] presents an interesting listing of the mythical fallacies associated with the diagnosis of cancer.

◇ All people with cancer are depressed:

◇ Depression in a person with cancer is normal.

◇ Treatments are not helpful.

◇ Everyone with cancer faces suffering and a painful death.

As cancer and its therapy causes changes in the human body, it also affects feelings and emotions. Psychiatrists state that upwards of 50 percent of patients with cancer have some degree of psychiatric disorder which, if untreated, can severely compromise the patient's quality of life.

Depression, anxiety, and delirium are the three clinical syndromes most often encountered. Depression may vary from the sadness found in everyday life to severe psychological and physical symptoms. The psychological signs and symptoms include sadness, crying, mood swings, withdrawing from friends and family, loss of pleasure, guilt, anger, low esteem, and even thoughts of death and suicide. The physical symptoms often include sleep disorders (too much or too little), diminished concentration, agitation or withdrawal, appetite change (increased or decreased), and fatigue.

Emotional signs of anxiety include excessive fear or worry, dread, trouble concentrating, anticipating the worst, restlessness, irritability, and discontent. Physical signs of anxiety may be sweating, dizziness, pounding heart, headaches, fatigue, insomnia, muscle tension, and dizziness.

If these symptoms persist more than two weeks, they must be seriously examined and treated appropriately.

Many patients may have underlying psychiatric disorders, and they will be more prone to major anxiety and depression; others may have malignancies, such as a brain tumor, and pancreatic cancer that may have depression as a presenting symptom of the cancer itself. Furthermore, certain drugs and therapies in general use are associated with psychiatric disorders, and among these are barbiturates, B-blockers, benzodiazepines that can cause depression, brain radiation, cytokines (interferons), opioids, procarbazine, steroids (associated with mania), and tamoxifen.

The treating physician must be aware of all these variables and then select out the appropriate therapy.

At the outset, a person experiencing excessive anxiety and depression should be evaluated by a healthcare professional, a psychologist or psychiatrist, and a therapist used to working with patients with cancer. Discussion may allay many of the anxieties and depression, or, in addition, the therapist may feel that the individual might have too many or too few of certain chemicals in the brain. In this case, antidepressants or anti-anxiety medications may be indicated. But it should be understood that taking these types of medications is not often a panacea for these symptoms, and also that these medications, in and of themselves, have many side effects, and that starting or stopping their usage should not be taken lightly.

Several benzodiazepines are used for anxiety and are of two types, short and long-acting. The short-acting, alprazolam and lorazepam, have short duration but can be used to treat panic attacks and intermittent anxiety. They cannot, however, be stopped abruptly; they must be withdrawn gradually. The longer-acting benzodiazepines, clonazepam and diazepam, are for persistent anxiety, and, because of their longer action, they do not wear off quickly when stopped. These two latter ones may not, however, be suitable for older people or anyone with kidney or liver disease.

In addition, low doses of antipsychotic medications can be used for anxiety, including haloperidol (Haldol), olanzapine (Zyprexa), quetiapine (Seroquel), and risperidone (Risperdal).

The older, most common, antidepressants are called SSRIs (selective serotonin reuptake inhibitors), and they affect serotonin release in the brain. The most common of these are citalopram (Celexa), escitalopram (Lexapro), fluoxitone (Prozac, Sarafem), paroxetine, and sertraline. However, these all have the side effects of mild nausea (temporary), significant sexual dysfunction with decreased libido, impotence, and anorgasmia (inability to have an orgasm), jitteriness, and insomnia. The newer antidepressants are bupropion (Wellbutrin) that increases norepinephrine in the brain and may improve attention, plus duloxetine (Cymbalta), mirtazapine (Remeron), and venlafaxine (Effexor), all of which affect the metabolism of serotonin as well as norepinephrine. They may also cause significant sexual dysfunction and occasional hot flashes. Many physicians use psychostimulants, such as dextroamphetamine (Dexedrine), methylphenidate (Ritalin), and pemoline (Cylert).

There are many complementary therapies for anxiety and depression that are effective but are not in the standard Western armamentarium. The Ayurvedic approach stresses two main causes of depression: an imbalance of the three doshas—vata, pitta, kapha—and a lack of awareness of one's deeper self. A patient would need a consultation with a Ayurvedic healer to discuss this type of therapy and determine the appropriateness of its use with depression and anxiety related to cancer.

More common herbal remedies include ginkgo biloba, ginseng, and St. John's Wort; these may be effective with minor depression, but they should not be first line of therapy for cancer patients with severe depression, and consultation with a physician is important to prevent potential suicidal reactions.

Recommended Chinese modalities are acupuncture, herbs, such as astragalus, dong quai, licorice, and Siberian ginseng, certain teas, healing sounds, and lifestyle changes. A comprehensive discussion of Chinese herbal therapies is available in the discussion by Jake Fratkin, CMD, in his article *New Chinese Herbal Formulas for Treating Depression.*[3]

## Genetic Testing and Counseling

Cancer develops as the result of an accumulation of genetic changes within a normal cell that allows uncontrolled cell growth. Most cancers are not inherited but result from one or several of the environmental or biological events previously described. There are, however, some malignancies that appear to be inherited, resulting from some abnormal gene passed down through a family. The most common inherited cancers include breast, colon, endometrial, ovarian, pancreatic, and prostate.

When a physician or a patient maps a family history of cancer, a determination can be made as to whether further studies are indicated. The general rule is to evaluate first- or second-degree relatives for the following history.

◇ A BRCA 1 or BRCA 2 mutation

◇ A rare cancer (such as male breast cancer)

◇ Cancer at a young age (before age fifty)

◇ Cancer occurring in paired organs—breasts, kidneys, ovaries

◇ Specific ethnic background (i.e., Ashkenazi Jewish)

◇ The same type of cancer

◇ Two or more cancers in the same person

When there is a strong family history of cancer in conjunction with the above characteristics, this creates a need to look into possible inherited origins. At this juncture a physician may recommend genetic counseling and this may lead to genetic testing.

Genetic counselors are specially trained individuals who will do an in-depth study of your family and help determine your odds of having a genetic mutation, estimate your cancer risks, and determine whether further studies, including genetic testing (that involves having blood drawn), should be done. Your counselor will discuss the pros and cons of this study, and that includes emotional and family concerns, marriage and childbearing concerns, as well as decisions about further procedures, or even surgery. Some individuals have been concerned about the insurance liability of such a test, although laws now in effect are intended to eliminate the possibility of discrimination on the basis of genetic test results (that should be private but often aren't).

Genetic counselors can provide assistance with all hereditary cancers, but their main expertise is with the following.

◇ Breast and ovarian cancers

◇ Colorectal cancer, especially nonpolyposis cancers

◇ Diffuse stomach cancer

◇ Endocrine cancers: adrenal, gastrinoma, insulinoma, parathyroid, pituitary, thyroid

◇ Genes have been discovered that are responsible for Burkitt's lymphoma, chronic myelocytic leukemia, retinoblastoma, and Wilm's tumor.

◇ Male breast cancer

◇ Syndromes: Basal cell, Cowden, hereditary diffuse gastric cancer, juvenile polyposis, Li-Fraumeni, nevus (Gorlin's), Peutz-Jegher's, von Hippel–Lindau (These are all complex syndromes beyond the scope of this book.)

When confronted with positive results, people may become angry, depressed, or anxious and require further counseling to determine what course of action should be taken. This can include vigorous surveillance, or even surgery, as in breast cancer, where a patient may opt for mastectomies and reconstruction, or colon, where a subtotal colon removal may be indicated or recommended.

## Cancer Rehabilitation

In 1972, the National Cancer Institute (NCI) sponsored the National Cancer Rehabilitation Planning Conference that identified four objectives in the rehabilitation of patients with cancer. These were psychosocial support, optimization of physical functioning, vocational counseling, and optimization of social functioning. From this beginning, most cancer centers have established comprehensive programs to deal with these situations and improve the quality of life for patients with cancer. Among their objectives are helping the cancer patient adjust to actual, perceived, and potential losses due to cancer, helping them become more independent and less reliant on caregivers, improving their physical strength, guiding them with nutritional programs, reducing any sleep problems, and thereby decreasing the need for recurrent hospitalizations. The prime objectives are to maintain or improve the quality of life of patients with varying stages of cancer, ascertaining a patent's overall status, and addressing the following conditions.

◆ Emotional well-being            ◆ Satisfaction with treatment

◆ Family well-being               ◆ Sexuality and intimacy issues

◆ Functional ability              ◆ Social functioning

◆ Physical concerns               ◆ Spiritual well-being

Rehabilitation services are usually coordinated under a cancer rehabilitation team staffed by a specially trained group of healthcare professionals. These include the following.

◆ Physicians. Oncologists, surgeons, radiation therapists who, along with a case manager or care coordinator, organize and manage the team. There will usually be a physiatrist or rehabilitation medical specialist who treats pain management, injuries, and illnesses that affect the way a person moves.

In addition, the following specialists are part of the team.

◇ A rehabilitation nurse who is expert in assisting people with chronic illness

◇ A physical therapist who restores mobility and physical functioning

◇ An occupational therapist for self-care issues—i.e., bathing, meal preparation, homemaking, dressing, and modification of the home environment

◇ A recreational therapist who reduces stress, anxiety, and depression with games, arts and crafts, music, and exercise

◇ A dietitian who evaluates nutritional needs and designs a healthy diet

◇ A psychologist or psychiatrist who deals with mental health issues

◇ A social worker who counsels the patient and the family

◇ A prosthetist who is in charge of artificial limbs

◇ A home health aide who provides personal care—i.e., bathing, dressing, toilet care, and mobility

◇ A vocational counselor who helps with finding a satisfying job

◇ A clergy member for spiritual guidance

◇ A speech/language pathologist who evaluates and treats communication deficits

◇ A dentist who manages oral and teeth problems due to cancer or therapy

The objective of all the members is to follow a program of therapy that identifies four categories:

**1** **Preventive.** To lessen the effects of expected disabilities and emphasize patient education in order to prevent further problems

**2** **Restorative.** To return patients to their previous levels of functioning

**3** **Supportive.** To teach the patient how to accommodate their conditions and minimize debility, and to educate in self-care and self-management.

**Palliative.** To give comfort and support in advanced disease through pain control, and prevent bedsores and unnecessary deterioration

A number of complementary programs are often used, including Ayurvedic herbal therapies, traditional Chinese medicine (TCM), holistic approaches, and naturopathic therapies that can be a productive part of a rehabilitation program. Therapies would also include acupuncture, acupressure, aromatherapy, massage, and meditation. A number of alternative dietary and herbal therapies may augment a comprehensive rehabilitation program.

## Cancer in Older People

In an article by Nathan Berger, the abstract mentions that, "as the population expands over the period from 2000 to 2050, the number and percentage of Americans over age 65 is expected to double. This population expansion will be accompanied by a marked increase in patients requiring care for disorders with high prevalence in the elderly. Since cancer incidence increases exponentially with advancing age, it is expected that there will be a surge in older cancer patients that will challenge both healthcare institutions and healthcare professionals."[4]

It has often been stated anecdotally that the seventy-year-old American today has the physiological age of a fifty-year-old from thirty years ago because of medical care, better nutrition and hygiene, and better treatment modalities. In view of this, many articles use the ages sixty to seventy-four as *young-old* and seventy-five to ninety as *old-old*, and many focus on the necessity of eliminating age bias in determining cancer care for these individuals. Rather than focus on age alone, the direction is to evaluate on the basis of health and tolerance of therapy. The older population is now into diet and exercise and maintaining youthfulness, and studies have shown that they often tolerate cancer treatment much the same as the younger patients. Of course, percentage-wise there will be more older patients diagnosed with cancer, as in the case of prostate and breast cancers, but data seems to indicate that precluding coexisting morbidities, such as severe heart, lung, or CNS disease (Alzheimer's, severe dementia), they tolerate treatment very well. Older individuals will be treated vigorously, with no consideration of their being *old folks dying of cancer,* as had been the practice fifty years ago when dealing with patients over the age of sixty-five years.

There are five things you need to be aware of in regard to cancer in older people.

1 One third of cancer is found in patients above seventy-five years of age and yet there has been a tendency to underevaluate and undertreat these people solely because of their age. This will change in the coming years.

2 Older people are becoming more visible advocates for their own treatment, stressing the need for equal and adequate vigorous treatment, demanding second opinions, and not being content to undergo second-class therapy because of their age. Instead of equating aging with cancer and pain, this population is realizing that their care and management deserves the same vigorous approach as the individual forty years younger.

3 Older individuals are now being encouraged to look for spiritual, as well as medical, support in returning to productive and vigorous lives after cancer.

4 Promoting increased energy and positive attitudes will decrease the anxiety and depression often found in those older people who have cancer.

5 Just because a cancer patient is advanced in age does not mean she or he has been handed a terminal diagnosis. These patients will learn to *live* with cancer, not die with cancer.

## Cancer Information in the Computer Age

With the vast amount of medical information accumulating each day, published medical and scientific texts are usually outdated by the time they are printed. In the computer age, the physician and the patient now have access to hitherto unknown up-to-date information via the Internet. Electronic knowledge sources have become the standard in all areas of medicine and even extend to medical records, protecting against inappropriate dosing of medications by a pharmacist or physician, as well as providing simply written descriptions of every disease entity for the general public.

Along with this, however, is a lot of *inexpert* expert advice and very little control over what can be found on the Internet. Patients and physicians are presented with much information, and, unlike the standard medical journals, there is little room for expert critique or any comparable standard to protect the public against false, spurious information. There are, however, many websites available to look up excellent information and some are listed in the back matter. An even more complete and comprehensive list of oncology-related websites is given in Dr. Vincent DeVita's medical text, *Cancer, Principles and Practice of Oncology*.[5]

## How to Find Competent Alternative and Complementary Specialists

There are many alternative and complementary specialists offering services throughout the United States. Many are fully trained in their specialty, whether it be traditional Chinese medicine (TCM), Indian Ayurvedic medicine, holistic medicine, or a whole host of other modalities. Whether or not you believe or adhere to the principles that are espoused by these traditions, it is important to select a practitioner who adequately represents the best of her/his specialty. There are many inadequately trained specialists and often there is not adequate documentation and licensure for their particular medical calling, according to establishment medicine's guidelines. In the Recommended Online Articles section, under Competent Alternative and Complementary Medical Specialists, I have listed several excellent resources for the cancer patient who wishes to seek out second or third opinions after consulting the oncologist. Hopefully, with a broader understanding of alternative therapies, a system of licensure and regulation that satisfies standard allopathic medicine will be established to receive their approval and widen acceptance of this important, forward-looking group of healthcare specialists.

## Hospice

The good news is that life is indeed a blessing, and everyone should enjoy every day. The bad news is that no one is going to get out of it alive. Making the transition can be a terrifying and tragic experience, or it can be one with love, kindness, and compassion. Hospice care has been established as a philosophy of end-of-life care that focuses on alleviating the dying patient's symptoms, along with providing emotional, spiritual, and social support.

The British have long had hospice programs and these were brought to the United States in the 1970s. Over the past forty years, they have expanded exponentially, and understanding their function and working with hospice-care workers is now an integral part of the oncologist's, internist's, and surgeon's work in taking care of terminally ill patients with cancer and other diseases.

Hospice programs are covered by insurance (mostly Medicare) when the physician can state that the patient has less than six months to live and is utilized by 1.5 million Americans every year (one-third of the dying population). Most patients are in hospice for around thirty days, but those who survive six months or more are accommodated by the system.

When an individual arrives at that point in the progression of his/her disease where the terminal nature of the disease is understood, and where living at home with some degree of pain and suffering is apparent, then hospice needs to be instituted. Often the patient (usually with the family) has decided not to continue life-supporting services and has decided not to receive CPR (cardio-respiratory resuscitation) if the heart stops or breathing ceases. The use of further chemotherapy or radiation is declined, although other modalities are certainly welcomed. Although this book focuses on cancer, it should be understood that hospice care can apply to many noncancerous terminal diseases. While more than 80 percent of the hospice patients in the United States are older than sixty-five, there are many in the pediatric age group with cancer or other developmental problems and the program is of great benefit to the family as well as the patient.

The hospice business has become very competitive and families should look for the best care possible. To receive government funding, the hospice must be certified by the Centers for Medicare and Medicaid Services.

Hospice team members include a director, physician, nurse, social worker, counselor, home health aide, pharmacist, and volunteers. Hospice care has four levels—**Routine** home care, **Continuous** home care, **Inpatient** care, and **Respite** inpatient care.

◇ In **Routine** home care, a provider will supply services, such as medical equipment and medications, and such incidentals as bed pads, diapers, and skin care, and must be available on call twenty-four hours as needed.

◇ **Continuous** care (usually for a short duration) is needed when a patient has ongoing severe needs and the time is usually for a minimum of eight hours or throughout the entire day at home.

◇ **Inpatient** care is provided at a hospital or special care unit where symptoms have progressed and death is imminent in days rather than weeks or months.

◇ **Respite** care is actually directed toward a family or caregiver where someone needs a break in caring for the dying individual. During brief periods the patient is transferred from home to a care facility, but this is limited to five days in any given benefit period.

# GLOSSARY

## A

**AA.** Alcoholics Anonymous. A twelve-step program of recovery

**Achalasia.** Failure of muscles to relax at the gastroesophageal junction

**Actinic.** Relating to exposure to ultraviolet radiation

**Acupressure.** Finger pressure at certain points on the body to treat disease symptoms

**Acupuncture.** A system of treatment using fine needles in the skin at certain points on the body

**Adenocarcinoma.** Cancer arising from glands—breast/colon/lung

**Adenopathy.** Enlargement of lymph nodes

**Adjuvant chemotherapy.** Chemotherapy given along with radiation or surgery

**Aflatoxins.** Toxic compounds produced by aspergillus that can lead to cancer

**Alkaline phosphatase.** Blood enzyme related to liver and bile duct function

**Alkylating agent.** Anticancer drug affecting cancer-cell DNA and preventing cell division

**ALL.** Acute lymphoblastic leukemia

**Allogeneic.** Of the same species, different genetic constitution—from a donor

**Allopurinol.** Drug to lower uric acid and prevent kidney damage during chemotherapy

**Alopecia.** Hair loss

**Alpha-fetoprotein.** Blood protein elevated with some liver and testicle cancers

**Alternative medicine.** Therapy used instead of conventional treatment; considered integrative when used in combination with conventional treatment or with complementary medicine, including acupuncture, diets, enemas, herbs, massage, meditation, and spiritual healing

**Amelanotic.** Unpigmented

**Amenorrhea.** Lack of menstrual periods

**Amino acids.** Building blocks of proteins

**AML.** Acute myelogenous leukemia

**Analgesic.** Drug to relieve pain

**Anaplastic.** Cancer that does not resemble its tissue of origin

**Anastomosis.** Connecting two bowel loops or organs together

**Androgens.** Male hormones

**Anemia.** Lower than normal blood level

**Angiogenesis.** Development of blood vessels

**Angiography.** X-ray of blood vessels

**Anorexia.** Loss of appetite

**Anthracyclines** (daunomycin, doxorubicin, epirubicin, et al). Chemotherapeutic class of drugs prone to cause cardiac complications

**Antibody.** A protein made in response to an antigen

**Antiemetic.** Drug to prevent nausea

**Antigen.** Substance causing activation of the immune system

**Antimetabolite.** Drug that interferes with normal metabolism

**Antrum.** First portion of the stomach

**Aphasia.** Inability to talk

**Apoptosis.** Cell death

**Aromatherapy.** Inhaling certain oils that affect mood and hormonal system

**Ascites.** Abnormal fluid in abdomen

**Ataxia.** Abnormal muscular coordination

**Atypical.** Not ordinary

**Autologous.** From the patient's own body, self

**Autosomal.** Non-sex-linked inheritance

**Axilla.** Armpit

**Ayurveda—the knowledge of life.** Called the science of living well, this ancient Hindu medical science uses yoga, breathing, nutritional guidance, meditation, herbs, and physical activity, based on types of energy (doshas).

## B

**Barium enema.** X-ray of colon using barium liquid

**Basal-cell cancer.** Slow-growing tumors that arise from the basal cells of the skin

**B-cell.** Type of lymphocyte involved in immune response

**BCG (bacillus-calumet-guerin).** Material from dead TB bacteria used in cancer treatment

**Benign.** Not cancerous

**Bilateral.** Both sides

**Bile.** Substance produced by liver that helps removal of toxic material and helps digestion

**Biliary.** Pertaining to bile or bile ducts

**Bilirubin.** Yellowish substance in bile secreted by liver from breakdown of blood—breakdown products in urine include urobilin that makes urine yellow and stercobilin that makes the stool brown

**Biofeedback.** System teaches control of involuntary bodily functions, including heart rate, muscle tension, breathing

**Bioflavonoids.** Brightly colored compounds found in plants

**Blastic.** Bone disease with increased calcium

**Bone marrow.** Soft substance inside bone containing various cells, often blood-producing

**Bone scan.** Pictures of bones in body using radioactive materials

**BPH (benign prostatic hypertrophy).** Noncancerous enlargement of the prostate

**Brachytherapy.** Use of radioactive material (seeds) directly at the site of treatment

**Brain parts.** *Cerebral cortex,* outer layer of brain–thought, voluntary movement, language, reasoning; *Cerebellum,* behind the brain–movement, balance, posture; *Brain stem,* area above spinal cord—breathing, heart rate, blood pressure; *Hypothalamus,* base of brain, the size of a pea—body-temperature control; *Thalamus,* relay center–receives/sends sensory information from brain and spinal cord; *Limbic system*—controls emotional responses; *Basal ganglia*—coordination of movement; *Midbrain*—vision, hearing, eye movement, body-movement control

**BRCA.** Inherited gene sometimes found in relation to breast, ovarian, and prostate cancer

**Bronchogenic.** Related to the lung

**Bronchogenic carcinoma.** Cancer of the lung

**Bronchoscopy.** Examination of lung using fiberoptic scope

# C

**Cachexia.** Weakness and wasting, usually due to chronic disease and cancer

**Carbohydrate.** A sugar molecule

**Carcinogenesis.** Creation of cancer

**Carcinoma.** Cancer developing from epithelial tissue or lining tissue

**Cataract.** Opacity or clouding of the lens of the eye

**CAT scan (computerized axial tomography).** A type of x-ray creating cross-section pictures of the body

**CEA (carcinoembryonic antigen).** Tumor marker in blood for certain cancers

**Cells.** Basic building blocks of tissue

**Central venous line.** Special catheter inserted into large vein for feeding or therapy

**Cervical nodes.** Lymph nodes in the neck

**Chemoembolization.** Administration of anticancer drugs into an artery supplying a tissue

**Chemosensitivity assay.** Testing a cancer for sensitivity to a certain drug

**Chemotherapy.** Treatment with drugs that kill cancer cells

**ChIVPP (chlorambucil, vinblastine, procarbazine, prednisone).** A chemotherapy combination

**Cholecystectomy.** Removal of the gallbladder

**CHOP (cyclophosphamide–Cytoxan, Doxorubicin or adriamycin, vin-cristine–Oncovin, and prednisolone).** A combination of chemotherapy drugs

**Chromosomes.** Strands of genetic material (i.e., **DNA)**

**Cirrhosis.** Noncancerous inflammation of liver

**Clinical trial.** Testing a drug in humans

**CLL.** Chronic lymphocytic leukemia

**CML.** Chronic myeloid leukemia

**Colitis.** Inflammation of the colon

**Colonoscopy.** Examining the colon using a fiberoptic scope

**Colostomy.** Intestine brought out through the skin's surface

**Concavalin-A.** Protein used to stimulate T-cells (mitogen)

**Contralateral.** Oposite side

**COPP (cyclophosphamide, vincristine, procarbazine, prednisone).** A chemotherapy combination

**Core biopsy.** Removal of tissue using a special needle

**Cortisone.** Corticosteroid hormone produced by the adrenal glands

**Cranial nerves. I.** Olfactory—transmits sense of smell **II.** Optic—vision **III.** Oculomotor—eye movement **IV.** Trochlear—eye movement **V.** Trigeminal—facial sensation and chewing movement **VI.** Abducens—eye motion **VII.** Facial—movement facial expression, taste front of tongue **VIII.** Vestibulocochlear—sense of sound, rotation, gravity **IX.** Glossopharyngeal—taste back of tongue, secretion by parotid, swallowing **X.** Vagus—swallowing, voice, visceral nerves **XI.** Accessory muscles—movement upper back and neck sternomastoid m. and trapezius m. **XII.** Hypoglossal—movement of tongue

**Cruciferous.** Vegetables high in B-carotene

**Cryotherapy/Cryosurgery.** Treatments using extreme cold to kill cancer by freezing

**CSF.** Cerebrospinal fluid

**Cushing syndrome.** Disorder of the adrenal gland cortex, characterized by obesity, hypertension, diabetes mellitus, etc.

**Cutaneous.** Pertaining to the skin

**Cystoscopy.** Examination of the bladder with a fiberoptic scope

**Cytogenetics.** Study of chromosomes

**Cytokine.** Immune system substance that signals other immune cells

**Cytology.** Microscopic examination of cells

## D

**Debulking.** Removing a large amount of cancer tissue with surgery

**DES (diethylstilbestrol).** Hormone used in past that can cause vaginal cancer

**Desquamation.** Shedding of surface skin cells

**Dialysis.** Use of an artificial kidney machine to excrete waste when the kidneys are impaired or have failed, temporarily or permanently

**Diplopia.** Double vision

**Diuretic.** Drug causing increased urination

**DNA (deoxyribonucleic acid).** Building block of genetic material

**Double-blind study.** Treatment trial where some patients receive a drug, others a placebo

**Dysgeusia.** Severe alteration of taste

**Dysphagia.** Difficulty swallowing

**Dysplasia.** Abnormal development of tissue

**Dyspnea.** Shortness of breath

**Dysuria.** Painful urination

## E

**Edema.** Fluid accumulation in tissue

**EEG (electroencephalogram).** Measurement, reading of electrical brain waves

**Effusion.** Fluid in a body cavity–abdominal (peritoneal), chest cavity (pleural)

**EGD (esophago-gastro-duodenoscopy).** Fiberoptic exam of the upper intestinal system

**EGFR (epidermal growth factor receptor).** Protein on surface of some cancer cells

**Electrolytes.** Body chemicals–Na (sodium), K (potassium), Cl (chloride)

**Emboli.** Blood clots or tumors that can travel via blood vessels to brain, lung, or other tissue

**Emesis.** Vomiting

**EMG (electromyelogram).** Measuring electrical conduction of nerves and muscles

**Encephalitis.** Inflammation of the brain

**Endocrine.** Gland that secretes its hormone directly into the blood

**Endoscopy.** Exam using a fiberoptic scope

**Epidemiology.** Population studies; Study of incidence and distribution of disease

**Epidermis.** Skin

**Epistaxis.** Nosebleed

**Epstein-Barr virus.** Virus causing mono, some cancers

**ERCP (endoscopic retrograde cholangiopancreatography).** Fiberoptic scope exam of bile ducts

**Estrogen.** Female hormone

**Estrogen receptor assay.** Test to determine if breast cancer is stimulated by estrogen

**Etiology.** Cause of a disease or condition

**Excision.** Surgical removal

**Exocrine.** Gland that secretes hormone into intestine via a duct

**Exophytic.** Growing outward

**Extracellular.** Outside the cell

**Extravasation.** Leakage of fluid, as from a damaged vein, infusion site, or surgical site

## F

**Fine needle aspiration.** Biopsy using fine needle (i.e., for thyroid biopsy)

**Fistula.** Abnormal passage or opening

**Flow Cytometry.** A technique for identifying and sorting cells and their components (as DNA)

**Foramen.** Normal opening

**Frozen section.** Quick study of tissue by a pathologist at time of surgery

**Fungating.** Description of tumor—growing like a fungus, globular, swelling

## G

**Gamma knife.** A type of radiation therapy for cancer

**Gammopathy.** Abnormal proliferation of cells that produce immuno-globulins

**Gene.** A basic unit of DNA, transmitting characteristics from parent to child

**Genome.** Complete set of chromosomes, entire genetic information for a cell

**Gleason score.** Microscopic grading system for prostate cancer

**Glioma.** A type of brain tumor that originates in the glial cells in the brain

**Graft-versus-host reaction.** Reaction of host to grafted material (i.e., bone-marrow transplant)

**Gray.** Measure of ionizing radiation in radiation therapy

**Gynecomastia.** Noncancerous enlargement of the male breast

## H

**H-pylori.** Bacteria causing some stomach cancer

**Hematocrit.** Measure of red blood cells

**Hematoma.** Collection of blood in tissue

**Hematopoietic.** Blood-forming organ (bone marrow)

**Hematuria.** Blood in urine

**Hemoglobin.** Measure of red blood cells

**Hemophilia.** Bleeding-tendency disease

**Hemorrhage.** Loss of blood

**Hepatic.** Pertaining to liver

**Hepatomegaly.** Enlargement of liver

**Her-2/neu.** Gene that controls certain cell growth

**Histology.** The study of the microscopic structure of plant and animal tissues

**HIV (human immunodeficiency virus).** Virus that causes AIDS

**HL.** Hodgkin's lymphoma

**Homeopathy.** System of treatment using highly diluted remedies from natural sources

**Hormonal therapy.** Cancer therapy using hormones (i.e., some breast and prostate cancers)

**Hospice.** Facility for care of dying patient, for comfort, symptom control, emotional support

**Hyperalimentation.** Intravenous high-calorie feeding

**Hypercalcemia.** Increased calcium in blood

**Hyperplasia.** Excessive proliferation of abnormal cells

**Hypnotherapy.** Visualization and guided imagery—promotes relaxation or hypnosis

**Hypoglycemia.** Decreased blood sugar

**Hysterectomy.** Removal of the uterus

**I**

**Ileostomy.** Small intestine brought to skin surface

**Immune system.** Body mechanisms that resist disease, infection, tumor

**Immunosuppression.** Decreased immunity due to disease (i.e., cancer, poor nutrition)

**Immunosuppressive drug.** Drug that alters the immune response, as after a transplant, to prevent rejection

**Immunotherapy.** Cancer therapy that stimulates the immune system

**Induction.** Initial chemotherapy treatment

**Indurated.** Hardened

**Infusion.** Putting fluids in a vein or artery

**Inguinal.** Groin area

**In situ.** Early stage of cancer, cancer growing in local area and not yet able to spread

**Interferon.** Substance produced naturally or artificially to fight cancer

**Interleukins.** Chemicals that convey messages between cells, used in cancer treatment

**Interventional radiologists.** Radiologists who use radiological techniques/invasive procedures for diagnosis and treatment (i.e., drain fluid collections, place stents in vessels and other tubular structures)

**Intra.** Inside of

**Intravenous.** Administration of fluid or drug into a vein

**Invasive cancer.** Cancer able to spread locally or distally, as opposed to in situ

## J

**Jaundice.** Yellowing of skin and eyes due to increased bilirubin—a sign of liver or bile-duct disease

**Jejunum.** A portion of the small intestine

## K

**Keratosis.** Very thick growth

## L

**Laparoscopy.** Examination of abdomen with a fiberoptic camera through a tiny hole

**Laparotomy.** Surgical opening into the abdomen

**LDH (lactic dehydrogenase).** Liver function test

**Leucopenia.** Decreased white cell count

**Leukocytosis.** Elevation of white blood-cell count

**Leukoplakia.** White plaque in mouth and gums

**Ligation.** Tying off a blood vessel

**Linear accelerator.** Radiation therapy machine

**Lobectomy.** Removal of one portion of an organ (liver, lung)

**Lumpectomy.** Removal of breast cancer by taking only part of the breast

**Lymphedema.** Swelling of arm or leg due to lymphatic obstruction

**Lymph nodes.** Oval organs containing lymph and lymphocytes, the drainage portals of the body

**Lynch syndrome.** Inherited colon polyps with increased risks for colon and other cancers

**Lysis.** Destruction of a cell

**Lytic.** Bone area with less calcium than normal

## M

**Macrophages.** White blood cells that devour invading organisms

**Malignant.** Cancerous

**MALT.** Mucosal associated lymphoid tissue lymphoma

**Mediastinum.** Central part of the chest with the heart, esophagus, trachea, aorta, and vena cava

**Melena.** Dark or black stools, indicating blood

**Menarche.** Onset of menstruation

**Meningioma.** A benign brain tumor

**Menopause.** Cessation of menstruation

**Metaplasia.** Cells that look abnormal under the microscope but are not cancerous

**Metastasis.** Spread of cancer

**Mitogen.** Substance that induces cell division

**Mitomycin.** Antitumor antibiotics produced by streptomyces bacteria

**Mitosis.** Cell division and reproduction

**Monoclonal antibodies (MAbs).** Antibodies, many made in the laboratory, for treatment of certain cancers; useful for fighting diseases because they can be designed specifically to target only a certain antigen, such as one found on cancer cells

**MOPP (mechlorethamine, vincristine [oncovin], procarbazine, prednisone).** A chemotherapy combination

**MRI (magnetic resonance imaging).** Images of the body using a magnetic field instead of x-rays

**Mucosa.** Mucous membrane lining hollow organs in the body

**Mutagen.** Substance causing a genetic mutation

**Mutation.** Permanent change in a cell's DNA

**MVPP (cyclophosphamide, vincristine, procarbazine, prednisone).** A chemotherapy combination

**Myeloid.** Pertaining to bone marrow

**Myeloma.** Cancer of plasma cells

**Myelosuppression.** Decrease in blood counts due to chemotherapy or radiation therapy

## N

**Narcotic.** Synthetic or natural pain-relieving substance

**Nasopharynx.** Part of the nasal cavity behind the nose

**Natural killer cells (NK cells).** Lymphocytes (white blood cells) normally found in body that kill cancer cells

**Naturopathy.** A system of healing, using natural methods and substances, but no drugs

**National Cancer Institute.** Major research center in Bethesda, Maryland

**Necrosis.** Death of tissue

**Needle biopsy.** Removing tissue for examination by inserting a needle into a tumor

**Neoadjuvant chemotherapy.** Chemotherapy given before surgery or radiation treatment

**Neoplasm.** A tumor, cancerous or benign

**Nephrotoxic.** Damaging to the kidney

**Neuropathy.** Damage to nervous tissue causing pain, numbness, weakness, or paralysis

**Neurosurgery.** Surgery on the brain and nervous system

**Neutropenia.** Low white-blood count

**NHL.** Non-Hodgkin's lymphoma

**Nitrosamines.** Cancer-causing substances with chemical makeup N-N:O

**No code.** Order in chart not to resuscitate a patient under certain carefully defined conditions

**Nocturia.** Excessive urination at night

**Nodule.** Lump or tumor, benign or malignant

**NSABP (National Surgical Adjuvant Breast/Bowel Project).** A large cooperative group of researchers

**NSAID.** Nonsteroidal anti-inflammatory drug

**NSCLC.** Non-small-cell lung cancer

**Nystagmus.** Involuntary rapid movement of the eyeballs

## O

**Omentum.** A fatty intra-abdominal fold of tissue extending downward from the stomach

**Oncogene.** A gene directing cell growth that may cause cancer when altered

**Oncologist.** Cancer therapy specialist

**Oophorectomy.** Removal of ovary

**Orchiectomy.** Removal of testicle

**Oropharynx.** Part of the throat between the soft palate and the epiglottis

**Osteolytic.** Causing dissolution of bone, seen by x-ray

**Ostomy.** Opening in abdominal skin for drainage of fecal material or urine

**Otalgia.** Pain in the ear

## P

**P-53 gene.** A tumor-suppressor gene that inhibits tumor growth and may be altered with cancer

**Palate.** Roof of mouth

**Palliative.** Treatment, not for cure, but to relieve symptoms or control cancer growth

**Paracentesis.** Removing fluid from the abdomen with a needle

**Paraneoplastic syndrome.** Signs and symptoms indirectly caused by the presence of cancer

**Paraplegia.** Paralysis of the lower half of the body

**Parenteral nutrition.** *See* hyperalimentation

**Paresthesia.** Abnormal skin sensation of pain, burning, itching, etc.

**Pathologist.** Physician studying tissue and laboratory tests

**Pathognomonic** (often misspelled as *pathognomic* and sometimes as *path-omnemonic*). Term often used in medicine that means *characteristic for a particular disease*; a pathognomonic sign is a particular sign whose presence means that a particular disease is present beyond any doubt; labeling a sign or symptom pathognomonic represents a marked intensification of a diagnostic sign or symptom.

**PDQ (physicians data query).** Online database by the National Cancer Institute at www.cancer.gov/cancertopics/pdq

**PEB.** Chemotherapy with (platinum-based) cisplatin, etoposide, bleomycin

**Perineum.** Area of the body between the anus and the genitals

**Periosteum.** Tissue covering the bones

**Peripheral stem-cell transplant.** Cells injected into bone marrow to help it recover after high-dose chemotherapy for cancer

**Peritoneal cavity.** Inside the abdomen

**PET scan (positron-emission tomography).** A scan to detect living and growing cells in cancer evaluation

**Phagocytosis.** Ingestion of bacteria and substances by certain cells

**Phrenic.** Relating to the diaphragm

**Phytochemicals.** Natural chemical substances found in plants

**Placebo.** Inactive substance used in some research as a comparison to the active tested drug

**Plasma.** Clear part of blood

**Platelet.** A part of blood important in formation of blood clots

**Pleura.** Thin layer of tissue covering the lungs

**Pneumonectomy.** Removal of a lung

**Polycythemia.** High red blood-cell count

**Polyp.** Mushroom-shaped growth

**Port a Cath.** Venous access device

**Postprandial.** After eating

**Precancerous.** Abnormal-appearing cells that may become cancerous

**Primary cancer.** Site of origin of a cancer

**Proctoscopy.** Direct examination of the rectum

**Progesterone receptor assay.** Test to evaluate cancer sensitivity to progesterone

**Protein.** Body structure made up of amino acids

**PSA (prostate-specific antigen).** A blood substance from the prostate that may indicate cancer

**Pulmonary embolism.** A blood clot traveling to lungs from vein in leg or pelvis

**Purpura.** Reddish/purple spots on skin, often from bleeding

**Purulent.** Containing pus

## Q

**Qi.** Energy in traditional Chinese medicine (TCM)

**Qigong.** Slow, meditative Chinese exercise

**Quercetin.** A phytochemical (flavonoid) ) in colored fruits that beneficially sensitizes breast-cancer cells to chemotherapy

## R

**Radiation.** The directed guidance of energy particles, as in treatment of disease

**Radiation fibrosis.** Scar tissue resulting from radiation therapy

**Radiation oncologist.** Physician specializing in radiation therapy

**Radiation therapy.** Treatment of cancer using high-energy radiation

**Radical mastectomy.** Removal of entire breast, underlying muscles, and axillary lymph nodes

**Radioactive isotope.** Radioactive substance used for cancer therapy

**Radiofrequency ablation.** Procedure to generate heat to destroy a tumor

**Radiologist.** Physician who specializes in x-rays and other investigative imaging techniques

**Radiosensitive.** A cancer that responds to a given therapy

**Radiosensitizer.** A substance that makes a cancer more responsive to a radiation therapy

**Ras gene.** Gene that may cause cancer when altered

**Recurrence.** Reappearance of a cancer after it has been treated and disappeared

**Regression.** Shrinkage of a cancer

**Remission.** Partial or complete dissolution of a cancer

**Renal.** Related to the kidney

## S

**Sarcoma.** Cancer of connective tissue

**Sclerosis.** Hardening of tissue due to radiation, infection, or tumor

**Secondary malignancy.** Cancer that occurs due to chemotherapy or radiation for a primary malignancy

**Sentinel node.** First lymph node draining a given area

**Sepsis.** Spread of infection to the blood

**SGOT (serum glutamic oxaloacetic transaminase).** Liver enzyme test

**SGPT (serum glutamic pyruvic transaminase).** Liver enzyme test

**SIADH.** Syndrome of inappropriate anti-diuretic hormone

**Sigmoidoscopy.** Examination of the lower colon and rectum with lighted tube

**Spleen.** Organ adjacent to stomach for filtering and producing blood

**Squamous-cell cancer.** Cancer arising from skin or certain lining surfaces

**Stem cell.** Primary or early cells found in bone marrow, blood, umbilical cord, and certain blood vessels

**Stent.** A tubular structure placed inside a vessel or hollow organ to keep it open

**Stereotactic biopsy.** Tissue sample taken under CT or x-ray guidance

**Steroids.** Substances, including cortisol and sex hormones, occasionally used for cancer therapy

**Stoma.** An opening

**Stomatitis.** Inflammation of the mouth

**Subcutaneous.** Just beneath the skin

**Supraclavicular.** Above the clavicle or breast bone

# T

**Targeted therapy.** Drug that targets a specific stage of cancer growth or cell, sparing normal cells

**T-cell.** Lymphocyte involved in immunologic competency (*See* B-cell)

**Thoracentesis.** Removing fluid from the chest with a needle

**Thoracic.** The chest

**Thoracotomy.** Surgical opening of the chest

**Thrombophlebitis.** Inflammation of a vein, often with blood clots

**Thrombosis.** Blood-clot formation in a blood vessel

**TKI (tyrosine kinase inhibitor).** New class of anticancer drugs (i.e., ima-tinib–Gleevac, erlotinib–Tarceva)

**TNM classification.** T=tumor, N=node, M=metastasis

**TPN (total parenteral nutrition).** High-calorie intravenous infusion

**Tracheostomy.** Opening in the neck and trachea and insertion of breath-ing tube

**Traditional medicine.** In the alternative/complementary world, the word traditional always refers to medicine going back centuries before the era of drugs, and it is so used in this book; it does not refer to twentieth-century mainstream, allopathic medicine

**Tumor.** Benign or malignant mass

**Tumor necrosis factor.** Natural protein that may induce tumor shrinkage

**Tumor-suppressor genes.** Genes that suppress cancer growth

**Tylosis.** Formation of a callous

## U

**Ulcer.** A pitted sore

**Ultrasound.** Diagnostic aid using sound waves to create an image

**Undifferentiated.** Cancer not resembling tissue of origin

**Ureter.** Tube going from kidney to bladder

**Urethra.** Tube from bladder to outside

**Urological.** Pertaining to the urinary tract

## V

**Vaccine.** A substance that stimulates the body to produce antibodies

**Varicocele.** Enlarged collection of veins in spermatic cord and scrotum

**Vascularity.** Presence and amount of blood vessels

**Vasectomy (male sterilization).** Tying off and dividing the vas deferens

**VEGF (vascular endothelial growth factor).** A substance that stimulates cells to produce blood vessels—blocking this substance blocks cancer's ability to develop and spread

**Venipuncture.** Inserting a needle into a vein

**Vertebral subluxation.** This occurs when one or more of the bones of your spine, the vertebrae, move out of position and create pressure on, or irritate, spinal nerves.

**Vessicant drugs.** Chemotherapy drugs that have the capacity to cause severe tissue damage if leaked from injection site

**Virus.** Infectious agent made up of RNA or DNA

## W

**Wart.** Benign, horny skin growth

**Well-differentiated.** A cancer that resembles normal tissue under the microscope

**White blood cells.** Cells that fight infection—chemotherapy and radiation cause a decrease in these cells

# APPENDIX

# SOME COMMON CHEMOTHERAPEUTIC AGENTS

*Listings are for general usages*

## Monoclonal Antibodies (mab Suffix)

Alemtuzumab. B-cell CLL

Bevacizumab. Breast and colorectal cancer, NSCLC

Cetuximab. Colorectal and head and neck cancer

Panitumumab. Colon cancer

Rituximab. Non-Hodgkin's lymphoma

Trastuzumab. Breast cancer

## Molecularly Targeted Therapies (Ib Suffix)

Bortezomib. Multiple myeloma

Dasatinib. ALL, CML

Erlotinib. Pancreatic cancer, NSCLC

Gefitinib. NSCLC

Imatinib. CML, GIST

Lapatinib. Breast cancer

Nilotinib. CML

Sorafenib. Kidney cancer

Sunitinib. Kidney cancer, GIST

Temsirolimus. Kidney cancer

## Antimetabolites

### Folate Analogs

Methotrexate. Breast, GI, leukemia, lung ALL, NHL

Pemetrexed. Mesothelioma, NSCLC

### Purine Analogs

Fludarabine. AML, CLL, NHL

Mercaptopurine. ALL, AML, CML

Thioguanine. Colorectal, myeloma, ALL, AML, CML

### Adenosine Analogs

Cladribine. Hairy cell leukemia, AML, CLL, CML, NHL

Pentostatin. Hairy cell leukemia, ALL, CLL

### Pyrimidine Analogs

Capecitabine. Breast, colorectal, GI

Cytarabine. Leukemia, AML, ALL, CML, CNS, NHL

DepoCyt. Leukemia, CNS

Floxuridine. Biliary, breast, colon, pancreas, GI

Fluorouracil. Colon, head/neck, ovary, pancreas, rectal, stomach

Gemcitabine. Bladder, breast, lung, ovary, pancreas

### Alkylating Agents

### Nitrogen Mustards

Bendamustine. CLL

Chlorambucil. Lymphosarcoma, ovarian cancer, CLL, HL, NHL

Cyclophosphamide. Breast, lung, ovary, testicle, ALL, AML, CLL, HL

Estramustine. Kidney, prostate

Ifosfamide. Germ-cell, lung, sarcoma, NHL

Mechlorethamine. Lung, CLL, CML, HL, NHL,

Melphalan. Breast, lung, myeloma, ovary, sarcoma, testicle

### Aziridine

Thiotepa. Many cancers—bladder, breast, ovary, CLL, CML, HL

### Alkyl Sulfonate

Busulfan. Leukemias, lymphomas, CML

### Nitrosoureas

Carmustine. Brain, melanoma solid tumors, myeloma, HL, NHL

Lomustine. Brain, GI, HL, NSCLC

Streptozosin. Carcinoid, colon, islet cell, liver, pancreas, HL, NSCLC

### Platinum Complexes

Carboplatin. Breast, endometrial, head and neck, leukemia, ovarian, NHL

Cisplatin. Bladder, cervix, lung, ovary, sarcoma, squamous, testicle, NHL

Oxaliplatin. Colorectal, ovary

### Nonclassic Alkylators

Altretamine. Breast, cervix, lung, ovary, NHL

Dacarbazine. Melanoma, neuroblastoma, sarcoma, HL

Procarbazine. Brain, lung, HL, NHL

Temozolomide. Astrocytoma, kidney, melanoma

### Substituted Urea

Hydroxyurea. Head/neck, leukemia, melanoma, ovary, CML

## Antitumor Treatments

### Antitumor Antibiotics

Bleomycin. Cervix, head/neck, penis, sarcoma, skin, testicle, vulva

Dactinomycin. Ewing's, testicle, Wilm's

Danorubicin. AML, ALL

DaunoXome. Kaposi's sarcoma

Doxorubicin. Bladder, breast, ovary, stomach, Wilm's, ALL, AML

Doxil. Kaposi's sarcoma, ovary

Idarubicin. ALL, AML, CML

Mitoxantrone. Breast, ovary, prostate, ALL, AML, CML

Mitomycin. Breast, cervix, colorectal, pancreas, stomach, uterus

Valrubicin. Bladder

### Epipodophyllotoxins

Etoposide. Hodgkin's lymphoma, lung, testicle, AML, NHL

Teniposide. Lung, ALL

### Microtubule Agents

Docetaxel. Breast, esophagus, head/neck, ovary, pancreas, prostate

Paclitaxel. Breast, colon, Kaposi's, lung, ovary, stomach, uterine

Vinblastine. Bladder, breast, Hodgkin's, Kaposi's, kidney, NHL

Vincristine. Breast, myeloma, Rhabdo, sarcoma, ALL, HL, NHL

Vinorelbine. Breast, head/neck, Hodgkin's, lung, ovary

### Camptothecan Analogs

Irinotecan. Cervical, colorectal, lung, ovarian

Topotecan. Cervical, lung, ovarian

### Enzyme

Asparaginase. ALL, AML, CML

(From: Pazdur, Wagman, Wamphausen, and Hoskins. *Cancer Management: A Multidisciplinary Approach.* CMP Medica, 1069–1079.)

# ONLINE RESOURCES

**Websites for Alternative/Complementary Associations**

Acupuncture Society of America, Inc.: acupuncturesociety.org

American Association of Naturopathic Physicians: www.naturopathic.org

American Chiropractic Association: www.acatoday.org

American Herbalists Guild: www.healthy.net/herbalists/

American Holistic Medical Association: www.holisticmedicine.org

Beth Israel Medical Center, NY: www.healthandhealingny.org/

Divyajyot Foundation, Inc: www.divyajyot.org/

Harvard University: www.bidmc.harvard.edu/medicine/camr

Minneapolis Medical Research Foundation: www.mmrf.org

National Center for Complementary and Alternative Medicine: www.nccam.nih.gov

National Center for Homeopathy: www.healthy.net/nch/

Stanford University: www.stanford.edu

University of California Irvine: www.ucihs.uci.edu/com/samueli/

University of California San Francisco: www.ucsf.edu

University of Texas (MD Anderson): www.mdanderson.org/departments/cimer/dindex.cfm?pn=6EB86A59-EBD9–11D4–810100508B603A14

**Websites for Additional Associations**

American Cancer Society: www.cancer.org

AIDS Clinical Trial Information Service: www.actis.org

American Board of Medical Specialties: www.abms.org

American Institute for Cancer Research: www.aicr.org

American Lung Association: www.lungusa.org

American Society of Clinical Oncology ASCO: www.asco.org

American Society for Therapeutic Radiology and Oncology: www.astro.org

Bone Marrow and Transplant Information Network: www.bmtinfonet.org/

Brain Tumor Society: www.tbts.org

Breast Cancer Awareness: www.tricaresw.af.mil/breastcd/index.html

Cancer Care: www.cancercare.org

Cancernet: www.cancer.gov/search/geneticsservices/

Cancer Research Institute: www.cancerresearch.org

Cancer Trials: cancer.gov/clinicaltrials

Centers for Disease Control: www.cdc.gov

Children's Oncology Group: http://nccf-cares.org

Environmental Protection Agency (EPA): www.epa.gov

FDA Guide to Choosing Medical Treatments:
    www.fda.gov/oashi/aids/fdaguide.html

FORCE (Facing Our Risk of Cancer Empowered): www.facingourrisk.org/

Gene tests: www.genetests.org

Hospice Association of America: www.nahc.org

Hospice Foundation of America: www.hospicefoundation.org

Joint Commission on Accreditation of Healthcare Organizations (JCAHO):
    www.jcaho.org

Leukemia and Lymphoma Society: www.leukemia-lymphoma.org

Lung Cancer Alliance: www.lungcanceralliance.org

Medicare Helpline: www.medicare.gov

Mayo Clinic: www.mayohealth.org

National Alliance of Breast Cancer Organizations (NABCO):
    www.nabco.org

National Association for Home Care: www.nahc.org

National Brain Tumor Foundation: www.braintumor.org

National Breast Cancer Coalition: www.natlbcc.org

National Cancer Institute: www.cancer.gov

Live Help—National Cancer Institute. https://livehelp.cancer.gov/

National Coalition for Cancer Research: www.cancercoalition.org

National Comprehensive Cancer Network: www.nccn.org

National Institute of Health: www.nih.gov

National Kidney Cancer Association: www.nkca.org

National Lymphedema Network: www.lymphnet.org

National Society of Genetic Counselors: www.nsgc.org

Ronald McDonald House Charities: www.rmhc.org

Susan B. Komen Breast Cancer Foundation: www.komen.org

United Ostomy Association: www.wocn.org

Y-Me National Breast Cancer Organization: www.yme.org

# RECOMMENDED
# ONLINE ARTICLES

### Acute Myelogenous Leukemia

Acute Myelogenous Leukemia. Mayo Clinic Staff. www.mayoclinic.com/
health/acute-myelogenous-leukemia/DS00548/DSCTION=alt

### Adrenal Cancer

Acupuncture Herbal. www.masterole.com/Adrenal/html

Adrenal Cancer.
www.healthline.com/channel/adrenal-cancer_alternativetherapies

Adrenal Cancer Hope, How Is Adrenal Cancer Treated.
www.adrenalcancerhope.org/default.asp?pg=treatment

Adrenal Cortical Cancer Overview. www.cancer.org/cancer/adrenalcortical
cancer/overviewguide/adrenal-cortical-ca

Adrenal Gland Cancer. www.cancercenter.com/adrenal_cancer.cfm

Ayurvedic Treatment. Natural Remedies for Adrenal Fatigue.
http://ayurvedic-treatment.com/natural-remedies-for-adrenalfatigue/

Goh, J. Imaging in Adrenal Metastases.
http://emedicine.medscape.com/article/376585-overview

How Is Adrenal Cancer Treated?
www.localhealth.com/article/adrenalcancer/treatments

Howell, N. Alternative Treatments for an Adrenal Tumor.
www.ehow.com/way_5511102_alternative-treatments-adrenal-tumor.html

Metastases to the Adrenal Gland. http://endocrinediseases.org/adrenal/
metastases.shtml. www.ehow.com/way_5511102_alternative-treatments-
adrenal-tumor.html

Wikipedia, Adrenal Tumor. http://en.wikipedia.org/wiki/Adrenal_tumor

317

## Alternative Cancer Treatment Centers

Hingle, Lynette. About Alternative Cancer Treatment Centers. www.ehow
.com/about_5107910_alternative-cancer-treatment-centers.html

New Hope Cancer Center. www.newhopemedicalcenter.com/

## American Board Of Holistic Medicine

Board Certification.
www.holisticmedicine.org/content.asp?pl=4&sl=53&contentid=53

## Anal Cancer

Anal Cancer, May Clinic, Alternative Medicine. www.mayoclinic.com/
health/anal-cancer/DS00852/DSECTION=alternative-medicine

## Avastin.

What You Should Know About Avastin. www.avastin.com/avastin/
patient/lung/avastin/?cid=ava_we_F001059_P000517&c

## Bladder Cancer

Chinese Medicine Treatment of Bladder Cancer.
http://17today.com/Cancer/7548.html

Mayo Clinic Staff. Bladder Cancer. www.mayoclinic.com/health/
bladder-cancer/DS00177/METHOD=print&DSECTI

Roe, L. Alternative Treatments for Bladder Cancer.
www.ehow.com/way_5234277_alternative-treatments=bladder-cancer.html

Schoenstadt, A. Alternative Bladder Cancer Treatment. http://cancer.emedtv
.com/bladder-cancer/alternative=bladder-cancer-treatment.html

## Bone Cancer

Bone Cancer. www.cancertutor.com/Other/Bone_Cancer.html

Bone Cancer. www.medicinenet.com/bone_cancer/article.htm

Bone Tumors. www.ncbi.nlm.nih.gov/pubmedhealth/PMH0002210/

Callabro, S. Complementary and Alternative Medicine for Bone Cancer.
www.everydayhealth.com/bone-cancer-alternative-medicine.aspx

Chinese Medicine and Metastatic Bone Cancer.
www.chineseherbs.com/?action-viewnews-itemid-22

Flaws, B. Chinese Medicine and Metastatic Bone Cancer.
http://bluepoppy.com/cfwebstorefb/index.cfm?fuseaction=feature
.display&feature_id+1115

Ivey, G. Chinese Herbs for Bone Cancer.
www.ehow.com/facts_5554817_chinese-herbs-bone-cancer.html

Mayo Clinic Staff. Bone Cancer.
www.mayoclinic.com/health/bonecancer/DS00520/METHOD+print

Wikipedia. Bone tumor. http://en.wikipedia.org/wiki/Bone_cancer

## Brain Cancer

ANSHIBO Cancer Research Institute. New drug for the treatment of
brain tumors Anbol. www.anshibo.org/en_home.asp

Brain Tumor. Wikipedia. http://en.wikipedia.org/wiki/Brain_tumor

Complementary Therapies for Brain Tumors.
www.everydayhealth.com/brain-tumor/complementary

Davis, C. Brain Cancer Symptoms, Causes, Treatment.
www.medicinenet.com/brain_cancer/page2.htm

Mayo Clinic Staff. Brain Tumor. http://mayoclinic.com/health/brain
-tumor/DS00281/METHOD=print&DSECTION

Programme for Brain Tumors. www.canceractive.com/cancer-active
-page-link.aspx?n=3058?Title=Complementa

Saper, J. Summary of Some Recent Research on Brain Tumors and
Chinese Herbs. www.eastmountain.ca/btumorresearch.html

## Breast Cancer

Ayurveda For Women. Breast Cancer, An Ayurveda Approach.
http://ayurvedaforwomen.wordpress.com/2011/12/29/breast-cancer
-an-ayurveda-approach/

Complementary and Holistic Medicine for Breast Cancer.
www.breastcancer.org/treatment/comp_med/

Daly, M. National Comprehensive Cancer Network: Genetic/Familial
High Risk Assessment: Breast and Ovarian. Clinical Practice Guidelines
in Oncology 1, 2008. www.bing.com/search?q=Daly%2C+M%2C+
genetic%2Ffamilial+high+risk+assess

Gitundu, P. Alternative Breast Cancer Treatment. http://ezinearticles
.com/?Alternative-Breast-Cancer-Treatment

Kieu, A. Alternative Medicine in Breast Cancer.
www.med.ucla.edu/modules/wfsection/article.php?articleid=202

Liu, W. Chinese Herbal Approach to Breast Cancer. www.tcmpage.com
/hpbreastcan.html

Mayo Clinic Staff. Alternative Medicine. www.mayoclinic.com/health/
breast-cancer/DS00328/DSECTION=alternative-medic

Susan B Komen for the Cure. Understanding Breast Cancer–
Complementary Therapies. www.Komen.org/BreastCancer/
Chinesemedicine.html

Vinh-Hung V, Verschraegen, C. "Breast-conserving surgery with or without
radiotherapy." *Journal of the National Cancer Institute*. 96:115–121, 2004.
www.ncbi.nlm.nih.gov/pubmed/14734701

Wikipedia. Breast Cancer. http://en.wikipedia.org/wiki/Breast_cancer

Wong, Cathy. Complementary and Alternative Medicine and Breast
Cancer Prevention. http://altmedicine.about.com/od.cance1/a/breast
_cancer.htm

### Cancer

Cancer-Fighting Strategies.
http://cancerfightingstrategies.com?testimonies.html

Cancer-Fighting Strategies.
http://cancerfightingstrategies.com/methylglyoxal.html

Cancer-Fighting Strategies, 1–10. (oxygenation, pH levels, methylglyoxyl,
cancer-killers, immune system, fungus, detoxify, antioxidants, enzymes,
energetics, psychological). http://cancerfightingstrategies.com

Cancer History. www.rare-cancer.org/history-of-cancer.php

Cancer in Chinese Medicine. www.orientalhealthsolutions.com/
conditions_treated/cancer

Cancer Prevention. www.cdc.gov/cancer/dcpc/prevention

Cancer Prevention. www.medicinenet.com/cancer_prevention/article.htm

Fayed, Lisa. The History of Cancer.
http://cancer.about.com/od/historyofcancer/a/cancerhistory.htm

History of Cancer. http://medicineworld.org/cancer/history.html

Learn About Cancer. ww.cancer.org/Cancer/CancerBasics/what-is-cancer

Learn About Cancer.
www.cancer.org/cancer/cancercauses/geneticsandcancer/index

Liotta, LA. Cancer Invasion and Metastasis.
www.ncbi.nlm.nih.gov/books/NBK20786/

Mayo Clinic Staff. Cancer Prevention. www.mayoclinic.com/health/cancer
-prevention/CA00024

Metastasis. http://en.wikipedia.org/wiki/Metastasis

Sherratt, JA. Mathematical Modeling of Cancer Invasion. www.ma.hw.ac.uk/~jas/researchinterests/cancerinvasion.html

The History of Cancer. American Cancer Society. www.cancer.org

What Is Cancer? www.cancer.gov/cancertopics/cancerlibrary/what-is-cancer

What Is Cancer? www.medicalnewstoday.com/info/cancer-oncology

Wikipedia. Cancer. http://en.wikipedia.org/wiki/Cancer

Wikipedia. Oncology. http://en.wikipedia.org/wiki/Oncology

### Cancer Diagnosis

Cancer Diagnosis Methods. www.shh.org/hospital-services/cancer-care/cancer-diagnosis-methods.asp

Grouch, A. Cancer Diagnosis Methods. www.ehow.com/way5267249/cancer-diagnosis-methods.html

### Cancer in Older People

Alspaugh, L. 5 Things You Need to Know About Cancer in the Elderly. www.livestrong.com/article/9223-need-cancer-elderly/

Berger, NA. Cancer in the Elderly. Transactions of the American Clinical and Climatological Association. 117: 2006, 147–156. www.ncbi.nlm.nih.gov/pmc/articles/PMC1500929/

### Cancer Rehabilitation

Cancer Rehabilitation. www.yenoh93./medceu.com/index/index/courses/cancerrehab.htm

Kaplan, RJ. Cancer and Rehabilitation. http://emedicine.medscape.com/article320261-overview

Oncology Rehabilitation. www.cancercenter.com/complementary alternativemedicine/physicaltherapy

Rehabilitation. www.cancer.net/patient/Survivorship/Rehabilitation

### Cancer Support Groups

Support Groups. www.cancer.org/treatment/treatmentsandsidesffects/ complementaryandalternati

Wikipedia. Cancer Support Group. http://en.wikipedia.org/wiki/Cancer_support_group

## Cancer Treatment Centers

Cancer Center at Mayo Clinic. http://cancercenter.mayo.edu/

Cancer Treatment Centers of America.
http://en.wikipedia.org/wiki/Cancer_Treatment_Centers_of_America

City of Hope. www.cityofhope.org/pages/default.aspx

Fox Chase Cancer Center. www.fccc.edu/whyChoose/aboutHospital/
index.html

MD Anderson Cancer Center. www.mdanderson.org/about-us/facts-and
-history/institutional-profile

M.D. Anderson Cancer Center. www.mdanderson.org/about-us/index.html

Memorial Sloan-Kettering Cancer Center. www.mskcc.org/about

National Cancer Institute. http://cancercenters.cancer.gov/about/index.html

The Moffitt Cancer Center. www.moffitt.org/site.aspx?spid
=BDA2338677DE40A6BA99B704B1D9DC56

## Carcinoid Tumors

Alternative Treatment—Carcinoid. http://carcinoid-options.com/
glossary.html

Alternative Treatments for Carcinoid.
www.rightdiagnosis.com/c/carcinoid/alternative.htm

Mayo Clinic Staff. Carcinoid Tumors. www.mayoclinic.com/health/
carcinoid-tumors/DS00834/METHOD=print

Tebbi, C. Carcinoid Tumor.
http://emedicine.medscape.com/article/986050-overview

Wikipedia. Carcinoid. http://en.wikipedia.org/wiki/Carcinoid

## Cervical Cancer

Cervical Cancer—Ayurvedic Herbal Treatment. http://ezinearticles.com/?
cervicalcancerayurvedicherbaltreatment?id=1831884

Cervical Cancer Treatment—Know all About Herbal Cure.
www.womenhealthtips.net/cervicalcancertreatment=know-about
-herbal-cure.html

Mundewadi, A. Cervical Cancer—Ayurvedic Herbal Treatment. http://
ayurvedictreatment.com/cervical-cancer-ayurvedic-herbal-treatment/

Wikipedia. Cervical Cancer. http://en.wikipedia.org/wiki/cervicalcancer

## Chinese Medicine

39 MEDICAL CENTER. Chinese Medicine, Acupuncture and Herbs. www.39clinic.com/english/default.asp

Chinese Herb Remedies. www.livestrong.com/article/118257-chinese -herb-remedies

Chinese Medicine andCancer. http://healthphone.com/consump_english/healthcare_center/cancer/ cancer.htm

Dr. Shen. Chinese Herbs and Chinese Medicine for Fighting Cancer. www.drshen.com/chineseherbsforcancer.htm

Gateway to Chinese Medicine. www.thegatewayportal.com/ acupuncture.html

Kobayashi, S, Keishi-ka-kei-to, FA. Traditional Chinese Herbal Medicine Inhibits Pulmonary Metastasis of B16 Melanoma. www.ncbi.nlm.nih.gov/pubmed/9137420

Liu, W. Fighting Cancer with Soy and Other Popular Chinese Foods. www.tcmpage.com/hpcandidiasis.html

Walters, Richard. Traditional Chinese Medicine. www.healthy.net/scr/article.aspx?Id=2006

Walters, Richard. Chinese Medicine and Cancer. www.healthy.net/health/rtiacle/chinese_medicine_and_cancer/2006/1–4

## Chiropractic

Wikipedia. Chiropractic. http://en.wikipedia.org/wiki/chiropractic

## Clinical Trials

Cancer Clinical Trials. www.cancer.gov/cancertopics/factsheet/ information/clinical-trials

## Colon Cancer

Alternative and Complementary Therapies for Colon Cancer. www.johnshopkinshealthalerts.com/reports/colon_cancer/1926–1.html

Colon Cancer Alternative Treatment. www.coloncancerresource.com/colon-cancer-alternative-treatment.html

Earnest-Pravel, D. Colon Cancer and Alternative Medicine. www.ehow.com/facts_5530759_colon-cancer-alternative-medicine.html

Mayo Clinic Staff. Colon Cancer. www.mayoclinic.com/health/colon
   -cancer/DS00035/DSECTION=alternative-medi

Wikipedia. Colon Cancer. http://en.wikipedia.org/wiki/Colon_cancer

Complementary/Alternative Medicine Specialists

BSC Traditional Chinese Medicine Degree.
   www.mdx.ac.uk/courses/undergraduate/complementaryhealth

Chinese Medical Doctors Directory.
   www.locateadoc.com/doctors/chinese-medicine.html

Choosing an Alternative or Complementary Medicine Practitioner.
   www.amfoundation.org/practitioner.htm

Complementary and Alternative Medicine.
   www.allergyuk.org/themanagementofallergy/complementary

Flaws, B. Presentation and Questions and Answers for
   CFS-FMS-Holistic Discussion Group.
   www.holisticmed.com/cfs/flaws.html

How to Find a Top Natural Doc.
   www.drjakefelice.com/2011/03/how-to-find-a-top-natural-doc/

MCM Integrated Masters in Complementary Medicine (Ayurvedic
   Medicine) Degree. www.mdx.ac.uk/courses/undergraduate/
   complementaryhealth/integratedmasters

Traditional Chinese Medicine Healing Center.
   http://acupuncturelosangeles.net/html/acupuncturelosangeles-faq.html

Who Provides Complementary Therapies?
   http://familydoctor.co.uk/info/CAMwho-provides
   -complementary-therapies

## Complementary/Alternative Medicine

Alternative and Complementary Treatments for Cancer.
   http://cancer.about.com/od/alternativetreatmentscomplementaryand
   alternativetreat

Alternative Cancer Program.
   www.utopiaawaits.com/index.php?option=comcontyent&taskview&
   id86&Itemi

Alternative Cancer Treatments. www.alternativecancertreatments.com/

Ayurvedic Medicines. Cancer Cures.
   www.ayurvedicmedicines.com/cancer.html

Ayurvedic Medicine for Tumor.
   http://answers.myyog.com/question/ayurvedic-medicine-for-tumor-721–337

Complementary and Alternative Medicine.

www.cancer.org/treatment/treatmentsandsideeffects/
complementaryandalternati

Dr. Reddy Clinic. Five Day Treatment.
www.dreddyclinic.com/ayurvedic/ayuirvediccure/5daysayurveda
programs.htm

Dr. Eddy Clinic. Panchakarma Treatments.
www.dreddyclinic.com/ayurvedic/pancha_treatments.htm

Ernst, E. Complementary and Alternative Medicine Treatments (CAM).
www.uptodate.com/contents/patient-information-complementary-and
-alternative-me

Cassileth, B. High Prevalence of Complementary and Alternative
Medicine Use Among Cancer Patients: Implications for Research and
Clinical Care. http://jco.ascopubs.org/content/23/12/2590.full?etoc

Chew, CM. Complementary and Alternative Medicine in Cancer.
www.ehow.com/about_6542395_complementary-alternative
-medicine-cacer.html

Health and Alternative Medicine Resources. http://db.ancient
-future.net/health.html

Hughes, E. Complementary and Alternative Medicine. CMDT.
Chapter 42, 2007. www.123helpme.com/view.asp?id=52028

Mayo Clinic Staff. Complementary and Alternative Medicine.
http://www.mayoclinic.org/complementary-alternative-medicine/

Mayo Clinic Staff. Lung Cancer, Alternative Medicine.
www.mayoclinic.com/health/lung-cancer/DS00038/DSECTION
=alternative-medici

Natural Strategies to Kill Your Cancer.
http://cancerfightingstrategies.com/print.html

Naturopathic Clinic.
www.denvernaturopathic.com/news/cancerinvasion.html

Schachter, M. Complementary and Alternative Medicine.
www.alkalizeforhealth.net/Lschachter.htm

Wikipedia. Alternative Medicine.
http://en.wikipedia.org/wiki/Alternative_medicine

## Complications

Cancer.
www.mayoclinic.com/health/cancer/DS01076/METHOD=print&
DSECTION=all

## Cranial Nerves
Wikipedia. Cranial nerve. http://en.wikipedia.org/wiki/Cranial_nerves

## Depression and Anxiety
Ashtikar, D. Ayurvedic Treatment for Depression.
   www.onlymyhealth.com/ayurvedic-treatment-depression-1313747043
Caring for the Patient with Cancer at Home.
   www.cancer.org/treatment/treatmentandsideeffects/physicalsideeffects
   /dealing
Complementary Therapies for Managing Depression.
   www.holistichotline.com/remedies/depression/dep_editorial.htm
Complementary Therapies for Depression.
   www.johnshopkinshealthalerts.com/reports/colon_cancer/1926–1
   .html?type=pf
Complementary Therapies.
   www.shawnemission.org/cancer/complementary-therapies.html
Depression.
   www.holisticonline.com/Remedies/Depression/dep_herbs_1.htm
Depression.
   http://holisticonline.com/Remedies/Depression/dep_ayurveda.htm
Depression (PDQ). www.cancer.gov/cancertopics/pdq/supportivecare/
   depression/healthprofessional/pag
Depression and Anxiety.
   www.cancer.net/patient/coping/emotional+and+physical+matters/
   depression+and
Depression and Anxiety for Cancer Survivors.
   www.nccn.com/component/content/article/65/133-dfci-nccn
   -survivorship-depression=
Fratkin, JP. www.acupuncturetoday.com/mpacms/at/article.php?id=31447
Kelchner, L. Herbal Therapy for Depression.
   www.ehow.com/way_5434784_herbal-therapy-depression.html
Lin, J. Chinese Herbs and Depression.
   www.livestrong.com/article/98164-chinese-herbs-depression/
Nuri, S.
   www.ehow.com/way_5982876_chinese-treatment-gene-depression.html

## Esophageal Cancer
Mayo Clinic Staff. Alternative Cancer Treatments.
   www.mayoclinic.com/health/cancer-treatment/CM00002
Rodriguez, D. Alternative Therapies for the Treatment of Esophageal

Cancer. www.everydayhealth.com/esophageal-cancer/alternative
-therapy-treatments.aspx

TCMWELL. Chinese Medicine Treatment of Esophageal Cancer.
http://tcmwell.com/tcmdiseases/internalmedicine/chinese-medicine
-treatment-of-esopha

Wikipedia. Esophageal Cancer.
http://en.wikipedia.org/wiki/Esophageal_cancer

## Eye Cancer

Eye Cancer. www.cancer.net/patient/Cancer+Types/Eye+Cancer
?sectionTitle=Treatment

Eye Cancer. www.mdanderson.org/patient-and-cancer-information/
cancerinformation/cancer-type

Eye Neoplasm. http://en.wikipedia.org/wiki/Eye_cancer

Normal, W. Eye Tumors.
www.ehow.com/facts_6155885_eye-tumors.html

Rockwell, K. Herbal Topical Treatments for Eye Cancer.
www.livestrong.com/article/392949-herbal-topical-treatments-for-eye
-cancer/

## Gallbladder and Bile Ducts

Abou-Alfa, G. About Gallbladder and Bile Duct Cancers.
www.mskcc.org/cancer-care/adult/gallbladder-bile-duct/about
-gallbladder-bile-duct

Ayurvedic, Cholangiocarcinoma—Ayurvedic Herbal Treatment.
http://ayurvedic-treatment.com/tag/cholangiocarcinoma-treatment/

Bile Duct Cancer—Chinese Herbal.
www.4uherb.com/cancer/other/treat.htm

Fong, Y. Gallbladder and Bile Duct Cancer. Memorial Sloan Kettering
Cancer Center. www.mskcc.org/cancer-care/adult/
gallbladderbileduct/treatment

Gallbladder and Bile Duct Cancer.
http://symptomchecker.about.com/od/Diagnoses/gallbadder=and-bile
-duct-cancer.htm

Gerdes, H. Diagnosis and Staging Gallbladder and Bile Duct Cancers.
www.mskcc.org/cancer-care/adult/gallbladder-bile-duct/diagnosis
-staging

Olsen, K. Alternative Bile Duct Cancer Treatments.
www.ehow.com/way_5506542_alternative=bile-duct-cancer
-treatments.html

## Gene Therapy

Cross, D. Gene Therapy for Cancer Treatment: Past, Present and Future. www.ncbi.nlm.nih.govmc/articles/PMC1570487/

## Genetic Counseling and Testing

BRCA1 and BRCA2: Cancer Risk and Genetic Testing. www.cancer.gov/cancertopics/factsheet/Risk/BRCA

Cancer Genetics Risk Assessment and Counseling. www.cancer.gov/cancertopics/pdq/genetics/risk-assessment-and -counseling/healthpr

Cancer Genetics at Stanford. http://cancer.stanford.edu/patient_care/services/geneticCounseling/

Genetic Testing. www.answers.com/topic/genetic-testing

Who Needs Genetic Testing for Cancer? www.mdanderson.org/publications/focused-on -health/issues/2011october/genetics.

## Graft-Versus-Host-Disease

Graft-Versus-Host-Disease. Wikipedia. http://en.wikipedia.org/wiki/Graft-versus-host_disease

## Head and Neck Cancer

Wikipedia. Head and Neck Cancer. http://en.wikipedia.org/wiki/Head_and_neck_cancer

## Heart Complications

Bressler, L. Chemotherapy Induced Cardiac Toxicity. www.uic.edu/classes/pmpr/pmpr652/Final/bressler/chemocardiac.html

Cardiac Toxicity. www.caring4cancer.com/go/cancer/effects/ lesscommon/cardiac-toxicity.htm

## Herbs

Licorice. www.cancer.org/treatment/treatmentsandsideeffects/ complementaryandalternati

Milk Thistle. www.mayoclinic.com/health/silymarin/NS_patient-milkthistle

NCCAM. Dandelion. http://nccam.nih.gov/health/dandelion

## HIV/AIDS

Alternative, Complementary, and Traditional Medicine, and HIV. http:/www.avert.org/alternative-medicine-hiv.htm

**Ayurvedic Treatment of AIDS.**
www.lifepositive.com/body-holistic/asids/aids-drugs.asp

FACT SHEET CDC: HIV/AIDS and Alternative Therapies.
www.aegis.com/[pubs/cdc_fact_sheets/1994/CDC94033.html

HIV/AIDS. Herbal Cure, Ayurveda.
www.aidscureherbal.com/herbalindex.htm

HIV/AIDS. Alternative Medicine. www.mayoclinic.com/health/hiv
-aids/DS00005/DSECTION=alternative-medicine

**Hospice**
Wikipedia. Hospice Care.
http://en.wikipedia.org/wiki/Hospice_care-in_the_United_States

**Hypersensitivity Reactions**
Allergic Reactions and Chemotherapy. www.chemocare.com/
managing/allergic_reactions_and_chemotherapy.asp

Desensitization Protocol.
http://theoncologist.alphamedpress.org/content/9/5/546.ful

Gammon, D. Hypersensitivity Reactions to Oxaliplatin and the Application
of a Hypersensitivity Reaction to Chemotherapy. www.wellness.com/
reference/allergies/hypersensitivity-reaction-to-chemotherapy

Lenz, H-J. Management and Preparedness for Infusion and Hypersensitivity
Reactions. http://theoncologist.alphamedpress.org/content/12/5/601.full

**Immunotherapy**
Wikipedia. Cancer Immunotherapy.
http://en.wikipedia.org/wiki/Cancer_immunotherapy

**Increased Intracranial Pressure**
Medline Plus. Increased Intracranial Pressure.
www.nlm.nih.gov/medlineplus/ency/article/000793.htm

Wikipedia. Intracranial Pressure.
http://en.wikipedia.org/wiki/Intracranial_pressure

**Hair Loss**
Chemotherapy and Hair Loss.
www.mayoclinic.com/health/hair-loss/CA00037

Hair Loss Prevention During Chemotherapy. www.hairloss
-research.org/UpdateChemo10–07.html

### Hepatotoxicity (Liver)

Hepatotoxicity from Chemotherapy Treatment. www.mesothelioma
.web.org/mesothelioma/treatment/chemotherapy-side-effects/hepat

King, PD. Hepatotoxicity of Chemotherapy.
http://theoncologist.alphamedpress.org/content/6/2/162.full

### Hyperthermia Cancer Treatment

Hyperthermia Cancer Treatments.
www.valleycancerinstitute.org/?tag=head-and-neck-cancer

### Infusion Therapy

Infusion Therapy. http://en.wikipedia.org/wiki/Infusion_Therapy

What Is Infusion Therapy? www.widegeek.com/whatisinfusion-therapy.htm

### Infections in Patients with Cancer

Infections in People with Cancer.
www.cancer.org/treatment/treatmentsandsideeffects/infection

Rolston, K. Infections in Patients with Cancer.
www.ncbi.nlm.nih.gov/books/NBK20904/

### Kidney Cancer

Ayurvedic Research Foundation. Ayurvedic Herbal Kidney Cancer Cure.
www.ayurveda-cancer.org/cancerbysystem11.htm

Mayo Clinic Staff. Alternative Medicine for Kidney Cancer.
www.mayoclinic.com/health/kidney-cancer/DS00360/
DSECTION=alternative-med

McGee, F. Herbs for Kidney Cancer. www.ehow.com/way_5453953_herbs
-kidney-cancer.html.

Thornton, J. Chinese Herb Remedy Linked with Cancer of the Kidneys.
www.telegraph.co.uk/health/1343598/chinese-herb-remedy-linked-
with-cance-of-t

What You Need to Know about Kidney Cancer.
www.cancer.gov/cancertopics/wyntk/kidney/page7

Wikipedia. Kidney Cancer. http://en.wikipedia.org/wiki/Kidney_neoplasm

### Liver Cancer

Alternative Treatments for Liver Cancer.
www.tarunaoils.com/articles/alternative-treatmentslivercancer.asp

Ayurvedic Treatment of Liver Cancer. http://alwaysayurveda.blogspot.com/
2009/10/ayurvedic-treatment-for-liver-cancer.html

eMed TV. Alternative Treatments for Liver Cancer. http://cancer.emedtv
.com/liver-cancer/alternative-treatments-for-liver-cancer.html

Luk, JM. Traditional Chinese Herbal Medicines for Liver Disease.
http://onlinelibrary.wiley.com/doi/10.1111/j.1478-3231.2007.01527.x/full

Lytle, B. Alternative Treatments for Liver Cancer.
www.ehow.com/way_5217593_alternative-liver-cancer-treatment.html

Marks, J. Liver Cancer. www.medicinenet.com/livercancer/artyicle.htm

QWei. Blog introduction to TCM Chinese Medicine.

http://tcm-eblog.com/tcm/three-advantages-of-chinese-medicine
-treatment-of-liver-cancer

Silverman, S. Alternative Treatments for Liver Cancer.
http://livestrong.com/article/28929-alternative-treatments-liver-cancer/

Stuart, KE. Liver Cancer. www.medicinenet.com/livercancer/page1-16.htm

Sundstrom, K. Herbal Remedies for Fatty Liver.
www.ehow.com/factsherbalremediesfattyliver.html

Wikipedia. Liver Cancer. http://en.wikipedia.org/wiki/Liver_cancer

## Lung Cancer

Bunn, PA. Immune Therapy for Lung Cancer.
http://ajrcmb.atsjournals.org/cgi/content/full/21/1/10

Cameron, . Lung Cancer Treatment Alternatives.
www.ehow.com/list_5481589_lung_cancer_treatment_alternatives.html

CAM Therapies for Lung Cancer.
www.lungcanceronline.org/treatment-cam/topics.html

Dinh, T. Lung Cancer Surgery Complications.
www.livestrong.com/74798lungcancersurgerycomplications/

Eldridge, L. Lung Cancer, Lobectomy Complications and Prognosis.
http://lungcancer.about.com/od/treatmentoflungcancer/a/
lobectomycomplications.htm

Fayed, L. Top 5 Ways to Prevent Lung Cancer.
http://cancer.about.com/od/lungcancer/tp/preventcancer.htm

Flaws, B. An Integrated Chinese-Western Medical Treatment of
Non-Small Cell Lung Cancer.
www.townsendletter.com/June2004/chinesemedicine0604.htm

Hellesvig-Gaskell, K. Post Lung Cancer Surgery Complications.
www.ehow.com/about_5382043_post_lung_cancer_surgery_
complications.html

How to Prevent Lung Cancer with Vitamins.
www.ehow.com/how_4550430_prevent_lung_cancer_vitamins.html

Koskela, C. Gene Therapy: Targeting the Cause of Lung Cancer to Treat It.
www.caring.com/articles/lung-cancer-gene-therapy

Kris, M. Molecular Medicine. www.mskcc.org/cancercare/adult/lung/
molecularmedicine

Lung Cancer Treatment Options.
www.tarceva.com/patient/learning/treatment.jsp?tar_we_F0010355
_P000453&c=M

Wikipedia. Lung Cancer. http://en.wikipedia.org/wiki/Lung_cancer

## Lung Complications

Acute Pulmonary Toxicity (Lung Damage). www.caring4cancer.com/go/
cancer/effects/lesscommon/acute-pulmonary-toxicity.htm

Hamilton, S. Pulmonary Toxicity and Chemotherapy.
www.chemocare.com/managing/pulmonary_toxicity_chemotherapy.asp

Lung Damage (Acute Pulmonary Toxicity). www.texasoncology.com/
cancertreatment/sideeffectsofcancertreatment/lesscom

## Lymphoma

Flaws, B. Chinese Medical Treatment of Malignant Lymphoma.
www.acupuncturetoday.com/mpacms/at/article.php?id=28009

Mayo Clinic Staff. Non-Hodgkin's Lymphoma.
www.mayoclinic.com/health/non-hodgkins-lymphoma/DS00350

Mundewadi, AA. Ayurvedic Herbal Treatment. http://ayurvedic-
treatment.com/lymphoma-ayurvedic-herbal-treatment/

Wikipedia. Lymphoma. http://en.wikipedia.org/wiki/Lymphoma

## Melanoma

Amerman, D. Alternative Treatments for Melanoma.
www.ehow.com/way_5783514_alternative-treatments-malignant-
melanoma.html

Complementary and Alternative Therapies. www.cancer.org/cancer/
skincancer-melanoma/detailedguide/melanoma-skin-can

Five-Year Survival Rates of Melanoma Patients Treated by Diet. www.whale.to/cancer/gerson1.html

Hamsa, TP. Harmine Activates Intrinsic and Extrinsic Pathways of Apoptosis in B16F-10 Melanoma. www.cmjournal.org/content/6/1/11

How Is Melanoma Treated? www.bettermedicine.com/article/melanoma-1/treatments

Melanoma. www.cancer.net/patient/Cancer+Types/Melanoma?section Title=Treatment

Melanoma Staging. www.cancer.org/cancer/skincancermelanoma/ detailedguide.melanomaskincan

Melanoma Treatment, Spiritual Support. www.cancercenter.com/melanoma/spiritual-support.cfm

Mind Body Medicine for Melanoma. www.cancercenter.com/melanoma/mind-body-medicine.cfm

Naturopathic Medicine for Melanoma. www.cancercenter.com/melanoma/naturopathic-medicine.cfm

Nutrition Therapy for Melanoma. www.cancercenter.com/melanoma/nutritional-therapy.cfm

Roe, L. Alternative Melanoma Treatments. www.ehow.com/way_5206111_alternative-melanoma-treatments.html

Wikipedia. Melanoma. http://en.wikipedia.org/wiki/Melanoma

## Mesothelioma

Alternative Medicine/Mesothelioma. www.mesothelioma.com/glossary/alternative_medicine.htm

Alternative Mesothelioma Treatment Options. www.mesothelioma.com/treatment/alternative/

Complementary and Alternative Medicines for Mesothelioma. www.asbestos.com/treatment/alternative

Mayo Clinic Staff. Alternative Medicine for Mesothelioma. www.mayoclinic.com/health/mesothelioma/DS00779/DSECTION =alternative-medi

Mesothelioma. Ayurvedic Herbal Treatment. http://mesothelioma.com /mesothelioma-ayurvedic-herba;treatment/

Wikipedia. Mesothelioma. http://en.wikipedia/wiki/mesothelioma

## Metabolic Emergencies

Johns Hopkins. Metabolic Emergencies in Cancer Medicine.
www.hopkinsguides.com/hopkins/ub/citation/3736270/metabolic
_emergencies_in_c. http://en.wikipedia/org/wiki/Multiple_myeloma
Metabolic Emergencies. www.startoncology.net/site/index.php?
option=com_content&view=article&id=136

Thomas, CR. Common Emergencies in Cancer Medicine: Metabolic
Syndromes. www.ncbi.nlm.nih.gov/pmc/articles/PMC2627107/

## Multiple Myeloma

Wikipedia. Multiple Myeloma. http://en.wikipedia/org/wiki/multiple
_myeloma. http://en.wikipedia/org/wiki/Multiple_myeloma

## Myelodysplastic Syndromes

Mayo Clinic Staff. Myelodysplastic Syndromes. www.mayoclinic.com/
health/myelodysplastic-syndromes/DS00596/METHOD=print

## National Center for Complementary and Alternative Medicine (NCCAM)

Cancer and CAM. http://nccam.nih.gov/health/cancer/camcancer.htm

Health Topics A to Z. http://nccam.nih.gov/health/atoz.htm

## National Institutes of Health—NIH/NCCAM

Gorski, D. The National Center for Complementary and Alternative
Medicine (NCCAM).
www.sciencebasedmedicine.org/index.php/the-national-center-for
-complementary-

Wikipedia. National Institutes of Health.
http://en.wikipedia.org/wiki/National_Institutes_of_Health

## Nausea and Vomiting

Ayurvedic Home Remedies for Nausea.
www.ayurvediccure.com/home-remedies/homeremedies-nausea.htm

Cancer Treatment, Nausea/Vomiting, and Chemotherapy.
www.yalemedicalgroup.org/stw/Page.asp?PageID=STW025814

Herbal Remedies for Nausea.
www.ayurvedictalk.com/herbal-remedies-for-nausea/370/

Mayo Clinic Staff. Chemotherapy, Nausea and Vomiting.
www.mayoclinic.com/health/cancer/CA00030

Nausea and Vomiting. www.cancer.gov/cancertopicss/pdq/supportivecare/
nausea/patient/page1/AllPages/Print

Nausea/Vomiting and Chemotherapy.
www.memorialhealth.com/aci/healthinfo/content.aspx?pageis=PO7271

Nausea and Vomiting. www.nutritionvista.com/Cancer/Nausea/Default.aspx

Nausea/Vomiting and Chemotherapy.

Nausea and Vomiting. www.cancer.org/treatment/treatmentsandtidetffects/
thysicalsidetffects/nausea

Related Nausea. www.ncbi.nlm.nih.gov/pmc/articles/PMC2764274/

## Neurotoxicity

Azim, HA. Long-Term Toxic Effects of Adjuvant Chemotherapy in Breast
Cancer. http://annonc.oxfordjournals.org/content/22/9/1939.full

Brooks, D. Neurotoxic Complications from Chemotherapy.
www.livestrong.com/article/205026-neurotoxic-complications-from
-chemotherapy/

Central Neurotoxicity.
www.chemocare.com/managing/central_neurotoxicity_memory_loss.asp

Kuroi, K. http://lib.bioinfo.pl/pmid:14718800

## Nutrition and Cancer

Cancer and Naturopathic Medicine. www.healthcommunities.com/
cancer/alternativemedicine/naturopathicmedicine

Cancer Patient Nutrition Therapies.
www.lef.org/LEFCMS/aspx/PrintVersionMagic.aspx?CmsID=113912

National Cancer Institute, Nutrition in Cancer Care. www.cancer.gov/
cancertopics/pdq/supportivecare/nutrition/patient/page1/allpages/pr

Nutrition Therapy. www.cancercenter.com/complementary-alternative
-medicine/nutritional-therapy.cfm?

## Oncology Nursing

Become an Oncology Nurse. http://allnursingschools.com/nursing
-careers/career/oncology-nursing

Oncology Nurse. www.nursesource.org/oncology.html

## Organ Transplantation

Wikipedia. Organ Transplantation.
http://en.wikipedia.org/wiki/Organ_transplants

## Ovarian Cancer

Dharmananda, S. Estrogen-Dependent Tumors and Herbs. www.itmonline.org/arts/estdep.htm

Green Tea: An Effective Alternative Medicine against Ovarian Cancer. www.ovca.org/ovariancancertreatment/greenteaaneffectivealternativ-medicin

Johns Hopkins Medicine. Complementary and Alternative Medicine for Ovarian Cancer. www.hopkinsmedicine.org/kimmelcancercenter/centers/ovarian/patientinformat

Mundewadi, A. Ovarian Cancer, Ayurvedic Herbal Treatment. http://ezinearticles.com/?Ovarian-Cancer-Ayurvedic-Herbal-Treatment&id=1939255

Wikipedia. Ovarian Cancer. http://en.wikipedia.org/wiki/Ovarian_cancer

Wong, K. Alternative Medicine and Ovarian Cancer. http://altmedicine.about.com/od/cance1/a/alt_med_ovarian_cancer.htm

## Pain and Pain Management

Acupuncture in Cancer Pain. www.cam-cancer.org/CAM-Summaries/Alternative-Medical-Systems/Acupuncture-in

Cancer Pain. http://en.wikipedia.org/wiki/Cancer_pain

Cancer Pain Management. www.drugs.com/cg/cancer-pain-management.html

How to Use Holistic Medicine for Pain Management. www.ehow.com/how_2033027_use-holistic-medicine.html

Kessler, HA. Acupuncture and the Treatment of Cancer. www.scribd.com/InnoVision%20Health%20%Media/d/29287681-Acupuncture-and-the

Pain Management. www.cancercenter.com/complementary-alternative-medicine/pain-management.cfm

Pain Management. http://seniorhealth.about.com/library/weekly/aa051400a.htm

Pain Management. www.mdanderson.org/patientandcancerinformation/cancerinformation/cancer-topi

Pain Management—The Ayurvedic Way. http://ayurvedic-treatment.com/pain-management-ayurvedic-way/

Pain Management—Traditional Chinese Medicine.
www.39clinic.com/english/pain/default.asp

Zmuida, C. Cancer Pain Management.
www.ehow.com/about_5453344_cancer-pain-management.html

## Pancreatic Cancer

Liu, J. Chinese Herbal Medicine for Advanced Pancreatic Cancer.
www.cam-cancer.org/CAM-Summaries/Alternative-Medical-Systems/
Chinese-herba

Pancreatic Cancer—Alternative Treatments.
www.cancertutor.com/Other/Pancreatic_Cancer.html

What You Need to Know about Cancer of the Pancreas.
www.cancer.gov/cancertopics/ /pancreas/page1–10

Wikipedia. Pancreatic Cancer.
http://en.wikipedia.org/wiki/Cancer_of_the_pancreas

## Paraneoplastic Syndromes

Paraneoplastic Syndrome.
http://en.wikipedia.org/wiki/Paraneoplastic_syndrome

Paraneoplastic Syndromes.
www.ninds.nih.gov/disorders/paraneoplastic/paraneoplastic.htm

Pelosof, L. Paraneoplastic Syndromes.
www.ncbi.nlm.nih.gov/pmc/articles/PMC2931619/

## Pathology

Flow Cytometry. http://en.wikipedia.org/wiki/Flow_cytometry

Who Is the Pathologist?
www.thedoctorsdoctor.com/pathologists/who_is_the_pathologist.htm

Wikipedia. Pathology. http://en.wikipedia.org/wiki/Pathology

## Plasma Cell Disorders

Macroglobulinemia of Waldenstrom.
www.bloodindex.org/Macroglobulinemia-of-Waldenstrom.php

National Cancer Institute. Plasma Cell Neoplasms.
www.cancer.gov/cancertopics/pdq/treatment/myeloma/patient/page1.and2

## Prostate Cancer

Alternative Medicine for Prostate Cancer. http://prostatecancer.about.
com/od/treatment/a/Alternative-Medicine-For-Prostate-Cancer

Ancient Chinese Herbal Remedy Now Being Tested as Prostate Cancer Treatment Drug. www.healthcanal.com/alternative-therapies/22634-ancient-chinese-herbal-remedy

Bicher Cancer Institute. Alternative Prostate Cancer Treatment Options. www.vci.org/cancertreatmentsmiscell/prostatecancertreatment.htm

Gleason Score. http://gleasonscore.net

Natural Cancer Treatments. Prostate Cancer. www.cancertutor.com/Other/Prostate_Cancer.html

Prostate Cancer and Alternative Medicine. www.healthcommunities.com/prostate-cancer/alternative-medicine/naturopathy.shtml

Prostate Cancer Guide. Alternative Medicine. www.webmd.com/ prostate-cancer/guide/prostate-cancer-alternative-treatment

Prostate Cancer Research. Western Medicine and Chinese Medicine. www.shen-nong.com/eng/cm/cm4.html

Roe, L. Alternative Medicine for Prostate Cancer. www.ehow.com/way_5592470_alternative-medicine-proatate-cancer.html

Wikipedia. Prostate Cancer. http://en.wikipedia.org/wiki/Prostate_(cancer)

### Radiation Therapy

Radiation Therapy for Cancer. www.cancer.gov/cancertopics/factsheet/Therapy/radiation

### Second Opinion

Wikipedia. Second Opinion. http://en.wikipedia.org/wiki/Second_opinion

### Secondary Malignancies

Krishnan, B. Non-Hodgkin's Lymphoma Secondary to Cancer Chemotherapy. http://cebp.aacrjournals.org/content/16/3/377.full

Secondary Malignancies. www.texasoncology.com/cancertreatment/sideeffectsofcancertreatment/longterm

Secondary Malignancies. www.caring4cancer.com/go/cancer/effects/lesscommon/secondarymalignancies.htm

Secondary Malignancies. www.tnoncology.com/secondarymalignancies.html

### Sexual Dysfunction

Cancer Treatment for Men—Possible Sexual Side Effects. www.mayoclinic.com/health/cancer-treatment/SA00070/NSECTIONGROUP=2

Male Sexual Dysfunction. www.livestrong.org/get-help/learn-about-cancer/cancer-support-topics/physical-

Sexual dysfunction. www.umm.edu/altmed/articles/sexual-dysfunction-000150.htm

Sexual Dysfunction. www.shands.org/health/Complementary%20and%20Alternative%20Medicine/33/000

Sexual Dysfunction. http://health.rush.edu/healthinformation/complementary%20and%20alternative%20medic

## Skin Cancer

Daniel, T. Alternative Skin Cancer Treatment. http://ezinearticles.com/?Alternative-Skin-Cancer-Treatment&id=3618167

Stone, B. Alternative Skin Cancer Treatment Options. www.healthguideinfo.com/skin-cancer/p107369/

Waterworth, C. Alternative Treatments for Skin Cancer. www.livestrong.com/article/244103-alternative-treatments-for-skin-cancer/

Wikipedia. Basal-Cell Carcinoma. http://en.wikipedia.org/wiki/Basal-cell_carcinoma

Wikipedia. Squamous-Cell Carcinoma. http://en.wikipedia.org/wiki/Squamous_cell_carcinoma

## Small Intestines

Fingerote, RJ. Cancer of the Small Intestine. www.emedicinehealth.com/cancer_of_the_small_intestine/article_em.htm

Vipiwala, N. Cancer of the Small Bowel. www.oncolink.org/types/article.cfm?c=5&s=74&ss=778&id=9498

WebMD. Cancer of the Small Intestine. www.webmd.com/cancer/cancer-of-the-small-intestine?page=1–2

Wikipedia. Small Intestine Cancer. http://en.wikipedia.org/wiki/Small_intestine_cancer

## Soft-Tissue Sarcomas

Mayo Clinic Staff. Soft-Tissue Sarcomas. www.mayoclinic.com/health/soft-tissue-sarcoma/DS00601/Method=print&DSEC

Rau, ATK. Soft-Tissue Sarcoma. http://old.cjmed.net/html/2010353_482.html

Soft-Tissue Sarcoma.
www.cancer.gov/cancertopics/factsheet/sitestypes/soft-tissue-sarcoma

Traditional Chinese Medicine (TCM).
www.hnmrc.net/pd-216690408.html

Wikipedia. Soft-Tissue Sarcomas.
http://en.wikipedia.org/wiki/Soft_tissue_sarcoma

## Spinal-Cord Compression

Malignant Spinal-Cord Compression. www.macmillan.org.uk/
cancerinformation/livingwithandaftercancer/symptomsside

## Vacahni, C. Spinal-Cord Compression.

www.oncolink.org/resources/article.cfm?c16&s46&ss205&id897

## Stem-Cell Transplantation

Bone-Marrow Transplant.
www.cumc.columbia.edu/dept/medicine/bonemarrow/bmtinfo.html

Mayo Clinic Staff. Stem-Cell Transplant.
www.mayoclinic.com/health/stem-cell-transplant/MY00089/
METHOD=print

Wikipedia. Hematopoietic Stem-Cell Transplantation.
http://en.wikipedia.org/wiki/Hematopoietic_stem_cell_transplantation

## Steroids—Their Uses And Problems

The Truth about Steroids. www.globalchange.com/steroids.htm

Use of Steroids in Medicine.
www.healthcareveda.com/post/use.of.steroidsinmedicine.aspx

The Uses of Steroid Medication. http://john-richard-roberts
.suite101.com/the-uses-of-steroid-medication-a49424

## Stomach Cancer

Dr Reddy Clinic. Stomach Cancer.
www.dreddyclinic.com/findinformation/cc/stomachcancer.htm

Fong, B. Diet for Stomach Cancer.
www.livestrong.com/article/135281-diet-stomach-cancer/

Juhasz, F. The Best Foods for Stomach Cancer Patients.
www.livestrong.com/article/347508-the-best-foods-forstomach
-cancer-patients/

Marie, J. Ayurvedic Herbs for the Stomach.
www.livestrong.com/article/512053-triphala-for-ibs/

More about Stomach Cancer.
www.4uherb.com/cancer/stomach/treat.htm

Scott, F. Green Tea and Stomach Cancer.
www.livestrong.com/article/365335-green-tea-stomach-cancer/

Stomach Cancer. Ayurvedic Herbal Stomach Cancer Cure.
www.ayurvedacancer.org/cancerby system5.htm.

Stomach Cancer Chemotherapy.
http://cancer.emedtv.com/stomach-cancer/stomach-cancer
-chemotherapy.html

Stomach Cancer Naturopathic Medicine.
www.cancercenter.com/stomach-cancer/naturopathic-medicine.cfm

Stomach Cancer, Side Effects.
www.cancercompass.com/stomach-cancer-information/side-effects.htm

Stomach Cancer Treatments.
www.cancercenter.com/stomach-cancer/stomach-cancer-treatment.cfm

Suresh, J. Side Effects of Chemotherapy for Stage IV Gastric Cancer.
www.ehow.com/facts_4866371_chemotherapy=stage-iv-gastric-cancer.html

Wikipedia. Stomach Cancer.
http://en.wikipedia.org/wiki/Stomach_cancer

## Testicular Cancer

Alternative Treatments for Testicular Cancer.
www.rightdiagnosis.com/t/testicularcancer/alternative.htm

Ayurvedic Herbal Testis Cancer Cure.
www.ayurvedacancer.org/cancerbysystem15.htm

Home Remedies for Testicular Cancer.
www.homemademedicines.org/remedies/testicularcancer.html

Kuang, H. Testicular Cancer Herbal Treatment.
www.hnmrc.net/pd1118209292.html

Wikipedia. Testicular Cancer.
http://en.wikipedia.org/wiki/Testicular_cancer

## Thyroid Cancer

Ayurveda Herbal Thyroid Cancer Cure.
www.ayurveda-cancer.org/cancerbysystem20.htm

Alternative Treatment for Thyroid Cancer. http://cancer.emedtv.com/thyroid-cancer/alternativee-treatment-for-thyroid-cancer.html

Dharmananda, S. Treatments for Thyroid Diseases with Chinese Herbal Medicine. www.itemonline.org/arts/thyroid.htm

Thompson, T. Thyroid Cancer Alternative Treatment. www.nativeremedies.com/articles/thyroid-cancer-alternative-treatments.html

Thyroid Remedies. Natural Treatment. www.ayurvedicmedicines.com/thyroid.html

Wikipedia, Anaplastic and Follicular Thyroid Cancer. http://en.wikipedia.org/wiki/Anaplastic_thyroid-carcinoma

Wikipedia, Medullary Thyroid Cancer. http://en.wikipedia.org/wiki/Medullary_thyroid_carcinoma

Wikipedia. Papillary Thyroid Cancer. http://en.wikipedia.org/wiki/Papillary_thyroid_carcinoma

Wikipedia. Thyroid Cancer. http://en.wikipedia.org/wiki/Thyroid_Cancer

## Uterine Cancer

Cancer of the Uterus—Ayurvedic Herbal Treatment. http://ayurvedic-treatment.com/cancer-of-the-uterus-ayurvedic-herbal-treatment/

Holistic Treatment of Uterine Cancer. www.energytreatments.com/holistichealing/holistictreatmentofcancer/holistic

Uterine Cancer. www.altmd.com/Articles/UterineCancerEncyclopediaof

Uterine Cancer Mind Body Medicine. www.cancercenter.com/uterinecancer/mindbodymedicine.cfm

Wikipedia. Endometrial Cancer. http://en.wikipedia.org/wiki/Endometrialcancer.

# ENDNOTES

## Introduction

1. Cancer prevention: 7 tips to reduce your risk. www.mayoclinic.com/health/cancer-prevention/CA00024.

2. The M. D. Anderson Cancer Center provides definitions for many complementary/integrative methods on this site; for details, refer to web pages linked to the site www.mdanderson.org/education-and-research/resources-for-professionals/clinical-tools-and-resources/cimer/about-complementary-integra tive-medicine/index.html.

3. DeVita, VT, Lawrence, TS, Rosenberg, SA. 2011. *DeVita, Hellman, and Rosenberg's Cancer: Principles and Practice of Oncology.* 9th ed. Philadelphia, PA: Lippincott, Williams & Wilkins.

## Chapter 2

1. "Oral Contraceptives and Cancer Risk." National Cancer Institute. www.cancer.gov/cancertopics/factsheet/Risk/oral-contraceptives.

2. "The Immune System and Cancer—How your immune system can fight cancer." http://cancerfightingstrategies.com/immune-system-and-cancer.html.

3. Radon and Cancer. National Cancer Institute. http://cancer.gov/cancertopics/factsheet/Risk/radon.

4. Cancer and EMF:EMR (Electromagnetic Radiation), Powerline and Electric Fields and . . . www.ehso.com/ehshome/emf.htm.

5. A meta-analysis on depression and subsequent cancer risk. www.ncbi.nlm.nih.gov/pmc/articles/PMC2235847/.

6. Current Projects—Research-Center on Stress and Health. Stanford University. http://stresshealthcenter.stanford.edu/research/projects.html.

7. Harmful Substances—chemicals, pollution and cancer: Cancer Research UK; www.cancerresearchuk.org/cancer/info/healthyliving/harmfulsubstances/harmful-su.

8. Carcinogen-Wikipedia. http://en.wikipedia.org/wiki/Carcinogen.

9. Avoid 100 Dangerous Food Additives Causing ADHD, Asthma and Cancer; http://preventdisease.com/news/13/051213_100-Dangerous-Food-Additives-Causing-ADH.

10. http://news.cancerconnect.com/risk-of-thyroid-cancer-remains-elevated-among-survivors-.

11. www.cancer.org/cancer/cancercauses/sunanduvexposure/skincancerprevetionandearl.

12. www.cancer.ca/en/cancer-information/cancer-101/what-is-cancer/?region=on.

13. Omega-6 fatty acids—University of Maryland Medical Center. http://umm.edu/health/medical/altmed/supplement/omega6-fatty-acids.

14. Omega-3 Fatty Acids. www.cancer.org/treatment/treatmentsandsideeffects/complementaryandalternativeme.

15. Do Omega-3's and Antioxidants Fight Cancer? www.webmd.com/cancer/features/antioxidants-omega3s?spon=912345_0.

16. RGBG in Milk May Increase Your Breast Cancer Risk. http://articles.mercola.com/sites/articles/archive/2011/10/23/rgbh-in-milk-increases-risk-of.

17. 2005. "Dairy Product Consumption and the Risk of Breast Cancer." *Journal of the American College of Nutrition.* 24 (6): 556–568s.

## Chapter 4

1. Breast Cancer—Side Effects of Breast Cancer Treatments. www.empowher.com/breast-cancer/content/side-effects-breast-cancer-treatments-may.

2. Radiation Side Effects—Natural Treatment for Radiation Side Effects. http://altmedicine.about.com/od/cance1/a/radiation_side_effects.htm.

3. Selenium Supplements for alleviating the side effects of chemotherapy, radiotherapy . . . ; www.ncbi.nlm.nih.gov/pubmedhealth/PMH0013195/.

4. Alternative Medicine Can Alleviate Cancer Therapy Side Effects. http://personal liberty.com/2009/11/19/alternative-medicine-can-alleviate-cancer-therapy-si.

5. Gordaliza, M. "Natural products as leads to anticancer drugs." Departamento de Quimica Farmaceutica, Facultad de Farmacia, Universidad de Salamanca, Salamanca, Spain. mliza@usal.es. www.ncbi.nlm.nih.gov/pubmed/18158980.

6. Dach, J. *Anti-Cancer Activity from Natural Plants.* http://open.salon.com/blog/jeffrey_dach_md/2013/06/14anti-cancer_activ ity_from_natura.

7. Chrysin Natural Alternative to Toxic Breast Cancer Drugs. www.naturalnews.com/026086_cancer_drug_chrysin.html.

8. Sinclair, S. 1998. "Chinese herbs: a clinical review of Astragalus, Ligusticum, and Schizandrae." *Alternative Medicine Review.* 3(5): 338–344.

9. Liu, LF, Desai, SD, Li, TK, et al. 2000. "Mechanism of action of camptothecin." *Annals of the New York Academy of Sciences.* 922: 1–10. Source: Department of Pharmacology, UMDNJ–Robert Wood Johnson Medical School, 675 Hoes Lane, Piscataway, NJ 08854, USA. email: lliu@umdnj.edu.

10. Grossarth-Maticek, R, Kiene, H, Baumgartner, SM, et al. 2001. "Use of Iscador, an extract of European mistletoe (*Viscum album*), in cancer treatment: prospective non-randomized and randomized matched-pair studies nested within a cohort study." *Alternative Therapies in Health and Medicine.* 7(3): 57–66, 68–72, 74–76 passim. Source: Institute for Preventive Medicine, European Center for Peace and Development, United Nations, Heidelberg, Germany.

11. Kelly, GS. 1999. "Larch arabinogalactan: clinical relevance of a novel immune-enhancing polysaccharide." *Alternative Medicine Review.* 4(2): 96–103.

12. Chovatiya, K. Agnihotri College of Pharmacy, Wardha, Maharashtra, India. www.pharmatutor.org/articles/natural-anti-cancer-drugs-and-recent-development-in-it.

13. *Nutrition in Cancer Care.* National Cancer Institute. www.cancer.gov/cancertopics/pdq/supportivecare/nutrition/Patient.

14. Landrith, G. Psychologist, Health and Addiction Advisor, Spiritual Life Coach. www.theuniverselieswithin.com/DVD.aspx.

15. 2011. Xu, J, Murray, F. *Magic Needles.* Laguna Beach, CA: Basic Health Publications.

16. Email correspondence from Merkin, L., Chiropractor/Kinesiologist, April 18, 2013. docmerkin@gmail.com.

17. www.youtube.com/watch?v=1W_ikSAA7KU.

18. Quote from private correspondence with author.

19. Rand, WL. 2000. *Reiki—The Healing Touch*, Southfield, MI: Vision Publications. www.reiki.org.

20. Miles, P.. *Reiki—A Comprehensive Guide.* London, England: Penguin Books Ltd., June 19, 2005. www.reikiinmedicine.org

21. Keyes, R. 2012. *The Healing Power of Reiki—A Modern Master's Approach to Emotional, Spiritual and Physical Wellness.* Woodbury, Mn: Llewellyn Publications, a division of Llewellyn Worldwide Ltd. www.ravenkeyes.com.

22. Paul, NL. 2006. *Reiki For Dummies.* Indianapolis, IN: Wiley Publishing Inc.

## Chapter 5

1. Adrenal Disease Prevention and Adrenal Disease Screening, M.D. Anderson Cancer Center. www.mdanderson.org/patient-and-cancer-information/center-information/cancer-typ.

2. Can Adrenal Cancer be Prevented? www.cancer.org/cancer/adrenalcorticalcancer/ overviewguide/adrenal-cortical-cancer.

3. National Cancer Institute. Bone Cancer: Questions and Answers. 2002. www.cancer .gov/cancertopics/factsheet/Sites-Types/bone.

4. Hiraoka, K, et.al. 2001. "Osteosarcoma cell apoptosis induced by selenium." *Journal of Orthopaedic Research.* 19 (5): 809–814.

5. Li, BB, Yu, SF, Pang, SZ. 2005. "Effect of genistein on the proliferation, differentiation and apoptosis of the osteoblasts." *Chinese Journal of Stomatology.* 40 (3): 237–240.

6. Cell Phones and Cancer Risk. National Cancer Institute. www.cancer.gov/cancertopics/factsheet/Risk/cellphones.

7. Aspartame controversy. http://en.wikipedia.org/wiki/Aspartame_controversy.

8. The link between aspartame and brain tumors. www.naturalnews.com/011804 .html.

9. Davis, J. 1993. "Family Pesticide Use and Brain Cancer." *Archives of Environmental Contamination and Toxicology.* 24: 87–92.

10. Draper, G, et. al. 2005. "Childhood cancer in relation to distance from high-voltage power lines in England and Wales: A case control study." *British Medical Journal.* 330: 1290.

11. New brain tumours and EMF exposure. www.emfields.org/news/201110211-brain-tumours-powerlines.asp.

12. Magnetic Field Exposure and Cancer. www.cancer.gov/cancertopics/factsheet/ Risk/magnetic-fields.

13. Can penile cancer be prevented? American Cancer Society www.cancer.org/ cancer/penilecancer/detailedguide/penile-cancer-prevention.

14. Howell, N, eHow contributor. *Holistic Treatment of Carcinoid Cancer.* www .ehow.com/way_5510447_holistic-treatment-carcinoid-cancer.html.

15. Carcinoid Tumors: Alternative Medicine—Mayo Clinic.com www.mayoclinic .com/health/carcinoidtumors/DS00834/DSECTION=alternative-m.

16. Childhood Cancers Home Page—National Cancer Institute http://cancer.gov/ cancertopics/types/childhoodcancers.

17. Ref: American Cancer Society. www.cancer.org/cancer/colonandrectumcancer/.

18. Yeh, M. 2009. "Higher intakes of vegetables and vegetable-related nutrients are associated with lower endometrial cancer risks." *Journal of Nutrition.* 139 (2): 317–322.

19. Lian, Z. 2004. "Soybean isoflavones inhibit estrogen-stimulated gene expression in mouse uteri." *European Journal of Gynecological Oncology.* 25(3): 311–314.

20. Bhat, KP, Pezzuto, JM. 2001. "Resveratrol exhibits cytostatic and anti-estrogenic properties with human endometrial adenocarcinoma (Ishikawa) cells." *Cancer Research.* 61 (16): 6137–6144.

21. Futugami, M. 2001. "Effects of melatonin on the proliferation and cisdi-amminedichloroplatinum (CDDP) sensitivity of cultured human ovarian cancer cells." *Gynecologic Oncology.* 82 (3): 544–549.

22. Shi, M. 2006. "Antiproliferation and apoptosis induced by curcumin in human ovarian cancer cells." *Cell Biology International.* 30 (3): 221–226.

23. Drisko, JA, Chapman, J, Hunter, VJ. 2003. "The use of antioxidants with first-line chemotherapy in two cases of ovarian cancer." *Journal of the American College of Nutrition.* 22(2): 118–123.

24. Leukemia and Lymphoma Society. Disease information: Leukemia. 2006. www.leukemia-lymphoma.org/all_page?item_id=7030–32.

25. Baxa, DM, Luo, X, Yoshimura, FK. 2005. "Genistein induces apoptosis in T-lymphoma cells via mitochondrial damage." *Nutrition and Cancer.* 51 (1): 93–101.

26. Chen, D. 2005. "Dietary flavonoids as proteasome inhibitors and apoptosis inducers in human leukemia cells." *Biochmeical Pharmacology.* 69(10): 1421–1432.

27. Liu, CY. 2009. "Cured meat, vegetables, and bean-curd foods in relation to childhood acute leukemia risk: A population based case-control study. *BMC Cancer.* 9 (15).

28. Handa, K, Krieger, N. 2002. "Diet patterns and the risk of renal cell carcinoma." *Public Health Nutrition.* 5 (6): 757–767.

29. Weikert, S. 2006. "Fruits and vegetables and renal cell carcinoma: Findings from the European Prospective Investigation into Cancer and Nutrition (EPIC)." *International Journal of Cancer.* 118 (12): 3133–3139.

30. Hagmar, B, Ryd, W, Skomedal, H. 1991. "Arabinogalactin blockade of experimental metastases to liver by murine hepatoma." *Invasion Metastasis.* II (6): 348–355.

31. Lee, CY, Hsu, Y–C, Wang, J–Y, et al. 2008. "Chemopreventive effect of selenium and Chinese medicinal herbs on N-nitrosobis (2-oxopropyl) amine-induced hepato-cellular carcinoma in Syrian hamsters." *Liver International.* 28: 841–855. doi:10. 1111/j. 1478–3231.01698.x.

32. Wo, AJ. 2003. "A Summary of Treating 46 Cases of Non-Small-Cell Lung Cancer with Integrated Chinese-Western Medicine." *Hunan Journal of Chinese Medicine.* 11. http://discount.vip.sina.com/cancer/non-small-cell-lung-cancer-treatment/non-small-cell-lun.

33. (For Simon Fraser University, Burnaby, Canada) Dugoua, JJ, Wu, P, Seely, D, et al. 2010. "Astragalus-containing Chinese herbal combinations for advanced non-small-cell lung cancer: a meta-analysis of 65 clinical trials enrolling 4751 patients." *Lung Cancer: Targets and Therapy*. 1(Default), 85–100. http://dx.dol.org/ 10.2147/LCTT .S7780.

34. (For U. of Mainz) U. of Mainz—Chinese herbal. www.bing.com/news/search? q=lung+cancer%2c+U.+of+Mainz-chinese+herbal&qp.

35. Lung cancer: alternative medicine—Mayo Clinic.com. www.mayoclinic.com/ health/lung-cancer/DS00038/DSECTION=alternative-medicine.

36. UC San Diego Moores Cancer Center. "Gerson Therapy as an Alternative Cancer Therapy." http://cancer.ucsd.edu/treatments/cam/therapies/Pages/gerson-therapy.aspx.

37. Dharmananda, S. 1996. "Treatments for Thyroid Diseases with Chinese Herbal Medicine." Portland, OR: Institute for Traditional Medicine.

38. Ming, Ou. 1993. *An Illustrated Guide to Anti-Neoplastic Chinese Herbal Medicine*. Seattle, WA: Eastland Press. www.nutritionalwellness.com/nutrition/herbs/i/ isatis_leaf.php.

39. Tierra, M. 2003. *Treating Cancer with Herbs: An Integrative Approach*. Detroit, MI: Lotus Press. http://www.amazon.com/Treating-Cancer-Herbs-Integrative-Approach/dp/0914955934.

40. 1992. *Anticancer Medicinal Herbs* (English Edition), *Chang Minyi* (Chinese), Translator in chief: Bai Yongquan, Hunan Science and Technology House.

**Chapter 6**

1. Roscoe, JA, Bushunow, P, et al. 2009. "Accupressure Bands Are Effective in Reducing Radiation Therapy-Related Nausea." *Journal of Pain and Symptom Management*. 38 (3): 381–389.

2. National Cancer Institute. Depression. www.cancer.gov/cancertopics/pdq/supportive care/depression/Patient/page2.

3. Fratkin, J. "New Chinese Herbal Formulas for Treating Depression." http:// drjake fratkin.com/articles/new-chinese-herbal-formulas-for-treating-depression.

4. Berger, NA, Savvides, P, et al. 2006. "Cancer in the Elderly." *Transactions of the American Clinical and Climatological Association*. 117: 147–156.

5. www.lww.com/wcsstore/PEMR/images/product/128/9781451105452.gif. DeVita, VT, Lawrence, TS, Rosenberg, SA, et al. 2011. *DeVita, Hellman, and Rosenberg's Cancer: Principles and Practice of Oncology*. Eds: DeVita, VT, Lawrence, TS, Rosenberg, SA, DePinho, RA, Weinberg, R. 9th ed. Philadelphia, PA: Lippincott, Williams & Wilkins.

# ADDITIONAL REFERENCES

American Joint Committee on Cancer. 2002. *AJCC Cancer Staging Manual.* 6th edition. Berlin, Heidelberg. Dordrecht, New York. Springer Science and Business Media.

Arnot, R. 1998. *The Breast Cancer Prevention Diet.* Boston, MA: Little Brown, and Co., 304.

Badell, Colleen C. *A Simple Plan, Alternative Medicine Made Easy.* 2006. Turning Point Press, 264.

Block, KI. 2009. *Life Over Cancer.* New York: Bantam Books, 591.

Case, HS. 2012. *The Vitamin Cure.* Laguna Beach, CA: Basic Health Publications.

Coleman, C. Norman. 2006. *Understanding Cancer: A Patient's Guide to Diagnosis, Prognosis and Treatment.* 2nd ed. The Johns Hopkins University Press, 232.

Eyre, HJ. 2002. *Informed Decisions.* American Cancer Society, 2002, 768.

Figlin, RA. 2003. *Kidney Cancer.* Boston, MA: Kluwer Academic Publishers, 256.

Halstead, B. 2006. *The Scientific Basis of Chinese Integrative Cancer Therapy.* Berkeley, CA: North Atlantic Books.

Hartmann, LC. 2005. *Mayo Clinic Guide to Women's Cancers.* Mayo Clinic Health Information. New York, NY: Kensington Publishing Corp, 638.

Kaushal, SP. 2003. *Cancer and Herbs.* Bangalore, India: Vedic Cancer Research Center, 523.

Ko, A, Dollinger, M, Rosenbaum, EA. 1991. *Everyone's Guide to Cancer Therapy.* Kansas City, MO: Andrews McMeel Publishing Co.

Link, J. 2007. *Breast Cancer Survival Manual.* 4th ed. New York, NY: Henry Holt.

Mars, B. 2007. *The Desktop Guide to Herbal Medicine.* Laguna Beach, CA: Basic Health Publications.

McCabe, V. 2007. *The Healing Enigma . . . Demystifying Homeopathy.* Laguna Beach, CA: Basic Health Publications.

McLanahan, SA, McLanahan, D. 2002. *Surgery and Its Alternatives.* New York, NY: Twin Streams Imprimis, Kensington Publishing, Corp. 814.

Micozzi, MS. 2006. *Complementary and Integrative Medicine in Cancer Care.* St. Louis, MO: Saunders Imprimis of Elsevier Publ.

Mincolla, M. 2011. *Customized Healing, Blending the Best of Eastern and Western Medicine.* Laguna Beach, CA: Basic Health Publications.

Murray, M. 2003. *How to Prevent and Treat Cancer with Natural Medicine.* New York, NY: Riverhead Books, The Berkley Publ. Co., Div. of Penguin Group.

Nagi, B, Kumar, NB, Allen, K, et al. *Integrative Nutritional Therapies for Cancer.* Philadelphia, PA:. Facts and Comparisons Publishing Group—Division of Wolters-Kluwer Health, Lippincott, William & Wilkins, 2002, 165.

Ody, P. 2000. *Complete Guide to Medicinal Herbs.* New York, N.Y: Dorling Kindersley Publishers, 240.

Patt, RB, Lang, S. 2006. *The Complete Guide to Relieving Cancer Pain and Suffering.* New ed. New York, NY: Oxford University Press, 464.

Pazdur, R, Cola, L, Wagman, L. (eds.) 2008. *Cancer Management: A Multidisciplinary Approach.* Philadelphia, PA: F.A. Davis Co.

Pescatore, F. 2010. *The Medical Breakthrough in Natural Immunotherapy.* Laguna Beach, CA: Basic Health Productions.

Quillin, P. 2005. *Beating Cancer with Nutrition.* Encinitas, CA: Nutrition Times Press.

Runowicx, C. 2004. *The Answer to Cancer.* Emmaus, PA: Rodale Press, 290.

Schiller, C, Schiller, D. 2008. *The Aromatherapy Encyclopedia.* Laguna Beach, CA: Basic Health Publications.

Schofield, J, Robinson, W. 2000. *What You Really Need to Know About Moles and Melanoma.* Baltimore, MD: The Johns Hopkins University Press.

Volk, RM. 2007. *The Medical Library Association Guide to Cancer Information.* New York, NY: Neal Schuman Publishers-Imprimis of American Library Assoc., 31.

Waller, D. 2005. *Art Therapy and Cancer Care.* Berkshire, England: Open University Press, McGraw Hill Education, McGraw Hill-House, 256.

Weisman, R, Berman, B. 2003. *Own Your Health.* Deerfield Beach, FL: Health Communications, Inc., 471.

Yarbro, C, et al. 2005. *Cancer Nursing: Principles and Practice.* 6th ed. Burlington, MA: Jones and Bartlett, 1879.

# INDEX

# ABOUT THE AUTHOR

**Dr. Joel Berman** is a practicing general and vascular surgeon in Southern California with an M.D. degree from the State University of New York Upstate Medical Center, and a master's degree in surgery for breast cancer research. He has enjoyed a distinguished career as a chief of surgery, a director of a center for breast care, and an associate professor of surgery at the University of Southern California Medical Center in its affiliation with the Orange County Regional Cancer Center.

Among the more than twenty books he has published are several on medical/surgical topics, the balance being an appealing variety of fictional and non-fictional works and a recently published account of his father's experiences as a WWII surgeon.

Dr. Berman's wide scope of interests also includes the arts (music, books, and theater), studying languages, and history. He lives in Southern California with his wife Suzanne.

His website address is www.doctorjoelberman.com